"Knowing is not enough; we must apply.
Willing is not enough; we must do."
—Goethe

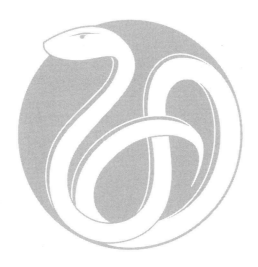

INSTITUTE OF MEDICINE
OF THE NATIONAL ACADEMIES

Adviser to the Nation to Improve Health

THE NATIONAL ACADEMIES
Advisers to the Nation on Science, Engineering, and Medicine

The **National Academy of Sciences** is a private, nonprofit, self-perpetuating society of distinguished scholars engaged in scientific and engineering research, dedicated to the furtherance of science and technology and to their use for the general welfare. Upon the authority of the charter granted to it by the Congress in 1863, the Academy has a mandate that requires it to advise the federal government on scientific and technical matters. Dr. Bruce M. Alberts is president of the National Academy of Sciences.

The **National Academy of Engineering** was established in 1964, under the charter of the National Academy of Sciences, as a parallel organization of outstanding engineers. It is autonomous in its administration and in the selection of its members, sharing with the National Academy of Sciences the responsibility for advising the federal government. The National Academy of Engineering also sponsors engineering programs aimed at meeting national needs, encourages education and research, and recognizes the superior achievements of engineers. Dr. Wm. A. Wulf is president of the National Academy of Engineering.

The **Institute of Medicine** was established in 1970 by the National Academy of Sciences to secure the services of eminent members of appropriate professions in the examination of policy matters pertaining to the health of the public. The Institute acts under the responsibility given to the National Academy of Sciences by its congressional charter to be an adviser to the federal government and, upon its own initiative, to identify issues of medical care, research, and education. Dr. Harvey V. Fineberg is president of the Institute of Medicine.

The **National Research Council** was organized by the National Academy of Sciences in 1916 to associate the broad community of science and technology with the Academy's purposes of furthering knowledge and advising the federal government. Functioning in accordance with general policies determined by the Academy, the Council has become the principal operating agency of both the National Academy of Sciences and the National Academy of Engineering in providing services to the government, the public, and the scientific and engineering communities. The Council is administered jointly by both Academies and the Institute of Medicine. Dr. Bruce M. Alberts and Dr. Wm. A. Wulf are chair and vice chair, respectively, of the National Research Council.

www.national-academies.org

DEDICATION

This report is dedicated to the memory of Christopher Reeve, whose tireless efforts galvanized the spinal cord injury research community and raised awareness of the issues involved in the care and cure of spinal cord injury and other chronic disabilities. His perseverance also gave hope to individuals with spinal cord injuries and caregivers. Continuing to advance toward curing spinal cord injuries is the ongoing challenge.

REVIEWERS

This report has been reviewed in draft form by individuals chosen for their diverse perspectives and technical expertise, in accordance with procedures approved by the National Research Council's Report Review Committee. The purpose of this independent review is to provide candid and critical comments that will assist the institution in making its published report as sound as possible and to ensure that the report meets institutional standards for objectivity, evidence, and responsiveness to the study charge. The review comments and draft manuscript remain confidential to protect the integrity of the deliberative process. We wish to thank the following individuals for their review of this report:

Thomas F. Budinger, Lawrence Berkeley National Laboratory
Diana Cardenas, University of Washington
Howard L. Fields, University of California, San Francisco
Ralph F. Frankowski, University of Texas Health Science Center at Houston, School of Public Health
Zach W. Hall, Keck School of Medicine of the University of Southern California
Julian T. Hoff, University of Michigan
Daniel P. Lammertse, CNS Medical Group
Oswald Steward, Reeve-Irvine Research Center
Steven M. Strittmatter, Yale University School of Medicine
Paul Tobin, United Spinal Association
Mark H. Tuszynski, University of California, San Diego

William D. Whetstone, University of California, San Francisco
Charles B. Wilson, Health Technology Center

Although the reviewers listed above have provided many constructive comments and suggestions, they were not asked to endorse the conclusions or recommendations, nor did they see the final draft of the report before its release. The review of this report was overseen by **Elena Nightingale,** National Academies, and **Enriqueta Bond,** Burroughs Wellcome Fund.
Appointed by the National Research Council and Institute of Medicine, they were responsible for making certain that an independent examination of this report was carried out in accordance with institutional procedures and that all review comments were carefully considered. Responsibility for the final content of this report rests entirely with the authoring committee and the institution.

PREFACE

How suddenly life can change—nowhere more dramatically than with a spinal cord injury: the robust young football player suddenly lying immobilized on the field; the child confined for life to a wheelchair after diving into a shallow pond; the vacationing family with a parent or child forever paralyzed after a skiing, bicycle, or car crash; the soldier left quadriplegic after a sniper shot to his neck; or anyone's accidental tumble down stairs or from a ladder. We have all witnessed the tragedy of spinal cord injuries. It sometimes results from risky behavior, but most injuries result from unforeseen accidents in an active, healthy life.

The time has come that we may be able to make a major change in how we deal with this frightening personal and public health problem. Survival from severe spinal cord injuries became a reality during and after World War II with the introduction of antibiotics that controlled the infections of the urinary tract and skin that had proved fatal in prior years. Subsequently, improved management with neck stabilization to minimize further damage and better respiratory support, autonomic regulation, and other supportive measures reduced the damage and improved the outlook for survival. The invention of mechanical devices improved independence and quality of life. These advances were largely in the fields of neurosurgery, intensive care, and physical medicine.

These were significant advances, but they were made in an era when we could not dream of actually addressing repair and regeneration. Those of us who were trained in the 1950s and 1960s were taught that "the neurons you are born with are all you ever get," that axonal regeneration and remyelination occurred only in the peripheral nervous system and not in the central nervous system, and that damage to the spinal cord was irreversible. New studies of regeneration and repair in the brains and spinal cords of experimental animals have challenged these dogmas. Central nervous system remyelination was recognized in the 1960s, the extension of central axons was observed in the 1980s, and neurogenesis in adult life was discovered in recent years. Enhancement of regeneration in the brain and spinal cord has become a rational goal, but not an easy one. The processes of regeneration are complex; there will likely be no magic bullet—such as antibiotics—to lift us over this next barrier.

Nerve cells will need to be saved or replaced, the growth of their axons will need to be not only stimulated but also guided, and connections to distant neurons or muscle fibers will need to be assisted or preserved. In addition, barriers or scars will need to be prevented or penetrated to permit this regeneration. Solutions will require novel and creative thinking. It is a great and, indeed, exciting challenge to the neurobiologists whose studies show increasingly greater promise. However, translation of the findings from these cell culture studies and studies with laboratory animals to humans with spinal cord injuries will need a new cadre of clinician-investigators recruited from diverse clinical backgrounds—neurology, clinical pharmacology, biomedical engineering, transplantation medicine, neurosurgery, and rehabilitation medicine. Talent will need to be joined to undertake these new tasks.

This report examines the field of spinal cord injury research and makes recommendations on future directions for the field in general and for the sponsors of the study, the New York State Spinal Cord Injury Research Board, in particular. The committee consisted of individuals with diverse backgrounds and opinions, but we all agreed that the problems were great and that knowledge has advanced to a level where opportunities abound.

Dedicated work on the part of every committee member contributed to this report. Further, the committee benefited from the expertise of the consultants to the committee, Jesse Cedarbaum, Gerald Fischbach, and Wise Young. Experts from across the country volunteered to speak in symposia and give advice informally. The public and voluntary organizations participated. However, the acquisition of expertise in the field, the compiling and sorting of data, the tireless organization and reorganization of contents, and the optimistic enthusiasm of Catharyn Liverman, Bruce Altevogt, Janet Joy, Kathleen Patchan, and Lora Taylor of the Institute of Medicine staff were remarkable; they made this report possible. On behalf of every committee member, I salute them.

Richard T. Johnson, M.D., *Chair*

ACKNOWLEDGMENTS

The committee acknowledges with appreciation the individuals who provided information to the committee. These individuals include Maria Amador, The Miami Project to Cure Paralysis; Doug Anderson, University of Florida College of Medicine; Michael Beattie, Ohio State University; Andrew R. Blight, Acorda Therapeutics, Inc.; John Bollinger, Paralyzed Veterans of America; Pak Chan, Stanford University; Moses V. Chao, New York University; Dennis W. Choi, Merck & Company, Inc.; Dalton Dietrich, The Miami Project to Cure Paralysis; V. Reggie Edgerton, University of California, Los Angeles; Alan Faden, Georgetown University; Marie Filbin, Hunter College of the City University of New York; Ralph Frankowski, University of Texas at Houston; Z. Alexander Gentle; William Heetderks, National Institute of Biomedical Imaging and Bioengineering; Maura Hofstadter, Reeve-Irvine Research Center; Susan Howley, Christopher Reeve Paralysis Foundation; Claire Hulsebosch, University of Texas Medical Branch; Naomi Kleitman, National Institute of Neurological Disorders and Stroke; Congressman James Langevin, Rhode Island; Fausto Loberiza, Jr., Medical College of Wisconsin; Curtis Meinert, Johns Hopkins University; Lorne Mendell, University of New York at Stony Brook; Geoff Raisman, National Institute for Medical Research, London; Cynthia Rask, Food and Drug Administration; Rajiv Ratan, Burke/Cornell Medical Research Institute; Jeffrey D. Rothstein, Johns Hopkins University; Evan Snyder, Burnham Institute, San Diego; Oswald Steward, University of California, Irvine; Paul J. Tobin, United Spinal Association; Lynne Weaver, Robarts Research Institute; Irving Weissman, Stanford University; and Scott Whittemore, Kentucky Spinal Cord Injury

Research Center, University of Louisville School of Medicine. This study was sponsored by the New York State Spinal Cord Injury Research Board. We appreciate their support and especially thank Martin Sorin for his efforts on behalf of this study. We also thank Judy Estep for all of her expertise in formatting the report for publication.

CONTENTS

APPENDIXES

EXECUTIVE SUMMARY

Spinal cord injuries occur unexpectedly. The normal events of life—driving a car, diving into a lake, or walking down stairs—can suddenly result in a life-changing injury with physical and lifestyle constraints that totally reconfigure the realities of daily life. An estimated 11,000 spinal cord injuries occur each year in the United States, and 247,000 Americans are currently living with a spinal cord injury.

In the past several decades there has been significant progress in improving patient survival and emergency care and in expanding the range of rehabilitative options. During this same time period, the breadth and depth of neuroscience discoveries relevant to spinal cord injury have widely expanded the horizons of potential therapies. What once was dogma—that the central nervous system cannot regenerate—has been dismissed. This newly discovered potential for central nervous system (CNS) regeneration and repair has opened up numerous therapeutic targets and opportunities. Many current avenues of research suggest that a concerted research effort on spinal cord injuries could result in important gains in restoring function and improving quality of life.

Recognizing this wealth of new opportunity, the New York State Spinal Cord Injury Research Board asked the Institute of Medicine (IOM) to examine future research directions in spinal cord injury. The IOM was asked not just to advise New York State on its research program, but to look more broadly at research priorities for funders of spinal cord research—federal and state agencies, academic organizations, pharmaceutical and device companies, and nonprofit organizations. To accomplish this task the IOM appointed a 13-member committee with expertise in basic

1

and clinical neuroscience research, trauma surgery, health care, biomedical engineering, clinical research methods, and research management.

This report by the IOM Committee on Spinal Cord Injury provides a broad overview of the current status of spinal cord injury research, examines the research and infrastructure needs, and provides recommendations for advancing and accelerating progress in the treatment of spinal cord injuries with particular attention to issues regarding translational research. The committee also addresses the contributions that the New York State program can make to complement the scientific efforts of other state, federal, and private supporters of research in this area.

DEFINING A CURE

Defining what constitutes a "cure" is an integral part of discussions on future directions for spinal cord injury research. In large part, the general public's perception of a cure for spinal cord injury has been the restoration of motor function, that is, restoration of the ability to walk. However, a spinal cord injury affects many systems and functions of the body that are vital to the health and well-being of the injured person. Neural control of motor, sensory, autonomic, bowel, and bladder functions is compromised, often leading to pain, pressure sores, infection, and diminished physiological well-being.

After carefully considering input from the community of individuals with spinal cord injuries, researchers, and clinicians, the committee decided to take a broad approach to "defining a cure" and to frame its definition around alleviating the multiple disabilities that result from spinal cord injury.

Spinal cord injury research should focus on preventing the loss of function and on restoring lost functions—including sensory, motor, bowel, bladder, autonomic, and sexual functions—with the elimination of complications, particularly pain, spasticity, pressure sores (decubitus ulcers), and depression, with the ultimate goal of fully restoring to the individual the levels of activity and function that he or she had before injury.

By setting forth a set of goals for spinal cord injury research, the committee wishes to emphasize the different stages of the injury during which interventions are needed and the multiple health impairments that affect an individual's daily quality of life and that require the development of effective therapeutic interventions.

IDENTIFYING RESEARCH DIRECTIONS

Spinal cord injury results in a cascading biological response ranging from the changes in blood pressure and blood volume and hypoxia (reduction of oxygen supply) immediately after the injury is sustained to the subsequent edema, inflammation, and necrotic and apoptotic cell death and, later, to the formation of a glial scar, which can be a barrier to axon regeneration. To regain sensory and motor function, to prevent and eliminate pain, and to retrain and relearn motor tasks will almost certainly demand different treatment strategies and a combination of therapies.

A number of therapeutic interventions for spinal cord injuries have been explored over the past several decades. Advances have been made in emergency medical treatment and in rehabilitation efforts, and there is an increased understanding of the specific mechanisms and pathways that are targets for therapeutic interventions. Additionally, recent advances in neuroscience research are opening up new opportunities for the development of therapeutic approaches. Research toward addressing the consequences of spinal cord injuries focuses on a natural progression of strategies: preventing further tissue loss, maintaining the health of living cells, replacing cells that have died through apoptosis or necrosis, growing axons and ensuring functional connections, and strengthening and reestablishing synapses that restore the neural circuits required for functional recovery. These strategies lead to a range of therapeutic targets and priorities for spinal cord injury research (Table ES-1), each of which could theoretically be pursued together with others. For example, cell therapies that replace myelin could be combined with agents such as neurotrophic factors that promote axon regrowth.

One of the major challenges in developing combination therapies is determining those specific therapies that are safe for use in combination and that, in concert, will provide the greatest efficacy for the treatment of spinal cord injuries. Although it is possible for different combinations of drugs to be combined by trial and error, greater progress can be made if specific research efforts are devoted to developing and implementing a mechanism to select the most likely components that will be required for combination therapies. This requires a strategic approach to screening and assessing the potentials of the compounds and therapies to be used as components of combination therapies.

Much remains to be learned about the basic biology of spinal cord injuries and the numerous potential therapeutic targets involved in the complex processes of maintaining cell and tissue viability and promoting axonal growth and synaptic integrity that will result in improved and appropriate function in individuals with spinal cord injuries. Adding to the body of knowledge on neurological circuitry and mechanisms will be of benefit not only to improving function after a spinal cord injury but also to developing therapies for other neurological diseases and conditions.

TABLE ES-1 Priorities for Spinal Cord Injury Research

Develop neuroprotection therapies: identify interventions that promote neuroprotective mechanisms that preserve the spinal cord.

Promote axonal sprouting and growth: enhance understanding of the molecular mechanisms that promote and inhibit axonal regeneration—including the roles of glia (astrocytes and oligodendrocytes), scar formation, and inflammation and inhibitory molecules—and develop therapeutic approaches to promote growth.

Steer axonal growth: determine the molecular mechanisms that direct axons to their appropriate targets and regulate the formation and maintenance of appropriate synaptic connections.

Reestablish essential neuronal and glial circuitry: advance the understanding of the molecular mechanisms that regulate the formation and maintenance of the intricate neuronal and glial circuitry, which controls the complex multimodal function of the spinal cord, including autonomic, sensory, and motor functions. Increase knowledge of the mechanisms that control locomotion, including the differences in the central pattern generator between bipeds and quadrupeds.

Prevent acute and chronic complications: develop interventions that prevent and reverse the evolution of events that lead to the wide range of outcomes that result from chronic injury and disability after a spinal cord injury.

Maintain maximal potential for recovery: expand the understanding of the requirements for proper postinjury care and rehabilitation that are needed to maintain the maximal potential for full recovery.

Recommendation 5.1:[1] *Increase Efforts to Develop Therapeutic Interventions*
The National Institutes of Health, other federal and state agencies, nonprofit organizations, and the pharmaceutical and medical device industries should increase research funding and efforts to develop therapeutic interventions that will prevent or reverse the physiological events that lead to chronic disability and interventions that are applicable to chronic spinal cord injuries. Specifically, research is needed to

   • improve understanding of the basic mechanisms and identify suitable targets to promote neuroprotection, foster axonal growth, enhance axonal guidance, regulate the maintenance of appropriate synaptic connections, and reestablish functional neuronal and glial circuitry; and

---

[1]For ease of reference, the committee's recommendations are numbered according to the chapter of the main text in which they appear followed by the order in which they appear in the chapter.

- enhance understanding of proper postinjury care and rehabilitation, such as retraining, relearning, and the use of neuroprostheses, to create the groundwork required to maintain and enhance the maximal potential for full recovery.

Recommendation 5.2: *Develop a Strategic Plan for Combination Therapeutic Approaches*
The National Institute of Neurological Disorders and Stroke should develop a strategic plan to screen and assess the potential for compounds and therapies to be used in combination to treat acute and chronic spinal cord injuries.

BOLSTERING THE RESEARCH INFRASTRUCTURE

Progress in spinal cord injury research depends on adequate research funding and an adequate physical infrastructure for research; well-trained and innovative investigators with career development opportunities; translational efforts that move the findings of preclinical studies to clinical trials with humans, as safe and appropriate; and an environment that promotes and encourages interdisciplinary collaboration. Foundations and other nonprofit organizations, state and federal governments, academic institutions, and others are attempting to fund and conduct research on spinal cord injuries. The National Institute of Neurological Disorders and Stroke supports an extensive extramural research program in spinal cord injuries and should continue to devote resources to both extramural and intramural research programs to build on these efforts. The pressing issue is how best to improve the current organization of basic and clinical research—the research infrastructure—to nurture and accelerate progress.

Key to accelerating progress in the treatment of spinal cord injuries is the development of a coordinated, focused, and centralized network that connects individual investigators, research programs, and research centers; facilitates collaborative and replicative research projects; incorporates relevant research from diverse fields; and builds on the unique strengths of each research effort to move toward effective therapies. A research network is of particular importance in spinal cord injury research because of the emphasis on interdisciplinary research and the need for an organized and systematic approach to examining potential combination therapies. This dedicated focus on translational research would be spearheaded by the Spinal Cord Injury Research Centers of Excellence (discussed below) and would involve collaborations with all sites performing research relevant to spinal cord injuries. Although online technologies greatly enhance the nearly instantaneous sharing of ideas across the nation and globally, the research network envisioned by the committee would involve not only a strong virtual component but also a structured plan for periodic and regular meetings and workshops to set priorities and strengthen interactions.

As a basis for this network, the committee urges a strong commitment by the federal government to designate and support Spinal Cord Injury Research Centers of Excellence. This would involve the establishment of new centers of excellence and the designation of several current spinal cord injury research programs as Centers of Excellence. Several multidisciplinary spinal cord injury research centers already exist, including the Miami Project to Cure Paralysis, the Kentucky Spinal Cord Injury Research Center, the Reeve-Irvine Research Center, and research centers funded by the National Institutes of Health. The translational capacities of existing research centers should be strengthened, and two to three additional research centers of excellence should be established and sustained. Centers should be developed regionally to facilitate clinical trial networks. It is important that the centers interface not only with state research programs and nonprofit organizations but also with U.S. Department of Veterans Affairs spinal cord injury research centers as well as the Model Spinal Cord Injury Care System clinics and patient care centers to broaden the potential research base for clinical trials. A national effort to prioritize translational research on spinal cord injuries would expand the capacity to explore and develop therapeutic approaches.

Spinal cord injury is a multidisciplinary problem, and thus, spinal cord injury research requires collaborations among scientists and clinicians with diverse backgrounds. Therefore, a key component of the proposed Spinal Cord Injury Research Centers of Excellence should be the capacity to provide an environment that encourages comprehensive interdisciplinary research. The centers should bring together and support investigators from multiple fields, including, but not limited to, neuroscience, cellular and molecular biology, systems biology, immunology, engineering, bioengineering, biostatistics, epidemiology, and clinical medicine.

Recommendation 7.2: *Establish Spinal Cord Injury Research Centers of Excellence*
The National Institutes of Health should designate and support five to seven Spinal Cord Injury Research Centers of Excellence with adequate resources to sustain multidisciplinary basic, translational, and clinical research on spinal cord injuries. This would involve establishing two to three new Centers of Excellence and designating three to four current spinal cord injury research programs as Centers of Excellence.

Recommendation 7.3: *Establish a National Spinal Cord Injury Research Network*
The National Institutes of Health should be appropriately funded to establish a National Spinal Cord Injury Research Network that would coordinate and support the work of an expanded cadre of researchers.

STRENGTHENING NEW YORK STATE'S RESEARCH PROGRAM

Currently, 14 states have enacted legislation to fund spinal cord injury research at an annual total level of funding of about $27 million. Many of the states that fund spinal cord injury research do so through surcharges on fines for traffic violations. Some state programs provide funding to specific academic institutions to conduct research, and other states have developed or have contributed to funding extensive spinal cord research centers in their states. There is much that the states can learn from one another in developing and strengthening their spinal cord injury research programs.

In 1998, New York State passed legislation to establish a new program whose ambitious mission is to support research "towards a cure for [spinal cord] injuries and their effects." Funding for the program comes from a surcharge on traffic violations, which is directed to the newly created Spinal Cord Injury Research Trust Fund. The estimated annual funding of $8.5 million is the largest amount of state-designated funding for spinal cord injury research. Its size and scope place the program in the position to become a leader in spinal cord injury research. Furthermore, New York has a strong biomedical and neuroscience research infrastructure that could be drawn upon to build a strong research program in spinal cord injuries.

The program possesses several features that bode well for future progress, including a sophisticated grant review structure (two tiered) and scientific board, a strong translational component, multiple types of grants, and an expansion capacity that could be realized by drawing on the unique strengths of New York State's biomedical research and clinical research programs.

Opportunities to strengthen New York State's program, to reduce the administrative bureaucracy, and to bolster its impact also exist. The committee's recommendations focus on the following four areas:

• building and strengthening New York State's research infrastructure,
• developing a regional clinical trials center,
• restructuring the research funding and oversight processes, and
• ensuring independent evaluation of the progress that has been made toward the stated mission of the New York State Spinal Cord Injury Research Board.

ACCELERATING PROGRESS

Progress in spinal cord injury research offers the potential to make significant improvements in the lives of individuals with spinal cord injuries. The challenges are to move research efforts forward in such a way as to accelerate the translation of the findings from research in the laboratory to clinical trials and then into clinical practice while ensuring patient safety and effectiveness. Although few therapeutic interventions are ready for clinical trials, the body of knowledge on the mechanisms underlying neuronal injury and repair is increasing rapidly, and many potential therapies show promise in in vitro studies and in studies with animals.

The committee believes that accelerating progress in spinal cord injury research involves the following three key efforts that, in addition to the recommendations for the New York State program, are the focus of the committee's recommendations (Box ES-1) and highlight the need for a concerted national priority effort to find the best treatments for spinal cord injuries.

Focus on increasing knowledge of basic neurobiology and therapeutic approaches. Many research avenues remain to be examined in understanding the biochemical mechanisms responsible for spinal cord injuries and thus the targets of therapeutic interventions. Research is needed on the processes involved in maintaining cellular viability and the therapeutic targets for those processes, the mechanisms that promote and inhibit axon regeneration, and the processes by which axons are directed to their appropriate targets and that regulate the formation and maintenance of appropriate and functional synaptic connections and circuitry. As no one solution for spinal cord injuries likely exists, strategies need to be developed to provide an organized approach to testing and evaluating therapies in combination.

To conduct this research, new and refined technologies are needed. In addition, assessment measures need to be standardized to provide insights into potential therapeutic interventions. Efforts are needed to improve animal models and assessment techniques, increase training efforts on the use of standardized research tools and techniques, identify biomarkers that can be used to monitor the progression of injury and recovery, improve imaging technologies to provide a real-time means to assess spinal cord injuries, and standardize outcome measures for preclinical studies.

Emphasize and coordinate translational multidisciplinary research and clinical trials. Research on spinal cord injuries is now at the point at which the biological targets and pathways that can be the focus of interventions can be identified. The development of regional clinical trial networks, the bolstering of collaborative efforts between basic and clinical researchers through the development of research centers, as well as the development of a structured and focused research network will provide the opportunities to develop safe and effective therapeutic interventions. It is important for the pharmaceutical industry to be involved in these efforts and for collaborative approaches to be developed among industry, academic, nonprofit, state, and federal resources. Furthermore, it is critically important that ongoing efforts in patient care and rehabilitation be coordinated with efforts directed toward the development of therapeutic interventions for spinal cord injuries.

Strengthen the research infrastructure and enhance training. High-quality neuroscience research has resulted in significant advances in understanding neuronal injury and repair. By improving and bolstering the research infrastructure through the development of research centers of excellence and enhanced training efforts, scientists will be encouraged to collaborate in efforts to accelerate research progress. It also offers the opportunity to draw a large cadre of young basic neuroscientists into the field of spinal cord injury research. Furthermore, it is important to establish a research network that can provide the structure for collaborative initiatives and multicenter clinical trials. Strengthening the research infrastructure will attract additional top-notch researchers and their students to contribute to research on these complex issues.

In acknowledging the opportunities ahead for spinal cord injury research, care must also be taken not to minimize the challenges. Treating spinal cord injury, particularly in the near term, will involve improving functional deficits and quality of life. The complexity of the nervous system, the varied nature of spinal cord injuries, and the severity of the loss of function present real and significant hurdles to be overcome to reach the ultimate goals of restoring total function. The urgent need to cure this devastating condition should not tempt overly optimistic predictions of recovery or time frames that cannot be met.

Neither the scientific community nor the community of individuals with spinal cord injuries is content with the limited therapeutic options currently available for the treatment of spinal cord injuries. There is an obvious and urgent need to identify and test new interventions and to accelerate the pace of research, particularly in moving laboratory findings to clinical practice. Spinal cord injury involves serious and traumatic adverse changes to the human body, and an extensive research effort is needed to develop treatment approaches for the range of health outcomes faced by individuals with spinal cord injuries.

BOX ES-1
Summary of the Committee's Recommendations

The following is a summary of the committee's recommendations. Complete text of each recommendation can be found in the corresponding chapters.

Focus on Increasing Knowledge of Basic Biology and Therapeutic Approaches

Increase Efforts to Develop Therapeutic Interventions (Recommendation 5.1)
Specifically, research is needed to:

- improve understanding of the basic mechanisms and identify suitable targets to promote neuroprotection, foster axonal growth, enhance axonal guidance, regulate the maintenance of appropriate synaptic connections, and reestablish functional neuronal and glial circuitry; and
- enhance understanding of proper postinjury care and rehabilitation, such as retraining, relearning, and the use of neuroprostheses, to create the groundwork required to maintain and enhance the maximal potential for full recovery.

Develop a Strategic Plan for Combination Therapeutic Approaches (Recommendation 5.2)
The National Institute of Neurological Disorders and Stroke should develop a strategic plan to screen and assess the potential for compounds and therapies to be used in combination to treat acute and chronic spinal cord injuries.

Bolster and Coordinate Research on Neuronal Injury and Repair (Recommendation 7.1)
The National Institutes of Health should increase the funding for mechanisms that encourage research coordination in neuronal injury and repair and should actively develop and support cross-institute and cross-disciplinary working groups, as outlined in the *NIH Blueprint for Neuroscience Research.*

Improve and Standardize Research Tools and Assessment Techniques (Recommendation 3.2)
Preclinical research tools and animal models should be developed and refined to examine spinal cord injury progression and repair and assess the effectiveness of therapeutic interventions. These preclinical tools and assessment protocols should be standardized for each type and each stage of spinal cord injury.

Increase Training Efforts on Standardized Research Tools and Techniques (Recommendation 3.1)
Spinal cord injury researchers should receive training in the use of standardized animal models and evaluation techniques.

Emphasize and Coordinate Translational Multidisciplinary Research and Clinical Trials

Facilitate Clinical Trials (Recommendation 6.1)
Mechanisms should be implemented that will facilitate the implementation of clinical trials while observing the established standards for the protection of human subjects in clinical research, including:

- coordinating existing facilities and resources in acute care, chronic care, and rehabilitation to support multicenter clinical trials,
- utilizing central institutional review board mechanisms,
- coordinating and expanding patient registries and databases to improve mechanisms to conduct clinical trials and facilitate patient recruitment,
- developing a set of standardized clinical outcome measures, and
- designing clinical trials that are a multidisciplinary effort and should incorporate, as appropriate, small "*n*" methodologies for early-phase clinical trials.

Increase Industry Involvement (Recommendation 6.2)
Mechanisms should be explored that can be used to link federal, state, academic, and nonprofit efforts with those of industry with the goal of increasing the investment and involvement of the private sector in the development of therapeutic interventions for spinal cord injuries.

Strengthen the Research Infrastructure and Enhance Training

Establish Spinal Cord Injury Research Centers of Excellence
(Recommendation 7.2)
The National Institutes of Health should designate and support five to seven Spinal Cord Injury Research Centers of Excellence with adequate resources to sustain multidisciplinary basic, translational, and clinical research on spinal cord injuries.

Establish a National Spinal Cord Injury Research Network
(Recommendation 7.3)
The National Institutes of Health should be appropriately funded to establish a National Spinal Cord Injury Research Network that would coordinate and support the work of an expanded cadre of researchers.

Increase Training and Career Development Opportunities
(Recommendation 7.4)
Resources should be designated to strengthen education programs for pre- and postdoctoral training in spinal cord injury research.

- The National Institutes of Health Office of Science Education and the National Institute of Neurological Disorders and Stroke should enhance training and develop a training module on the functional complexity of the spinal cord for neuroscience Ph.D. and medical students.

Continued

BOX ES-1 Continued

• The National Institutes of Health, state programs, and other research organizations should increase funding for training and career development opportunities for graduate and postdoctoral researchers interested in spinal cord injury research.

Strengthen New York State's Spinal Cord Injury Research Program

Build and Strengthen New York State's Research Infrastructure (Recommendation 8.1)
The New York State Spinal Cord Injury Research Board should increase its research infrastructure to meet the program's mission. The Board should:

• develop and sustain a vigorous recruitment and training effort for fundamental and translational research;
• establish a coordinated statewide research network;
• cultivate formal linkages with researchers, programs, and biopharmaceutical companies in the region to forge partnerships for basic, translational, and clinical research; and
• establish regional core laboratory facilities.

Develop a Regional Clinical Trials Center (Recommendation 8.2)
The state of New York should use its unique strengths to establish a regional clinical trials center. This center should:

• develop and coordinate multicenter clinical trials to examine therapies for the treatment of spinal cord injuries;
• sponsor a clinical trial of decompression as an early intervention and clinical trials of other therapies to be used during the acute phase of a spinal cord injury by using the special opportunities offered by New York City's geographic location and the unique resources of its trauma centers; and
• manage a clinical trials clearinghouse.

Restructure Research Funding and Oversight Processes (Recommendation 8.3)
The New York State Spinal Cord Injury Research Board should work with the state of New York to reduce administrative burdens, improve the approval and grant distribution processes, and establish a rapid-response funding mechanism to capitalize on new research ideas.

Ensure Independent Evaluation (Recommendation 8.4)
The New York State Spinal Cord Injury Research Board should establish an independent external review panel that meets periodically to rigorously assess the program's efforts toward its stated mission to cure spinal cord injuries.

1

INTRODUCTION

A teenager diving into a shallow lake, a young mother in a car accident on her way to work, a collapse of a workman's scaffolding, an elderly woman falling down a flight of stairs—spinal cord injuries can happen to anyone at any time. Going from daily routine to a life-changing spinal cord injury can put independent living in jeopardy and totally reconfigure the realities of daily life. The events that cause spinal cord injuries are sudden and unexpected; however, the resulting physical and lifestyle constraints and limitations remain lifelong challenges.

Although advances in medicine and neuroscience have resulted in limited progress in developing therapeutic interventions for spinal cord injuries, many current avenues of research suggest that a concerted research effort on spinal cord injuries could result in important gains in restoring function and improving quality of life. This report highlights the current status of spinal cord injury research, examines the research and infrastructure needs, and provides recommendations for advancing and accelerating progress in the treatment of spinal cord injuries.

The ancient Egyptians declared spinal cord injury as a condition "not to be treated." Early efforts to treat spinal cord injuries began to be developed by the Greek physician Hippocrates, who constructed several rudimentary forms of traction using a board or ladder to immobilize the patient's back (Eltorai, 2002). Development of antiseptics and sterilization techniques in the 1800s improved the rates of survival from surgery. However, it has been estimated that during World War I 90 percent of the individuals who sustained a spinal cord injury died within 1 year of the injury and only approximately 1 percent survived more than 20 years (Swain and Grundy, 2002). "Up until the 1940s, spinal cord injury was essentially a death sentence. If the injury itself didn't prove fatal, then the complications . . . became fatal" (Kreutz, 2004). Since then, the development of antibiotics, improvements in general medical care, and advances in rehabilitation medicine and in technologies such as respirators have resulted in gains in patient survival, care, and life expectancy. Although the life expectancy for an individual with a spinal cord injury has improved dramatically, it remains lower than that for the general population (Charlifue and Lammertse, 2002).

EXTENT AND COSTS

It is estimated that 11,000 spinal cord injuries occur each year in the United States and that 247,000 Americans are living with a spinal cord injury (NSCISC, 2004). Most individuals with spinal cord injuries are young adults, primarily males (78.2 percent of cases since 2000) (NSCISC, 2004). The average age at the time of injury has increased in recent years, from an average of 28.6 years in 1979 to the current average of 38 years. Explanations for this trend include greater numbers of injuries in the population over 60 years of age (the percentage of individuals older than 60 years of age at the time of injury increased from 4.7 percent before 1980 to 10.9 percent since 2000) and the general aging of the U.S. population (NSCISC, 2004). Only about 5 percent of spinal cord injuries occur in children, usually as a result of traffic accidents or falls (Swain and Grundy, 2002).

Historical trends in spinal cord injury incidence in the United States showed an increase from 22 per million population in the period from 1935 to 1944 to 71 per million population from 1975 to 1981. That rate has fallen, however, to the current rate of approximately 40 incidents of spinal cord injuries per million population each year, a rate that has remained stable for the past 20 years (Sekhon and Fehlings, 2001; DeVivo, 2002). These statistics indicate that unless new treatments or preventive measures are developed, spinal cord injuries will likely continue to be the source of severe disability and loss of function for thousands of Americans each year.

On the basis of reports to the National Spinal Cord Injury Statistical Center (NSCISC), the major causes of spinal cord injuries in the United States are motor vehicle crashes and traffic accidents (50.4 percent); followed by falls (23.8 percent); violent acts (11.2 percent), primarily gunshot wounds; and recreational sports activities (9.0 percent) (NSCISC, 2004). Recent trends, however, show a decrease in work-related causes of injuries and an increase in sports and recreational causes (Sekhon and Fehlings, 2001). Causes of injuries also vary between regions of the country and between urban and rural locations. Table 1-1 provides NSCISC demo-

TABLE 1-1 Demographics of Persons in the NSCISC Database by Year of Injury

	1973-1977	1995-1999
Gender (percent)		
Male	82.7	79.5
Female	17.3	20.5
Age at Injury (percent)		
1-15	7.7	3.0
16-30	61.6	42.1
31-45	17.7	28.1
46-60	8.8	15.1
61-75	3.6	8.5
76+	0.7	3.2
Mean Age (yr) at Injury	28.2	36.5
Race or Ethnicity (percent)		
Caucasian	76.8	62.2
African American	14.9	23.7
Hispanic	6.2	10.9
Asian American	0.8	2.2
Native American	1.3	0.3
Other Race	0.0	0.7

NOTE: The NSCISC database includes data from an estimated 13 percent of new spinal cord injury cases in the United States. As of July 2004, the database contained information on 22,992 individuals who had sustained traumatic spinal cord injuries. Since 1973, 25 federally funded Model Spinal Cord Injury Care Systems have contributed data to the NSCISC database. Although the database has a large sample size and geographic diversity, it is not population based.
SOURCE: Reprinted with permission, from DeVivo et al., 2002. Copyright 2002 by Demos Medical Publishing.

graphic data for individuals with spinal cord injuries occurring in the periods from 1973 to 1977 and 1995 to 1999.

The nature and extent of spinal cord injuries vary widely, depending on the site of the injury and its severity. Table 1-2 highlights the heterogeneous nature of the functional outcomes resulting from spinal cord injuries. Each individual's experience is unique in terms of the degree of paralysis and pain, the extent of spasticity, and the therapies involved in stabilizing autonomic system dysfunction. Therefore, how a spinal cord injury impacts a person's life is highly individualized. Injuries to the upper sections of the spine nearest the head can result in quadriplegia (also termed tetraplegia), with the individual losing motor and sensory functions in the arms and legs, as well as bowel, bladder, chest, abdominal, and diaphragm function. Injuries occurring in the lower areas of the spine may

TABLE 1-2 Activities of Daily Living, by Level of Spinal Cord Injury

Activities of Daily Living	Level of Injury			
	Cervical 1-3	Cervical 4	Cervical 5	Cervical 6
Respiratory control	• Ventilator dependent • Inability to clear secretions	May be able to breathe without ventilator	• Low endurance • May require assist to clear secretions	• Low endurance • May require assist to clear secretions
Bowel control	Total assist	Total assist	Total assist	Independent to total assist
Bladder control	Total assist	Total assist	Total assist	Some to total assist
Bed mobility	Total assist	Total assist	Some assist	Independent to total assist
Bed and wheelchair transfers	Total assist	Total assist	Total assist	Independent to total assist
Pressure relief and positioning	Total assist; may be independent with equipment	Total assist; may be independent with equipment	Independent with equipment	Independent with equipment
Eating	Total assist	Total assist	Total assist for setup, then independent eating with equipment	Independent

Dressing	Total assist	Total assist	• Lower extremity: total assist • Upper extremity: some assist	• Lower extremity: some to total assist • Upper extremity: independent
Grooming	Total assist	Total assist	Some to total assist	Some assist to independent
Bathing	Total assist	Total assist	Total assist	• Lower body: some to total assist • Upper extremity: independent
Wheelchair propulsion	• Manual: total assist • Power: independent with equipment	• Manual: total assist • Power: independent	• Manual: independent to some assist • Power: independent	• Manual: independent to total assist • Power: independent
Standing and ambulation	Total assist	Total assist	Total assist	Total assist
Communication	Total assist to independent	Total assist to independent	Independent to some assist	Independent
Transportation	Total assist	Total assist	Total assist to independent	Independent
Amount of assistance required	24-hour care	24-hour care	Home care: 6 hours/day Personal care: 10 hours/day	Home care: 4 hours/day Personal care: 6 hours/day

Continued

TABLE 1-2 Continued

Activities of Daily Living	Level of Injury			
	Cervical 7-8	Thoracic 1-9	Thoracic 10-Lumbar 1	Lumbar 2-Sacral 5
Respiratory control	• Low endurance • May require assist to clear secretions	Low endurance	Intact function	Intact function
Bowel control	Some to total assist	Independent	Independent	Independent
Bladder control	Independent to some assist	Independent	Independent	Independent
Bed mobility	Independent to some assist	Independent	Independent	Independent
Bed and wheelchair transfers	Independent to some assist	Independent	Independent	Independent
Pressure relief and positioning	Independent	Independent	Independent	Independent
Eating	Independent	Independent	Independent	Independent
Dressing	• Lower extremity: some assist to independent • Upper extremity: independent	Independent	Independent	Independent

Grooming	Independent	Independent	Independent	Independent
Bathing	• Lower body: some assist to independent • Upper extremity: independent	Independent	Independent	Independent
Wheelchair propulsion	Independent to some assist	Independent	Independent	Independent
Standing	Independent to some assist	Independent	Independent	Independent
Communication	Independent	Independent	Independent	Independent
Transportation	Independent	Independent	Independent	Independent
Amount of assistance required	Home care: 2 hours/day Personal care: 6 hours/day	Homemaking: 3 hours/day	Homemaking: 2 hours/day	Homemaking: 0-1 hour/day

SOURCE: Reprinted with permission, from Sie and Waters, 2002. Copyright 2002 by Demos Medical Publishing.

result in paraplegia (loss of movement and sensation in the lower body) or the loss of specific functions.

An injury is categorized as complete if the patient has no sensory or motor function below the level of injury and as incomplete if the patient has such function (see Chapter 2). Data from the Model Spinal Cord Injury System since 2000 show that the most frequent neurological category at discharge is incomplete quadriplegia (34.3 percent), followed by complete paraplegia (25.1 percent), complete quadriplegia (22.1 percent), and incomplete paraplegia (17.5 percent) (NSCISC, 2004). Depending on the extent of the injury, the individual can recover some function and sensation (Levi, 2004). Many patients with complete paraplegia at 72 hours postinjury do not regain any function (Maynard et al., 1979). Individuals with incomplete paraplegia or tetraplegia have higher rates of improvements in motor function (Ditunno et al., 2000). An important prognostic factor is the preservation of sensation, particularly in the anal area. In one study, 47 percent of patients with incomplete sensory function at 72 hours postinjury and 87 percent of patients with incomplete motor function at 72 hours postinjury recovered the ability to walk within a year (Maynard et al., 1979).

The economic costs of spinal cord injuries largely depend on the severity of the injury and the nature of the resulting disability. The costs are highest in the first year after injury, primarily because of emergency, hospital, and rehabilitation care costs. Data on hospital admissions show that the average length of hospital stay in the acute care unit for patients with spinal cord injuries declined from 25 days in 1974 to 15 days in 2002; over that same period similar decreases were seen for stays in rehabilitation facilities (a decrease from 115 days to 40 days) (NSCISC, 2004). An analysis of the potential impacts of these reductions was not provided.

In 1996, the total annual cost of spinal cord injuries in the United States was estimated to be $9.73 billion, including an estimated $2.6 billion in lost productivity (Table 1-3) (Berkowitz et al., 1998). Of the total cost, first year costs were estimated to be $2.58 billion. Individuals with spinal cord injuries also incur significant costs for home and vehicle modifications, equipment purchase, medications, and personal assistance services (Table 1-4), with an estimate of $244,000 for each individual's first-year medical and home modification costs (Berkowitz et al., 1998). Costs are higher for those with more disabling injuries (Table 1-4).

In discussing the health outcomes from spinal cord injuries and their associated costs, it is helpful to put these types of injuries into perspective with other diseases and health conditions (Table 1-5). Spinal cord injuries, although relatively infrequent health outcomes, impose heavy economic costs on society, particularly as they often affect young people and severely limit their productivity and quality of life. The economic costs to an indi-

TABLE 1-3 Costs of Spinal Cord Injuries to Society (1996)

Service	Costs ($ millions)
First-Year Costs	
First-year medical and related costs	2,366.57
Initial home modifications	221.58
Total first-year costs	2,588.15
Annual Costs	
Medical care (recurring)	1,624.86
Medications and supplies	449.02
Vehicle modifications	103.01
Home modifications (recurring)	67.83
Wheelchairs	235.60
Personal assistance	2,068.10
Total annual costs	4,548.42
Indirect Costs	2,591.11
Total Costs	9,727.68

SOURCE: Reprinted with permission, from Berkowitz et al., 1998. Copyright 1998 by Demos Medical Publishing.

TABLE 1-4 Average Yearly Individual Expenses (2004 dollars)

Severity of Injury	First-Year Expenses	Expenses for Each Subsequent Year
High tetraplegia (C1 to C4)	$682,957	$122,334
Low tetraplegia (C5 to C8)	$441,025	$50,110
Paraplegia	$249,549	$25,394
Incomplete motor function	$201,273	$14,106

NOTE: C1 to C8 refer to the site of the injury on the cervical section of the spinal column (see Chapter 2).
SOURCE: Reprinted with permission, from NSCISC, 2004. Copyright 2004 by NSCISC.

vidual over his or her lifetime can be as high as $2.7 million for someone with high tetraplegia who is injured at 25 years of age (NSCISC, 2004). On the other hand, the average age at diagnosis of many of the diseases that affect the nervous system is older, resulting in lower lifetime costs. For example, only 15 percent of those diagnosed with Parkinson's disease are younger than age 50. Of the individuals with Alzheimer's disease, 3 percent are between the ages of 65 to 74 at the time of diagnosis, whereas nearly

TABLE 1-5 Comparison of the Extent and Costs of Selected Neurological Conditions

Injury or Disease	Estimated Current Prevalence in the U.S. (number of cases)	Estimated Annual Incidence in the U.S. (number of new cases per year)	Estimated Annual Cost to Society, $ billions (year used as base estimate)[a]
Spinal cord injury	247,000	11,000	9.7 (1996)
Multiple sclerosis	400,000	10,400[b]	20.0
Epilepsy	2,300,000	181,000	12.5 (1995)
Parkinson's disease	500,000	50,000	5.6
Alzheimer's disease	4,500,000	377,000	100.0 (1991)
Stroke	5,400,000	700,000[c]	56.8

[a]The cost estimates were calculated by a variety of methods and with various years as their basis. Most of the estimates include direct and indirect costs. Where available the year used as the basis for the estimate is included in parentheses.

[b]This number is based on the National Multiple Sclerosis Society estimate that 200 individuals are diagnosed each week with multiple sclerosis.

[c]In any given year, 500,000 are first attacks and 200,000 are recurrent attacks.

SOURCES: Ernst and Hay, 1994; Berkowitz et al., 1998; Begley et al., 2000; Hebert et al., 2001, 2003; National Multiple Sclerosis Society, 2004; NINDS, 2004; NSCISC, 2004; American Heart Association, 2005.

half of those age 85 and older may have the disease (Alzheimer's Disease Education & Referral Center, 2004). The average age for those who suffer spinal cord injuries (28.6 years) is similar to that of individuals who are diagnosed with multiple sclerosis or who suffer a brain trauma.

These economic costs are only a hint of the enormously devastating physical, social, and emotional burdens that individuals and their families face after a spinal cord injury. To have limited or no ability to walk, pick up a coffee cup, or write with a pencil or pen and to face daily routines that take many times longer than before the injury are a fraction of the hardships and challenges that individuals living with spinal cord injuries continually encounter. With tenacity, creativity, and compassion, these challenges have been and continue to be overcome by individuals living with spinal cord injuries and their families. Furthermore, a number of nonprofit organizations work tirelessly to support individuals with spinal cord injuries and their families and caregivers.

SPECTRUM OF PREVENTION TO TREATMENT

In delineating the scope of this report, it is useful to consider the framework that has been developed in the field of injury prevention and control to represent the injury process. Injury events are attributable to the uncontrolled release of physical energy (kinetic, chemical, thermal, electrical, or radiation energy) (Haddon, 1968). In considering the events that result in an injury, there are three temporal phases of injury causation: pre-event, event, and postevent (Haddon, 1980). Each phase requires different types of interventions to prevent or treat the resulting injury. In the pre-event phase, efforts are focused on how to prevent the injury from occurring. Examples of pre-event interventions include highway design improvements and the construction of pedestrian crosswalks and overpasses. Research on interventions in the second phase, when the injury is occurring, is focused on the transfer of energy to the individual and the negation or minimization of the injury. Second-phase interventions include the installation of airbags in vehicles, the use of bicycle and motorcycle helmets, appropriate emergency medical services at the time of injury, and rapid transfer and evacuation to definitive care. These are active areas of research that have resulted in innovations that have saved lives and reduced the severities of injuries, including spinal cord injuries.

The third phase—the postevent phase of the injury—is the focus of this report. After the injury has occurred, the goal is to minimize the damage and restore the lost function and former quality of life. As described in greater detail in Chapter 2, the acute-care phase of the injury—the short period of time just after the injury has occurred—is a window of opportunity to minimize the injury and prevent further damage or loss of function from occurring. Once the patient is stabilized, there are opportunities for a range of therapeutic interventions to improve or restore the lost function. Developing acute and chronic care interventions is the challenge facing the spinal cord injury research community.

DEFINING A CURE

Defining what constitutes a "cure" is an integral part of discussions on future directions for spinal cord injury research. In large part, the general public's perception of a cure for spinal cord injury has been the restoration of motor function—to walk. However, a spinal cord injury affects many systems and functions of the body that are vital to the health and well-being of the injured person. Neural control of motor, sensory, autonomic, bowel, and bladder functions are compromised, often leading to pain, pressure sores, infection, and diminished physiological well-being.

After carefully considering input from individuals with spinal cord injuries, researchers, and clinicians, the committee decided to take a broad approach to "defining a cure" and to frame its definition around alleviating the multiple disabilities that result from spinal cord injury.

Spinal cord injury research should focus on preventing the loss of function and on restoring lost functions—including sensory, motor, bowel, bladder, autonomic, and sexual functions—with the elimination of complications, particularly pain, spasticity, pressure sores (decubitus ulcers), and depression, with the ultimate goal of fully restoring the activity and function of an individual to his or her preinjury levels.

By setting forth a set of goals for spinal cord injury research, the committee wishes to emphasize the different stages of the injury during which interventions are needed and the multiple health impairments that affect an individual's daily quality of life and that require the development of effective therapeutic interventions (Figure 1-1).

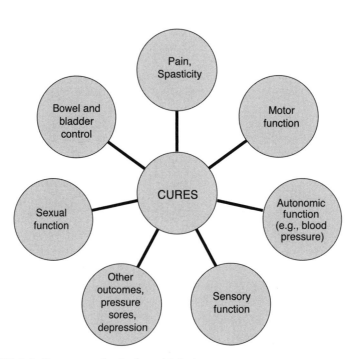

FIGURE 1-1 Outcomes of spinal cord injuries.

Walking again is not my "gold standard." If I could take a pill and be cured of paralysis and be able to walk, that is just fine. But I guarantee you that in this chair I could keep up with any one of you going down the street outside. My problem everyday is the little things. It is the pressure sore. It is the dexterity. It is that kind of thing that I wish that we could make progress as far as restoration of function is concerned.

— John Bollinger
Paralyzed Veterans of America

FROM CHALLENGES TO OPPORTUNITIES

Although breakthroughs in the biomedical sciences in the past 50 years have resulted in medications and interventions for the treatment of many health disorders and diseases, progress in treating spinal cord injuries has been slow and uneven. However, a confluence of factors (described below) now points to more rapid progress. Some of the hurdles that have stymied progress in the past are now being overcome and other opportunities are being realized. A few of these opportunities are highlighted below, and these and others are further discussed throughout the report.

• *Understanding the biology of the nervous system.* For years it was thought that neurons in mammals do not regenerate and that it was not possible to initiate axonal growth. However, beginning in the 1980s, the discovery that neurons in rat spinal cords could regenerate and make functional connections and that regeneration could be enhanced with changes in the environment of the damaged nerve cells opened possibilities to an array of research approaches to the treatment of spinal cord injuries. Other recent advances—including the ongoing elucidation of the biological blockers and promoters of nerve regeneration—have continued to accelerate research progress and move research closer toward clinical therapies

• *Emergency medical treatment.* Emergency care for individuals with spinal cord injuries has only recently reached a point at which rapid response, standardized protocols for the immobilization and treatment of neck injuries, and the training of emergency medical technicians have led to increased survival rates and decreases in the number of complete spinal cord injuries. More patients thus present to the emergency department with residual function. Furthermore, the challenges of conducting clinical trials of emergency care interventions may be beginning to be overcome with the development of networks of trauma centers and the development of protocols and standards for addressing informed-consent issues in emergency situations.

• *Research tools and imaging techniques.* Improved laboratory techniques and refined statistical methodologies are opening up opportunities for more closely monitoring the effects of potential therapeutic interventions. Furthermore, significant advances have made it possible to more closely visualize neuronal growth and alterations in vivo and to identify regions of damage to the spinal cord.

- *Leveraging progress in treating other conditions.* Progress in other fields of research may well be critical in advancing therapies for spinal cord injuries. Insights into neuronal injury and repair are being gained through research on neurodegenerative disorders, and research in other areas (such as understanding the role of stem cell biology in cancer) may prove important.

In acknowledging the opportunities ahead for spinal cord injury research, care must also be taken not to minimize the challenges. Treating spinal cord injury, particularly in the near term, will involve improving functional deficits and quality of life. The complexity of the nervous system, the varied nature of spinal cord injuries, and the severity of the loss of function present real and significant hurdles to be overcome to reach the ultimate goals of restoring total function. The urgent need to cure this devastating condition should not tempt overly optimistic predictions of recovery or time frames that cannot be met.

SCOPE AND ORGANIZATION OF THIS REPORT

In 1998 the state of New York established the New York State Spinal Cord Injury Research Trust to focus on funding and coordinating research on therapeutic interventions for spinal cord injuries (see Chapter 8). Monies for this fund are obtained from surcharges on fines for certain traffic violations, as well as from gifts and donations. In 2002, the New York State Spinal Cord Injury Research Board requested that the Institute of Medicine (IOM) examine the current state of research on spinal cord injuries and make recommendations on priorities for research efforts, particularly with a focus on translational research and strategies to accelerate progress in this field (Box 1-1).

The IOM appointed a 13-member committee with expertise in neuroscience, clinical research, trauma surgery, health care, physiology, and biomedical engineering. The committee met four times during the course of its work and held three workshops (Appendix A) to receive input on future directions for spinal cord injury research. Additionally, the committee received input from individuals with spinal cord injuries and from relevant nonprofit organizations.

This report provides the committee's recommendations for furthering spinal cord injury research. Written for a broad audience that includes

---

BOX 1-1
Statement of Task

Spinal cord injuries are a leading cause of major disability, and there is currently no cure for such injuries. However, over the last several decades there has been a steady flow of new scientific findings suggesting that spinal connections damaged by injury can be functionally restored.

An Institute of Medicine committee will identify approaches and strategies that offer the promise of accelerating the development of cures for spinal cord injuries. Particular attention will be paid to strategies for translating the advances in neuroscience and cell biology to clinical research and treatment. In addition, the study will provide recommendations to its sponsor, the Health Department of the State of New York and its Spinal Cord Injury Research Board, about how to best utilize its resources to facilitate progress in translational spinal cord injury research.

The committee will:

(1) Review the state of the science relevant to curing spinal cord injuries, including what is known about the postinjury pathophysiology in humans, as well as relevant basic science and clinical concepts. The focus of the study will be on methods to reduce paralysis and restore lost function, as opposed to rehabilitative methods limited to maintaining function remaining after injury.

(2) Identify the gaps in knowledge and technological barriers that exist, as well as areas that have the greatest potential to accelerate the development of cures for spinal cord injuries. Related fields that may provide insights or promote progress in the search for cures for spinal cord injuries will also be explored.

(3) Provide recommendations for short- and long-term strategies to fill the gaps that exist in research relevant to curing spinal cord injury. The portfolios of major funders of spinal cord injury research will be examined. The committee will identify those research directions that are likely to have near-term impact on the field, those efforts that are more likely to come to fruition at later times, and those efforts that are more speculative, but likely to pay off if they succeed. Mechanisms that can be used to encourage research in these areas will be explored and barriers to progress will be identified.

(4) Define the unique strengths of New York State's institutions and researchers in neurological, basic, clinical, and translational research on spinal cord injuries. The committee will provide recommendations that consider the distinctive contribution that can be made by New York's Spinal Cord Injury Research Board and Trust Fund to complement the efforts of other state, federal, and private supporters of research aimed at stimulating the search for cures for spinal cord injuries.

---

individuals with spinal cord injuries, advocates, policy makers, researchers, and clinicians, the report provides both broad overviews of the issues as well as specific details on the science of spinal cord injury. Chapter 2 introduces the biology of spinal cord injury and the state of the science. Chapter 3 focuses on advances in research technologies and tools. Chapter

4 describes the current status of therapeutic interventions for spinal cord injuries, and Chapter 5 provides an overview of the progress that is being made in neural repair and regeneration. Chapter 6 discusses the issues involved in moving research from the laboratory to the bedside and particularly addresses the challenges and opportunities for clinical trials on therapeutic interventions for spinal cord injuries. In Chapter 7, the committee examines the research infrastructure and proposes recommendations for accelerating progress in spinal cord injury research. Chapter 8 highlights the state programs in spinal cord injury research and provides recommendations to the New York State Spinal Cord Injury Research Board, the sponsor of this study.

REFERENCES

Alzheimer's Disease Education & Referral Center. 2004. *General Information*. [Online]. Available: http://www.alzheimers.org/generalinfo.htm#howmany [accessed November 11, 2004].

American Heart Association. 2005. *Heart Disease and Stroke Statistics—2005 Update*. Dallas: American Heart Association.

Begley CE, Famulari M, Annegers JF, Lairson DR, Reynolds TF, Coan S, Dubinsky S, Newmark ME, Leibson C, So EL, Rocca WA. 2000. The cost of epilepsy in the United States: An estimate from population-based clinical and survey data. *Epilepsia* 41(3): 342-351.

Berkowitz M, Harvey C, Greene CG, Wilson SE. 1998. *Spinal Cord Injury: An Analysis of Medical and Social Costs*. New York: Demos Medical Publishing.

Charlifue S, Lammertse D. 2002. Spinal cord injury and aging. In: Lin V, Cardenas DD, Cutter NC, Frost FS, Hammond MC, Lindblom LB, Perkash I, Waters R, eds. *Spinal Cord Medicine: Principles and Practice*. New York: Demos Medical Publishing. Pp. 829-838.

DeVivo MJ. 2002. Epidemiology of spinal cord injury. In: Lin V, Cardenas DD, Cutter NC, Frost FS, Hammond MC, Lindblom LB, Perkash I, Waters R, eds. *Spinal Cord Medicine: Principles and Practice*. New York: Demos Medical Publishing. Pp. 79-85.

Ditunno JF Jr, Cohen ME, Hauck WW, Jackson AB, Sipski ML. 2000. Recovery of upper-extremity strength in complete and incomplete tetraplegia: A multicenter study. *Archives of Physical Medicine and Rehabilitation* 81(4): 389-393.

Eltorai IB. 2002. History of spinal cord medicine. In: Lin V, Cardenas DD, Cutter NC, Frost FS, Hammond MC, Lindblom LB, Perkash I, Waters R, eds. *Spinal Cord Medicine: Principles and Practice*. New York: Demos Medical Publishing. Pp. 3-14.

Ernst RL, Hay JW. 1994. The US economic and social costs of Alzheimer's disease revisited. *American Journal of Public Health* 84(8): 1261-1264.

Haddon W Jr. 1968. The changing approach to the epidemiology, prevention, and amelioration of trauma: The transition to approaches etiologically rather than descriptively based. *American Journal of Public Health & the Nation's Health* 58(8): 1431-1438.

Haddon W Jr. 1980. Advances in the epidemiology of injuries as a basis for public policy. *Public Health Reports* 95(5): 411-421.

Hebert LE, Beckett LA, Scherr PA, Evans DA. 2001. Annual incidence of Alzheimer disease in the United States projected to the years 2000 through 2050. *Alzheimer Disease & Associated Disorders* 15(4): 169-173.

Hebert LE, Scherr PA, Bienias JL, Bennett DA, Evans DA. 2003. Alzheimer disease in the US population: Prevalence estimates using the 2000 census. *Archives of Neurology* 60(8): 1119-1122.

Kreutz D. 2004, October 17. Tucson quadriplegics live Reeve's battle. *Arizona Daily Star*. Pp. 2-4.

Levi ADO. 2004. Approach to the patient and diagnostic evaluation. In: Winn HR, Youmans JR, eds. *Neurological Surgery: A Comprehensive Reference Guide to the Diagnosis and Management of Neurological Problems*. Vol. 4. 5th ed. Philadelphia: W. B. Saunders. Pp. 4869-4884.

Maynard FM, Reynolds GG, Fountain S, Wilmot C, Hamilton R. 1979. Neurological prognosis after traumatic quadriplegia. Three-year experience of California regional spinal cord injury care system. *Journal of Neurosurgery* 50(5): 611-616.

National Multiple Sclerosis Society. 2004. *National Multiple Sclerosis Society*. [Online]. Available: http://www.nationalmssociety.org [accessed October 28, 2004].

NINDS (National Institute of Neurological Disorders and Stroke). 2004. *Parkinson's Disease: Hope Through Research*. [Online]. Available: http://www.ninds.nih.gov/disorders/parkinsons_disease/detail_parkinsons_disease.htm [accessed November 11, 2004].

NSCISC (National Spinal Cord Injury Statistical Center). 2004. *Facts and Figures at a Glance—August 2004*. [Online]. Available: http://www.spinalcord.uab.edu/show.asp?durki=21446 [accessed November 11, 2004].

Sekhon LH, Fehlings MG. 2001. Epidemiology, demographics, and pathophysiology of acute spinal cord injury. *Spine* 26(24 Suppl): S2-12.

Sie I, Waters RL. 2002. Outcomes following spinal cord injury. In: Lin V, Cardenas DD, Cutter NC, Frost FS, Hammond MC, Lindblom LB, Perkash I, Waters R, eds. *Spinal Cord Medicine: Principles and Practice*. New York: Demos Medical Publishing. Pp. 87-103.

Swain A, Grundy D. 2002. At the accident. In: Grundy D, Swain A, eds. *ABC of Spinal Cord Injury*. 4th ed. London: British Journal of Medicine. Pp. 1-4.

2

PROGRESSION OF SPINAL CORD INJURY

Injury to the spinal cord triggers a cascade of biological events that unfold within seconds and that proceed for months or even years. The events affect three major bodily systems: the nervous system, the immune system, and the vascular system. These systems interact dynamically as they respond to injury. Although some injurious responses heal and promote the recovery of function, others leave a wave of tissue damage that expands well beyond the original site of injury.

The choreography of tightly interwoven responses that lead to dysfunction is known as injury pathophysiology. The final outcome of serious spinal cord injury is shattering: loss of reflexes, loss of sensation, and paralysis (i.e., the loss of control over muscles and movement of the body). Although much has been learned about the progression of spinal cord injuries and the biochemical reactions and pathways that are involved in the process, much remains to be explored. With understanding of injury pathophysiology comes the ability to interfere with its progression, to harness the regenerative potential of the spinal cord, to improve therapies, and to create new ones.

This chapter on the biology of spinal cord injuries provides a broad overview of spinal cord anatomy, injury types, and injury classification. The chapter discusses the cellular and molecular events underlying the body's response to injury—both pathological and protective—and covers the biological basis of pain, as well as functional losses involving muscles, sensory organs, the bladder, and the bowel. The basic information in this chapter serves as a backdrop for later chapters on therapeutic approaches.

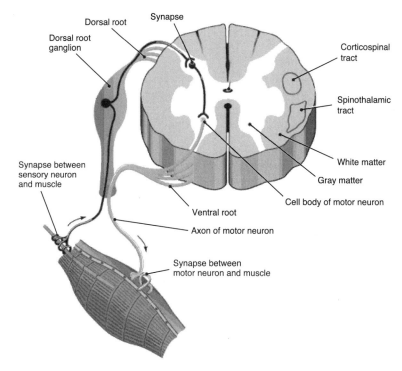

FIGURE 2-1 Cross section of the spinal cord.
SOURCE: Reprinted with permission, from Taber and Thomas, 1997. Copyright 2003 by F. A. Davis Company.

SPINAL CORD, NERVES, MUSCLES, AND THE SENSORY SYSTEM

The spinal cord is the elongated portion of the central nervous system (CNS) that connects the brain to all muscles of the body and most sensory nerves to the brain.[1] It is surrounded and protected by vertebrae, or the spinal column. The outer edge of the spinal cord is the white matter (Figure 2-1), which contains the branching portions of nerve cells known as axons. Wrapping around the axons is a fatty whitish substance called myelin, which speeds up the nerve impulses from the brain to the rest of the body. In addition to an axon, each nerve cell (or neuron) has a cell body, which is its control center housing the nerve cell genes and other parts needed to

---

[1]Except for the cranial nerves to the head and neck.

produce energy and to make proteins. The cell bodies of neurons cluster together in the gray matter of the spinal cord and are not located in the white matter. Two regions of the gray matter are of special interest: the ventral horn and the dorsal horn. The ventral horn contains the cell bodies of motor neurons, which induce muscles to contract. The dorsal horn contains the primary sensory pathways that transmit information from the skin and muscles into the spinal cord and up to the brain. The cell bodies of sensory neurons lie outside the spinal cord in a discrete cluster known as the dorsal root ganglion.

Spinal Cord Anatomy as the Basis for Injury Classification

The term "spinal column" refers to the vertebral bones and discs that collectively encase and protect the soft tissue of the spinal cord. The spinal cord is made up of nerve tracts carrying signals back and forth between the brain and the rest of the body. The spinal cord is traditionally divided into four levels, beginning with the highest (most rostral) portion and ending with the lowest (most caudal) portion: cervical, thoracic, lumbar, and sacral (Figure 2-2). Each of the four levels of the spinal cord controls the functions of a particular region of the body through a defined set of spinal nerves that enter and exit the spinal nerve roots (Figure 2-1) through particular openings in the vertebrae. Injury at one level can often lead to the loss of sensory and motor functions below that level because the injury disrupts nerve conduction to and from the brain (Table 2-1).

On the basis of pathology, there are at least three general types of spinal cord injuries: contusion, laceration, and solid cord injuries (Table 2-2). Contusion injuries, often of the cervical spine, are the most frequent and can be simulated in the most widely used animal models (see Chapter 3). The type of spinal cord injury, as well as its level and severity, dictates its functional impact and prognosis.

In an effort to systematize the classification of spinal cord injuries, the American Spinal Injury Association (ASIA) developed in 1992 a uniform and comprehensive way of assessing the level and extent of injury severity. The ASIA International Standards for Neurological Classification are based on the systematic examination of neurological function to assess any deterioration or improvement in neurological function throughout the course of the injury. The classification, which has prognostic, therapeutic, and research value, has four components: (1) sensory and motor levels, (2) the completeness of the injury, (3) the ASIA Impairment Scale, and (4) the zone of partial preservation for complete injuries (ASIA, 2000).

The **sensory and motor levels** refer to the spinal location of the injury and indicate the lowest (most caudal) segment with normal function. The sensory level is identified after extensive testing of skin areas via light touch

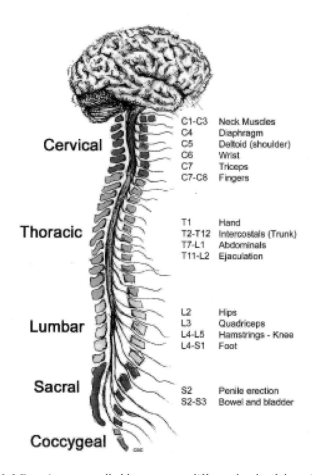

C1-C3	Neck Muscles
C4	Diaphragm
C5	Deltoid (shoulder)
C6	Wrist
C7	Triceps
C7-C8	Fingers

T1	Hand
T2-T12	Intercostals (Trunk)
T7-L1	Abdominals
T11-L2	Ejaculation

L2	Hips
L3	Quadriceps
L4-L5	Hamstrings - Knee
L4-S1	Foot

| S2 | Penile erection |
| S2-S3 | Bowel and bladder |

Cervical

Thoracic

Lumbar

Sacral

Coccygeal

FIGURE 2-2 Functions controlled by nerves at different levels of the spine. Damage at a particular level usually impairs the functions controlled by all nerves at lower levels.
SOURCE: Reprinted with permission, from CRPF, 2002. Copyright 2002 from CRPF.

and pinprick. Predefined regions of the skin covering the whole body, called dermatomes, are each scored as having normal, impaired, or absent sensation. Similarly, the motor level is determined by manual testing and grading of the strengths, on a scale of 0 to 5, of 10 muscle groups that control different motor functions, including limb, bowel, and bladder functions. Although the sensory and motor levels may differ somewhat, they both come under an umbrella "neurological level," which is defined as the most

TABLE 2-1 Spinal Cord Levels and Areas of Control

Spinal Cord Section	Spinal Cord Levels	Areas of Control[a]	Likely Condition After Injury
Cervical	C1-C8	Head, neck, diaphragm, arms	Tetraplegic
Thoracic	T1-T12	Chest, abdominal muscles	Paraplegic
Lumbar	L1-L5	Hips, legs	Paraplegic
Sacral	S1-S5	Bowel, bladder, groin, calves, buttocks, legs	Paraplegic

[a]An injury at a given level indicates that the portion of the spinal column beneath the site of injury will likely be affected.
SOURCES: El Masry et al., 1996; ASIA, 2000; Young, 2002.

TABLE 2-2 Types of Spinal Cord Injuries

Type of Spinal Cord Injury	Percentage of Total Injuries	Description
Contusion	25 to 40	Bruising, but not severing, of the spinal cord
Laceration	25	Severing or tearing of the spinal cord and introduction of connective tissue into the spinal cord, typically from gunshot or knife wounds
Solid cord injury	17	Axon injury and demyelination

SOURCES: Bunge et al., 1993, 1997; Harper et al., 1996; Hulsebosch, 2002.

caudal segment of the spinal cord with both normal sensory and motor functions.

The **completeness of the injury** gives a strong indication and prognosis of the severity of the injury, and it serves as the basis for the ASIA Impairment Scale (described below). A complete injury relies on the detection of any neurological function below the site of the injury (Levi, 2004), especially the loss of motor and sensory functions in the lowest sacral region of the spinal cord (S4 and S5), which supplies nerves to the anal and perineal regions. Few people with a complete spinal cord injury regain the useful function of this region (Levi, 2004). An incomplete injury, on the other

TABLE 2-3 ASIA Impairment Scale

ASIA Grade	Level of Impairment
A	No motor or sensory function preserved in the lowest sacral segments (S4 and S5)
B	Sensory but no motor function preserved, including the lowest sacral segments (S4-S5)
C	Motor function present below the injury, but the strengths of more than half of the key muscles are graded < 3 of 5
D	Motor function present below the injury, but the strengths of more than half of the key muscles are graded ≥ 3 of 5
E	Motor and sensory functions in key muscles and dermatomes are normal

SOURCE: Reprinted with permission, from ASIA, 2000. Copyright 2000 by ASIA.

hand, leaves a person with some sensory or motor function below the site of injury and in the lowest sacral region. It is important to assess sacral sensation when investigating the completeness of an injury, because there is the potential for partial function to be preserved in this area and this may be the only evidence of neurological function below an injury.

The **ASIA Impairment Scale** provides clinicians with a standard way of grading the functional severity of a spinal cord injury (Table 2-3). The scale has one grade for complete injuries (ASIA A), three others grades for incomplete injuries (ASIA B through ASIA D), and another for no impairment from the injury (ASIA E). To assign one of the three grades for incomplete injuries (ASIA B through ASIA D), clinicians determine the degree of muscle strength (on a scale from 0 to 5, with 0 being total paralysis and 5 being active movement against full resistance) of the key muscles below the neurological level of the injury. The assignment is based on the extent to which more than half of the key muscles have a muscle strength grade of 3 or higher.

The **zone of partial preservation** applies only to complete injuries (ASIA A). It refers to the area of the spinal cord that still retains some motor or sensory function above the level of S5 (and below the level of injury). For example, a person might be classified as having a zone of partial preservation at T1 to T3, meaning that he or she has some degree of sensory or motor function at that level of the thoracic spinal cord, even though the injury is complete. A zone of partial preservation is likely due to the presence of intact fiber pathways. About 65 percent of individuals with neurologically complete injuries show some amount of tissue and axonal sparing across the site of the lesion (Bunge et al., 1997).

THREE PHASES OF SPINAL CORD INJURIES

A spinal cord injury immediately injures or kills cells, but it also causes delayed damage and death to cells that survive the original trauma. The biological response to a spinal cord injury is divided into three phases that follow a distinct but somewhat overlapping temporal sequence: acute (seconds to minutes after the injury), secondary (minutes to weeks after the injury), and chronic (months to years after the injury). A general overview of the three phases is presented in Table 2-4. Diverse groups of cells and molecules from the nervous, immune, and vascular systems are involved in each phase. Most participating cells reside in the spinal cord, but others are summoned to the site of injury from the circulatory system (Table 2-5). To carry out many of their functions, the cells depend on changes in gene expression. As would be expected, injury triggers certain cells to up-regulate (increase expression) or down-regulate (decrease expression) genes responsible for a host of proteins involved in inflammation, neurotransmission, regrowth and repair, and other local responses to injury (Bareyre and Schwab, 2003). The final pattern of sensory and motor losses from the

TABLE 2-4 Major Features of the Three Phases of Injury

Acute (Seconds after Injury)	Secondary (Minutes to Weeks)	Chronic (Months to Years)
• Systemic hypotension and spinal shock • Hemorrhage • Cell death from direct insult or ischemia (disruption of blood supply) • Edema (swelling) • Vasospasm (reduction in blood flow) • Shifts in electrolytes • Accumulation of neurotransmitters	• Continued cell death • Continued edema • Continued shifts in electrolytes • Free-radical production • Lipid peroxidation • Neutrophil and lymphocyte invasion and release of cytokines • Apoptosis (programmed cell death) • Calcium entry into cells	• Continued apoptosis radiating from site of injury • Alteration of ion channels and receptors • Formation of fluid-filled cavity • Scarring of spinal cord by glial cells • Demyelination • Regenerative processes, including sprouting by neurons • Altered neurocircuits • Syringomyelia

SOURCES: Sekhon and Fehlings, 2001; Hulsebosch, 2002.

TABLE 2-5 Cell Types Involved in Spinal Cord Injuries

Cell Type	Function and Description
Neuron 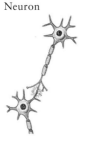	• Carries information within the brain to the rest of the body by conducting electrical signals from neuron to neuron • Several functional types: motor neuron, sensory neuron, autonomic neuron, and interneuron
Astrocyte	• A type of glial cell found in the CNS • Sequesters potassium ions during neural activity • Removes excess neurotransmitters (e.g., glutamate and γ-aminobutyric acid) • Reacts to injury with hypertrophy and cell division, an increase in protein filaments, and formation of a glial scar
Oligodendrocyte 	• A type of glial cell found in the CNS • Forms myelin that insulates the neurons' axons to expedite transmission of electrical signals • One oligodendrocyte myelinates multiple axons • Produces molecules, including Nogo-A, that inhibit neurite outgrowth
Schwann cell 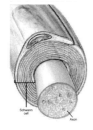	• Found in the peripheral nervous system • Forms myelin that insulates the neurons' axons to expedite transmission of electrical signals • One Schwann cell myelinates only one axon • Promotes neurite outgrowth • Migrates into the spinal cord after injury

Continued

TABLE 2-5 Continued

Cell Type	Function and Description
Endothelial cell 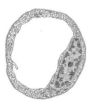	• Forms the lining of blood vessels • Upon injury, up-regulates cell adhesion molecules on the endothelial cell membrane, which helps to recruit inflammatory cells to the site • When injured, releases cytokines and chemokines, which contribute to inflammation
Neutrophil 	• Removes microbial intruders and tissue debris • Emits substances that activate other inflammatory cells and glial cells and that injure neurons
Monocyte	• Migrates to area of injury and differentiates into macrophages • Releases inflammatory cytokines and free radicals • Emits growth factors • Removes tissue debris
Microglia 	• Found in the CNS • Has actions similar to those of macrophages
T–lymphocyte	• Emits inflammatory cytokines • Kills cells (cytotoxic killing) • Neuroprotection in part by possible secretion of growth factors

SOURCES: Reprinted with permission, from Lentz, 1971. Copyright 1971 by Elsevier, Inc.; Dammann et al., 2001. Reprinted with permission from Elsevier; Reprinted with permission, from Stimson, 2001. Copyright 2001 by Muscular Dystrophy Association; Reprinted with permission, from Caceci and El-Shafey, 2002. Copyright 2002 by Caceci; Reprinted with permission, from Merck & Co., Inc., 2004. Copyright 2004 by Merck & Co., Inc.; Reprinted with permission, from Shier et al., 2004. Copyright 2004 by McGraw-Hill Higher Education.

three phases of injury depends on which nerve cells and fiber tracts die, which remain intact, and which regenerate or form new branching patterns to compensate for the losses.

The elucidation of the distinct phases of injury—and the cellular and molecular events underlying them—comes largely from animal models. As events unfold, many of the cellular and molecular events designed to heal the injury can paradoxically lead to further neuronal injury or death. The site of injury may spread to adjacent areas of the spinal cord, sometimes extending four spinal segments above and below the initial site (Crowe et al., 1997; Liu et al., 1997). The affected area becomes filled with immune cells, and a "scar" is formed. The details of the pathophysiology continue to evolve.

Acute Phase

The acute phase, which begins within seconds of the injury, is marked by systemic as well as local events (Tator et al., 1998; Hulsebosch, 2002). The foremost systemic event, after a fleeting increase in blood pressure, is a prolonged decrease in blood pressure (hypotension) that sometimes coincides with a decrease in blood volume. Systemic hypoxia, a reduction of the oxygen supply to the tissues, occurs if, during the injury, respiration is compromised by airway obstruction or by paralysis of diaphragm muscles. Failure of the spinal cord to function for the first 2 to 24 hours after injury, a condition known as spinal shock, results from inadequate flow of oxygen and nutrients into the tissue.

Numerous local events within the spinal cord occur immediately after the injury and also contribute to spinal shock. Direct trauma from injury causes necrosis (cell death) to spinal cord neurons and to the endothelial cells lining the blood vessels of the spinal cord. The surviving neurons at the site of injury respond with a procession of electrical impulses, known as action potentials. Because action potentials require the influx and efflux of ions across the neuron's membrane, the barrage of action potentials creates significant local shifts in ion levels. Higher ion levels are also produced by the mechanical shearing of nerve cells, causing their membranes to rupture and release their contents. Ion buildups can reach levels toxic enough to kill nearby neurons. Similarly, the barrage of action potentials causes the release of excess amounts of neurotransmitters, which then accumulate in the synapses between nerve cells. The accumulation of certain neurotransmitters (e.g., glutamate) can cause the death of nearby neurons through a mechanism called excitotoxicity (Faden and Simon, 1988). Neuron death, by whatever mechanism, contributes to the losses of sensory, motor, and autonomic functions that occur after spinal cord injury.

Direct trauma to the spinal cord causes its small blood vessels to hemorrhage, consequently disrupting the blood-spinal cord barrier, which normally helps protect the CNS. Rapid bleeding into the normal fluid-filled spaces of the spinal cord contributes to local edema. As the swelling within the confined space of the vertebral canal continues, it impinges on and further compromises nerve cells. Other important vascular changes are vasospasm, which is a narrowing of the blood vessels that often decreases blood flow by 80 percent (Anthes et al., 1996) and small-vessel thrombosis (Koyanagi et al., 1993). These vascular perturbations result in ischemia (i.e., deprivation of neurons and other cells of the oxygen and the other nutrients that they need to survive). Perhaps because it is more vascularized, the spinal cord's gray matter (which contains neuron cell bodies) is far more necrotic after injury than the white matter, which contains large tracts of myelinated fibers (axons) that traverse up and down the spinal cord (Wolman, 1965).

Secondary Phase

The secondary phase sets in minutes after injury and lasts for weeks. During this phase the area of injury markedly expands. The secondary phase features a continuation of some events from the acute phase—electrolyte shifts, edema, and necrotic cell death—as well as novel ones, including the formation of free radicals, delayed calcium influx, immune system response (inflammation), and apoptotic cell death.

Formation of Free Radicals

Free-radical formation, usually from oxygen atoms, gives rise to a series of pathological reactions inside cells, including the breakdown of lipids in the cell membrane, a process known as lipid peroxidation. The cell tolerates some degree of lipid peroxidation, but if it is substantial, the cell membrane becomes so disrupted that it bursts and dies. As it dies, the cell spills its contents into the extracellular space, which then threaten neighboring cells. For example, the spillage of the neurotransmitter glutamate can cause the death of nearby cells. If free radical attack does not lyse (burst) the cell membrane, it can invoke other types of damage. Free radicals, for example, can also attack membrane enzymes, distort ion gradients across the cell membrane, and damage genes.

The process of free-radical formation from oxygen begins in the mitochondria, a specialized portion of the cell devoted to converting oxygen into energy-rich molecules. Injury brings an influx of calcium into the cell, which can trigger the process of free-radical formation (Young, 1992). Oxygen atoms lose one of their outermost electrons and become highly reactive. To become more stable, they lure electrons from nearby atoms. In the case of lipid peroxidation, for example, free radicals draw an electron from a lipid molecule, which in turn becomes less stable, thus launching a chain reaction that ultimately leads to lysis of the membrane and death by necrosis.

Delayed Calcium Influx

Although neurons require some intracellular calcium for their normal function, too much calcium is injurious because it activates damaging enzymes and destructive processes and can trigger the formation of free radicals. Some calcium enters neurons at the time of injury and contributes to the acute phase of damage. An additional influx of calcium is triggered by the acute injury and continues for hours afterwards. A particularly powerful mode of calcium influx within injured axons in white matter involves an initial inward leakage of sodium due to the acute injury, which drives the sodium-calcium exchanger to import damaging levels of calcium; this multistage cascade has been demonstrated within myelinated axons of the optic nerve (Stys et al., 1992b) and the spinal cord (Imaizumi et al., 1997). This delayed calcium influx is an important target for interventions because, by blocking it, it is possible to reduce the degree of secondary damage to myelinated spinal cord axons (Stys et al., 1992a).

Immune System Response

The inflammatory response to injury involves four major categories of immune cells: neutrophils, monocytes, microglia, and T-lymphocytes (Schnell et al., 1999; Bareyre and Schwab, 2003). The neutrophils are the first immune cells to arrive at the site of injury. They are recruited there from the circulatory system, especially by vascular endothelial cells, which up-regulate and express adhesion molecules on their cell membranes to help guide neutrophils to the site of injury. Once the neutrophils have entered the spinal tissue, they remove microbial intruders and tissue debris. This is accomplished in many ways, especially through the release of toxic molecules and antibacterial agents (e.g., myeloperoxidase). Neutrophils also release cytokines, proteases, and free radicals, all of which activate other inflammatory and glial cells for the inflammatory cascade that can ultimately lead to neuron injury or death. Cytokines, which are soluble proteins released by most types of inflammatory cells, act as signals between immune cells and carry out immune functions. Neutrophils are the initial dominant cells involved in the immune response.

Over the next 24 hours, microglia respond in earnest. Monocytes begin to enter from the circulatory system and, after they penetrate the spinal cord tissue, differentiate into macrophages. Microglia, on the other hand, actually reside within the spinal cord. Once these cells are activated, they too remove degenerating fiber tracts and other tissue debris by phagocytosis. They also secrete numerous cytokines, free radicals, and growth factors, which, in turn, affect nearby cells in positive and negative ways (Lindholm et al., 1992; Schnell et al., 1999; Anderson, 2002). The growth factors are critical for neuron survival and tissue repair. However, free radicals and proinflammatory cytokines contribute to expansion of the lesion, worsening the impact of the injury. Activation of macrophages and microglia is sustained over the course of weeks.

The role of lymphocytes in spinal cord injuries is somewhat controversial. Some argue that one type of lymphocyte (autoreactive T-lymphocytes) have destructive properties: according to this schema they exacerbate injury to axons and induce demyelination, leading to functional loss (Popovich and Jones, 2003). Others argue that this lymphocyte is not pathological but, rather, confers protection to the myelin-insulated neurons (Schwartz and Kipnis, 2001; Kipnis et al., 2002). Protection of myelin also protects the integrity of the axon that it insulates.

Apoptotic Cell Death

During the acute phase, the mechanical trauma to the spinal cord causes cells to die instantaneously by necrosis, a process of cell swelling and then cell membrane rupture. Within hours, however, another type of cell death assumes center stage: apoptosis. This very active form of death afflicts neurons, oligodendrocytes, astrocytes, and other cells of the spinal cord after injury (Liu et al., 1997; Beattie et al., 2000). Apoptosis has been detected in humans (Emery et al., 1998) and lasts for about one month in animal models (Beattie et al., 2000). With apoptosis, cells do not swell before death; rather, they condense and break apart into small fragments in a very orderly process that requires energy and protein synthesis. These fragments of the apoptotic cell are engulfed by other cells in a process that prevents spillage of the dying cells' contents and avoids elicitation of an inflammatory response. Necrotic cell death, on the other hand, elicits inflammation and spills out neurotransmitters and other contents that build to levels toxic enough to harm or kill nearby cells.

What triggers apoptosis after spinal cord injury? An answer to this question would immediately open up new targets for treatments that could prevent apoptosis from occurring. A major trigger appears to be the injury-induced rush of calcium into cells (Young, 1992). Calcium influx activates key enzymes inside the cell—the caspases and calpain—that break down proteins in the internal cytoskeleton and membrane of the cell (Ray et al., 2003). With the destruction of its structural integrity, the cell dies. Yet, apoptosis of cortical motor neurons can occur after the axons centimeters away are severed by spinal cord injury, too far for the calcium to diffuse (Hains et al., 2003a). Therefore, besides calcium influx, there are likely other triggers of apoptosis in spinal cord injury.

Chronic Phase

The chronic phase of spinal cord injury sets in over a period of months to years. The chronic phase is marked by the emergence of new types of pathology at both the microlevel and the macrolevel (e.g., the formation of a fluid-filled cavity or a glial scar). At the microlevel, the death of oligodendrocytes has an amplifying effect. Because most oligodendrocytes myelinate (i.e., insulate) about 10 to 40 nerve axons, the loss of one oligodendrocyte can leave many healthy nerve axons without conduction capacity. If nerve conduction is stopped entirely, the spinal cord cannot transmit signals to the brain and body, even though axons may be intact. Axons undergo molecular changes, such as alteration of the ion channels that are normally responsible for propagating electrical impulses through nerves (Waxman, 2001; Hains et al., 2003b). The combination of myelin loss and altered ion channel function, among other changes, can lead to molecular changes in the surviving neurons that can produce chronic pain in animals with experimental spinal cord injuries. At the macrolevel, the lesion site becomes increasingly devoid of normal tissue and begins to form a fluid-filled cavity or a glial scar, or both. The cavity forms within a few weeks of injury in animal models and may extend several segments above and below the site of injury. The cavity creates a physical gap that blocks axon regrowth, whereas the glial scar contains substances that inhibit axon regrowth.

Glial Scar Formation

Glial scarring (also known as reactive gliosis) creates an environment that inhibits axon regeneration. The glial scar is an extracellular matrix that contains astroyctes, microglia, and oligodendrocytes. It grows in size over time, from weeks to months after the injury, but the groundwork is set within hours of the injury. That is when the remnants of the acute phase— myelin debris and damaged axons—begin to accumulate at the site of the injury. The remnants begin to attract an array of different types of glial cells, from oligodendrocytes and their precursors to activated microglia and astrocytes. Astrocytes are most commonly found in the scar, and they are tightly bound to one another (Fawcett and Asher, 1999). If the spinal cord has been penetrated, meningeal cells, which normally form a protective layer around the spinal cord, also accumulate at the lesion site. Each type of cell expresses and/or releases a host of inhibitory molecules (Table 2-6).

TABLE 2-6 Cells and Molecules That Inhibit Axon Regeneration

Cell Type	Inhibitory Molecule
Oligodendrocyte	NI-250 (Nogo-A)
	Myelin-associated glycoprotein (MAG)
	Oligodendrocyte myelin glycoprotein (OMGP)
	Tenascin-R
Oligodendrocyte precursor	NG2 (a proteoglycan)
	DSD-1 or phosphacan (a proteoglycan)
	Versican (a proteoglycan)
Astrocyte	Tenascin
	Brevican (a proteoglycan)
	Neurocan (a proteoglycan)
	NG2 (a proteoglycan)
Meningeal cell	NG2
	Semaphorins
Activated microglia	Free radicals
	Nitric oxide
	Arachidonic acid derivatives

SOURCE: Fawcett and Asher, 1999.

The collective action of these inhibitory molecules is the prevention of axon regeneration.

Oligodendrocytes, which are already at the scene because they myelinate axons, express a potent inhibitor of axon growth, Nogo-A, on the exterior surface of the cell membrane (Fournier et al., 2002). The vital importance of Nogo-A was revealed by studies with an animal model that showed that antibodies against this molecule, which block its action, promote some regeneration of severed axons (Schnell and Schwab, 1990). The first glial cells to arrive at the scene, within 3 to 5 days, are thought to be oligodendrocyte precursor cells, although no direct evidence of this has emerged. Oligodendrocyte precursors are immature oligodendrocytes that are destined, with further growth and differentiation, to become mature oligodendrocytes. At the scene they proliferate and release a variety of molecules that block axon growth. Astrocytes also arrive at the injury site and begin to undergo hypertrophy and divide.

Astrocytes form the bulk of the glial scar. In the scar, they are surrounded by an extracellular matrix made up of several types of proteoglycans, which are proteins on the outside of the cell membrane that have sugar moieties attached to them. Proteoglycans are up-regulated and secreted by astrocytes themselves, and they directly inhibit axon growth (Fawcett and Asher, 1999). The role of astrocytes has perplexed researchers because, in addition to their inhibitory role, they can also play a growth-promoting role under different circumstances (Jones et al., 2003).

Syringomyelia

Syringomyelia is a complication that arises as early as 2 months or as late as 30 years after the injury. It results from the formation of a cyst in the center of the spinal cord. This cyst expands and elongates over time, significantly damaging the center of the spinal cord. About 4 percent of individuals with spinal cord injuries develop syringomyelia (Schurch et al., 1996; Terre et al., 2000). Individuals with syringomyelia can present with multiple symptoms, including pain, weakness, headaches, and stiffness of the limbs and the back. The pathogenesis of syringomyelia, however, is not well understood. It may even lie dormant for many years before symptoms arise. Detection was especially difficult because of the wide range of other complications and sensory deficits that result from spinal cord injuries; however, the advent of magnetic resonance imaging (MRI) technologies has greatly enhanced the ability of clinicians to detect syringomyelia.

SPONTANEOUS HEALING

Often overlooked amid the litany of pathological changes that occur after a spinal cord injury is the natural ability of the spinal cord to heal itself. In fact, most individuals with spinal cord injuries, especially those with incomplete injuries, show some degree of functional recovery, and some show substantial degrees of recovery (Tator et al., 1998). Conventional wisdom had been that although some recovery is possible, it is limited in time and extent. A change of thinking has emerged in recent years, however. It is now well accepted that the spinal cord has the capacity to recover in several unforeseen ways starting at about 24 hours after injury and continuing for years. That capacity has become so well recognized that new treatments are being designed to marshal its potential.

Mature nerve cells lack the capacity to divide once they are injured. Whatever recovery of function that occurs naturally after a spinal cord injury is largely the product of plasticity in the surviving neurons. Plasticity is a generic term that denotes the body's natural capacity to react to changing conditions in numerous ways, from regrowth to gene up-regulation. The surviving neurons can adapt to compensate for injury; however, for many years it was thought that within limits the axons of neurons in mammals do not spontaneously regrow more than a few millimeters (Raineteau and Schwab, 2001). However, groundbreaking discoveries in the early 1980s established that CNS axons have the intrinsic capacity for regrowth over long distances, but they are actively inhibited by molecules in their extracellular environment (Aguayo et al., 1982). The extracellular environment may also lack molecules that promote or guide axon regrowth to its correct target site. Thus, CNS axons can regrow if their immediate environment is supportive. By contrast, peripheral nervous system axons can and do regrow spontaneously due to the growth-promoting molecules produced by Schwann cells.

Mechanisms Behind Natural Recovery of Function

After injury, the spinal cord can spontaneously recover to varying degrees through a variety of biological mechanisms (Table 2-7). The degree of recovery depends on numerous factors, including the severity of the injury, the individual's age, the area of the spinal cord affected, the degree of inhibition by astrocytes and oligodendrocytes, and other factors yet to be identified. Knowledge of the biological basis of functional recovery comes mostly from a host of animal models, although many of the intricate details are still unknown. As described in greater detail in Chapter 5, many strategies are being developed to facilitate these mechanisms of recovery, and these are areas of intense research.

Recovery of function is first apparent within days after injury as a result of recuperation from spinal shock. Some degree of remyelination within the spinal cord can occur and may have a clinical impact. Remyelination can occur in two different ways. The first is by Schwann cells, which are myelinating cells normally found in the peripheral nervous system, but after an injury they are able to migrate directly into the spinal cord, where they can myelinate regrowing axons (Bunge and Wood, 2004). Awareness of the role of Schwann cells has spawned an entire new line of research on therapies involving the transplantation of a variety of cell types (see Chapter 5).

The second means of possible remyelination is by oligodendrocyte precursor cells. Mature oligodendrocytes cannot divide or migrate. Yet, imma-

TABLE 2-7 Mechanisms of Spontaneous Recovery in the Spinal Cord

- Remyelination by Schwann cells entering the spinal cord after injury
- Remyelination by oligodendrocyte precursors
- Recovery of conduction in demyelinated axons
- Strengthening of existing synapses
- Regrowth and sprouting of intact axons to form new circuits
- Release of growth factors and guidance molecules
- Shift of function to alternate circuits

ture oligodendrocytes, already in the spinal cord, migrate short distances to the site of injury, where they can differentiate into mature oligodendrocytes and produce myelin (Gensert and Goldman, 1997). It bears remembering, however, that oligodendrocyte precursor cells can also mature into oligo-dendrocytes that do the opposite: inhibit axon regrowth through the release of inhibitory substances (see above). What triggers their development into inhibitory cells versus beneficial cells is not yet known.

It is also possible that demyelinated axons within the injured spinal cord may reorganize at the molecular level to acquire the ability to conduct nerve impulses without myelin insulation. This type of recovery is known to occur not only in animal models but also in humans with multiple sclerosis, in whom demyelinated spinal cord axons produce additional sodium chan-nels to support impulse conduction after damage to the myelin (Craner et al., 2004).

Limited regrowth of axons and sprouting of new branches from the tips of existing axons to form new synapses are part of yet another mechanism of functional recovery (Raineteau and Schwab, 2001). The fact that limited regrowth and sprouting do occur reveals that axons possess the capacity for some degree of regrowth, a capacity that can be cultivated with better knowledge of what governs it. Numerous studies with animals have dem-onstrated the ways in which axonal regrowth from central neurons can be improved, particularly across the area of injury. Research indicates that, after injury, the surviving cells continue to produce certain molecules and release them into the extracellular milieu that bathes the sprouting axons. Some of the molecules are growth factors—members of a family of mol-ecules called neurotrophins (Raineteau and Schwab, 2001). Others are guid-ance molecules that guide axons to their destination (Walsh and Doherty, 1997; Willson et al., 2002). This area of research is still in its early phases, and much of the information on axonal guidance gained to date involves the developing nervous system. Research is needed to determine if the same or similar mechanisms are involved in axon guidance following injury in the adult CNS.

BIOLOGICAL BASES OF FUNCTIONAL LOSSES

No daily activity can be taken for granted for someone with a spinal cord injury. A range of functions—getting out of bed, walking, dressing, eating, controlling the bladder and the bowel, and breathing—can be se-verely compromised, and their loss has a staggering effect. To develop the technological or medical means to restore function and to improve quality of life, it is vital to understand the neurological basis of dysfunction. The emphasis in this section is on the nervous system's role in generating move-ments and how injury to the spinal cord results in functional loss.

Spinal Cord Injury Disruption of Motor Pathways

The initiation and regulation of movements require a complex set of events that integrate information from many regions of the brain, brain stem, and spinal cord (Figure 2-3). When an action potential is generated in the brain, it travels along axons and down the spinal cord via the corticospinal tract to the motor neurons at speeds upwards of 100 meters per second, resulting in contraction of a muscle and a movement. However, before it reaches the motor neurons, the information is modulated by neurons found in the basal ganglia, cerebellum, and brain stem. When the signals finally reach the motor neurons, these specialized nerve cells provide the final conduit for the transmission of the signals to muscles throughout the body, stimulating muscles to contract. Thus, an injury or disruption to the motor pathways leading to and from the brain could cause a patient to lose motor function.

Differences in Degree of Cortical Control on Motor Function

The circuitry between the primary motor cortex and the motor neurons of the ventral horn of the spinal cord is very complex. Many regions of the CNS, including the basal ganglia, cerebellum, and brain stem, help regulate movements (Figure 2-3). The degree of cortical control varies depending on the motor function. For example, movement of the fingers requires more integration from the brain than gross movement of the legs, which relies more on circuitry confined to the spinal cord. The majority of the signals from the brain are transmitted along bundles of axons that make up the corticospinal tract, which connects the primary motor cortex in the brain to the motor neurons in the ventral horn of the spinal cord. The motor neurons in turn transmit the information from the ventral horn directly to the muscle. Motor control of most other body parts involves additional circuitry, or connections, between the primary motor cortex and the motor neurons. Signals are transmitted either from the primary motor cortex to intermediate layers within the spinal cord to modulate the tone or reflex gain and to cause direct contraction of the muscles or through intermediate processing stages in the midbrain or pons of the brain stem.

In addition to regulating voluntary movements, neurons in the descending motor tracts traveling from the brain down to the spinal cord are also responsible for regulating the smooth muscles of internal organs. Descending motor tracts also contain neurons associated with the autonomic nervous system, which regulates blood pressure, body temperature, and the body's response to stress.

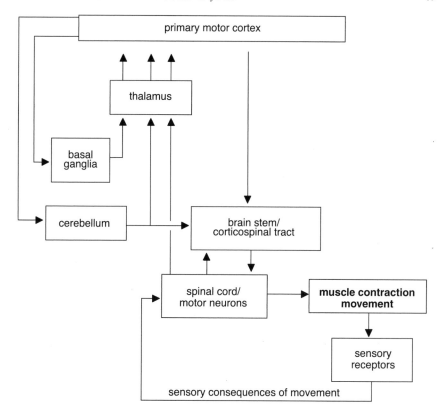

FIGURE 2-3 Initiation and regulation of movements.
Control of movements involves a complex network of connections. Signals commanding the initiation of a movement are generated in the primary motor cortex of the brain. These signals are modulated before they reach the muscle. They are modulated through an intricate circuit in the basal ganglia and thalamus, which regulate the initiation of movements and help coordinate movements. Information from muscle contractions is also transmitted back to the brain through sensory receptors. This information is also used to provide feedback and to modify the movements.
SOURCE: Adapted from Kandel et al., 1991.

Feedback Control of Movements

Critical feedback from sensory nerve endings located on muscles is transferred to the spinal cord via the sensory roots and dorsal horn to the brain, resulting in involuntary modulation of movements. This component of the sensory system is called proprioception. It is responsible for immediately varying the degree of muscle contraction in response to incoming information regarding external stimuli. When individuals lose their proprioception, they are unable to freely move and interact comfortably with the external environment (see Box 5-1).

A subset of the sensory neurons located in the spinal cord is also responsible for establishing the circuitry that controls simple reflex reactions, such as the knee-jerk reflex that doctors test by tapping a hammer on a patient's knee. This sensory information bypasses ascending information to the brain and is conveyed directly to lower motor neurons, resulting in involuntary or reflex movements.

Role of the Central Pattern Generator in Humans

Experiments performed by Shik, Severin, and Orlovsky in the 1960s provided evidence of a central pattern generator (CPG), which is a complex circuit of neurons responsible for coordinated rhythmic muscle activity, such as locomotion (Shik et al., 1969). In these experiments, the brain stem of a cat was transected so that no information could travel from the brain to the spinal cord. Surprisingly, following this surgery, cats were still able to stand on their own and could be induced to walk (Box 2-1). Similar results have been observed in rats and mice that have had their spinal cords transected. Therefore, it was concluded that the CPG is located in the spinal cord of these animals and does not require input from the brain.

If the CPG is located in the spinal cord and does not require any input from the brain, why is it that most individuals with spinal cord injuries and a complete transection of the spinal cord cannot walk? The function and control of the CPG in Old World primates and humans may be different from those in animals that walk on four feet, like cats and dogs (i.e., bipeds versus quadrapeds) (Vilensky and O'Connor, 1998). Humans and other bipeds may have more cortical dominance integrated into the locomotor circuitry than quadrapeds (Fulton and Keller, 1932), which may explain why the recovery of rhythmic locomotor activity is not commonly observed in primates and humans with complete spinal cord injuries (Kuhn, 1950; Bussel et al., 1996; Vilensky and O'Connor, 1998). However, because of the limitations of performing invasive experiments with primates and humans, it is difficult to verify the significance of the cortical circuitry. The complexity of the cortical regulation of the CPG in humans and primates compared with that in cats and rodents demonstrates a potential area of concern for the translation of the results from experiments performed with laboratory animals to humans.

Muscle Spasticity as a Result of Altered Activity in Motor Neurons

Spasticity is a state of increased muscular tone, often with heightened stretch reflexes. In severe cases, spasticity causes chronic pain, flexion

BOX 2-1
Rhythmic Motor Activity in Cats Is
Independent of Brain Stimulation

At the turn of the 20th century, Charles Scott Sherrington and T. Graham Brown published two seminal papers that demonstrated the capacity of the spinal cord in cats and dogs to generate rhythmic motor activity (Brown, 1914). Sherrington's experiment provided evidence that dogs and cats were still able to generate rhythmic movements elicited from their hind limbs weeks after their spinal cords were severed. Later, in the 1960s, further insight was garnered when the work of three Russian scientists, M. K. Shik, F. V. Severin, and G. N. Orlovsky, and one Swedish scientist, Sten Griller, showed that when a portion of the brain stem of a cat was cut across the middle—thus severing any connections between the brain and the spinal cord—the cat was still capable of standing. Furthermore, if a specific region of the brain stem was stimulated, the cats could be induced to walk on a treadmill, and alternating bursts of muscle activity could be recorded in extensors and flexors in conjunction with walking (Shik et al., 1966). These series of experiments led to the conclusion that each limb is controlled by a central pattern generator (CPG) in the spinal cord, which controls rhythmic motor activity, including walking.

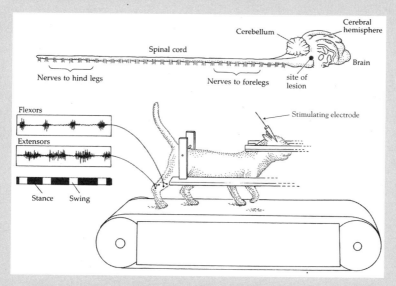

Shik and colleagues experimented with a cat whose brain stem was severed but that was still able to walk on a treadmill when a specific region of the brain stem was stimulated. The top of the figure shows the brain and the spinal cord. The muscle activity recorded from the flexors and extensors demonstrates that they are contracting and relaxing at opposite times from each other, consistent with normal function.

SOURCE: Reprinted with permission, from Dowling, 2001. Copyright 2001 by Sinauer Associates, Inc.

contractures, decubitus ulcers,[2] and bone fractures (Nance, 1999). Muscle spasticity frequently occurs after spinal cord injuries, with one study finding 78 percent of individuals experiencing spasticity after they were discharged from the hospital (Maynard et al., 1990).

The precise causes of muscle spasticity are not well understood. Most studies point to the greater excitability of motor neurons, with several possible causes (Burchiel and Hsu, 2001). One is thought to be decreased inhibitory input from the brain to spinal cord motor neurons through direct or indirect (via spinal cord interneuron) connections. For nearly a century, the lower motor neuron has been described as the "final common pathway" to muscles because of the thousands of neurons that converge on it. Some of those neurons are inhibitory, whereas others are excitatory. A single motor neuron can receive a direct or an indirect input from several regions of the brain and from sensory neurons. The array of inputs is critical for the modulation and fine-tuning of motor neuron control of muscles. If inhibitory input to the motor neuron is destroyed or reduced as a result of a spinal cord injury, the balance weighs in favor of heightened excitability and firing of motor neurons.

The spasticity that occurs with a spinal cord injury may also be produced by other mechanisms. One is a by-product of injury-induced sprouting. The new synapses formed by surviving axons (see below) may be too excitatory in nature. They might arise from motor pathways that descend from the brain, from ascending sensory pathways, or from the many synapses between the interneurons that form an intricate local circuitry within the spinal cord. Continual sensory feedback from muscles (such as for the detection of muscle length) is indispensable for the production of graded movements. If stretch reflexes are altered in individuals with spinal cord injuries, the lack of appropriate feedback may lead to spastic muscle contractions.

Spasticity may also be produced by pathological alterations in the electrical properties of the motor neurons themselves, including changes in sodium channel type, number, and distribution (Hiersemenzel et al., 2000) and alterations in neurotransmitter reuptake by glial cells.

Pain and Its Causation

Pain is a common and debilitating outcome of spinal cord injuries. Most studies find that 60 to 80 percent of individuals report chronic pain after a spinal cord injury. More precise estimates have been hindered by a

---

[2]Decubitus ulcers, or pressure ulcers, of the skin form over bony parts of the body, usually from prolonged pressure in patients and individuals who are not able to move around easily.

lack of uniform definitions and a comprehensive classification system (Burchiel and Hsu, 2001). The lack of definitions was addressed in 2000 with the release of a proposed scheme by the International Association for the Study of Pain for characterization of the pain associated with spinal cord injuries. By using those new definitions, a prospective study of 100 people found that 5 years after injury, 81 percent reported pain (of all types), and 58 percent reported that their pain was "severe or excruciating" (Siddall et al., 2003). The impact of chronic pain may be so great— deterioration of quality of life, ability to function, self-image, and care delivery—that depression and thoughts of suicide are common (Cairns et al., 1996).

The new classification system organizes spinal cord injury pain under two broad categories—nociceptive and neuropathic—along with five sub-classifications (each of which has further clinical subtypes and possible pathologies; see Table 2-8). Nociceptive pain arises from an external source (e.g., a noxious stimulus and consequent tissue damage), whereas neuro-pathic pain arises from the pathological changes occurring within sensory neurons or pathways. The two types of nociceptive pain—musculoskeletal and visceral—were reported by 59 and 5 percent of patients, respectively, in the prospective trial cited above (Siddall et al., 2003). Of the three types of neuropathic pain, 41 percent of patients reported at-level neuropathic pain, whereas 34 percent reported below-level neuropathic pain (Siddall et al., 2003).

Nociceptive pain is the dull and aching pains that one encounters when a limb is broken or when one has lower back pain. Painful stimuli are registered by specialized sensory cells known as nociceptors. Nociceptors, which are intact with this type of pain, respond to local damage to non-neural tissues (e.g., bone, muscles, and ligaments).

Neuropathic pain, on the other hand, is produced by direct damage to neural tissue. It is described as a sharp, shooting, burning, or electrical type of pain. Sensory neurons and pathways undergo physiological alterations; they may become exquisitely sensitive, firing off impulses out of proportion to the stimulus (hyperesthesia) or even without an external trigger whatso-ever. They may register the light touch of a feather as an unpleasant burn-ing sensation (dysesthesia) instead of a pleasant one.

Nociceptive pain and neuropathic pain have distinct causes and, as a result, distinct treatments. Because nociceptive pain arises from tissue dam-age and not from nerve pathology, it is often treated with standard thera-pies, most commonly physical therapy, various pain medications, and surgical therapy. Neuropathic pain is more difficult to treat, partly because its mechanisms are still being uncovered. The distinction between the two types of pain, however, is not always clear-cut (Bryce and Ragnarsson, 2002). Over time, nociceptive pain can lead to the sensitization of spinal

TABLE 2-8 Classification of Pain from Spinal Cord Injury

Broad Type (Tier 1)	Broad System (Tier 2)	Specific Structure or Pathology (Tier 3)
Nociceptive	Musculoskeletal	• Bone, joint, muscle trauma, or inflammation • Mechanical instability • Muscle spasm • Secondary overuse syndromes
	Visceral	• Renal calculus, bowel, sphincter dysfunction, etc. • Dysreflexive headache
Neuropathic	Above level of injury	• Compressive mononeuropathies • Complex regional pain syndromes
	At level of injury	• Nerve root compression (including cauda equina) • Syringomyelia • Spinal cord trauma or ischemia (transitional zone, etc.) • Dual-level cord and root trauma (double lesion syndrome)
	Below level of injury	• Spinal cord trauma or ischemia (central dysesthesia syndrome)

SOURCE: Vierck et al., 2000.

cord neurons, which leads to neuropathic pain. Sensitization represents an increased response to a standard stimulus, and it is manifest as hypersensitivity to pain (Woolf and Mannion, 1999).

Much of what is known about the pathophysiology of the pain that occurs after a spinal cord injury comes from studies with a host of animal models of different types of injuries. Although much remains to be learned, some of the intensively studied mechanisms underlying spinal cord pain include the following (Yezierski, 2000):

• loss or disruption of descending pathways from the brain that normally inhibit the sensory input as it enters the spinal cord;
• increases in pain neurotransmitter[3] or receptor levels through up-regulated gene expression;

---

[3]Neurotransmitters and neuromodulators commonly involved in excitatory pain pathways include glutamate, substance P, aspartate, galinin, brain-derived neurotrophic factor, and calcitonin gene-related peptide.

- changes in the types or numbers of ion channels in sensory neurons and pathways that render them more excitable (Hains et al., 2003b);
  - sprouting of sensory fibers entering the spinal cord;
  - alterations in post-receptor signal transduction mechanisms; and
- switching of the identities of sensory fibers from non-pain fibers to pain fibers (Bryce and Ragnarsson, 2002; Hulsebosch, 2002).

Many of these mechanisms also apply to other pain conditions not associated with spinal cord injuries (Woolf and Mannion, 1999).

The brain plays a large role in modulating and interpreting the sensation of pain, so much so that experts describe pain as an "experience" rather than a sensation. Multiple areas of the cerebral cortex process pain information relayed there by a certain tract in the spinal cord, which receives its information from incoming peripheral nerves. The brain, in turn, modulates the incoming messages through several descending pathways from nuclei in the midbrain, including the periaqueductal gray.

Biological Causes of Bladder Dysfunction

Three common types of bladder dysfunction accompany spinal cord injuries, depending on the level of the injury (Kaplan et al., 1991). Understanding of the types of dysfunction first requires some understanding of the anatomy of the bladder and its control by the spinal cord and the brain. Two main muscle groups surrounding the bladder control urination: the detrusor muscle, which controls bladder contraction, and the external sphincter muscles at the base of the bladder, which control bladder outflow. The two muscles normally work reciprocal to one another: the detrusor muscle contracts while the sphincter muscles relax, allowing urine to flow from the bladder. Because each is fed by separate nerves, their coordination—i.e., detrusor muscle contraction with sphincter muscle relaxation—is integrated at a higher level, which, in this case, is performed by the pons region of the brain. That portion of the brain sends its axons to the sacral region of the spinal cord (S2 and S3), which also receives sensory input from the bladder (via the pelvic nerve) about bladder distention. When the pelvic nerve conveys the message that the bladder is full, the information is relayed up to the pons, which then coordinates the motor messages necessary to empty the bladder. This process is called the voiding reflex.

In individuals with complete spinal cord injuries above the level of the sacral cord, disruption of the pathway from the spinal cord to the brain can lead to bladder problems related to the lack of coordination between the detrusor and the sphincter muscles (see below). If the sacral cord or the cauda equina is injured directly, the bladder detrusor muscle becomes flaccid—a condition known as areflexia. The detrusor muscle loses its ability to contract and can be readily stretched. Large volumes of urine overfill the bladder and back up to the kidneys (Kaplan et al., 1991).

Two common types of bladder conditions occur in individuals with spinal cord injuries at levels above the sacral cord. The first is detrusor hyperreflexia, in which the bladder is overreactive. As the bladder fills with small volumes of urine, the detrusor muscle contracts prematurely, causing frequent urination. Research with animals suggests that part of the pathological process occurs in the sensory nerves coming from the bladder. Sensory fibers normally carrying other types of information actually switch their functioning: they become sensitive to bladder distention and trigger bladder detrusor contraction (de Groat, 1995). This form of sensory plasticity is mediated by changes in electrical properties of C fibers, a particular type of sensory neuron (Yoshimura, 1999).

Less is known about the biological basis of the second type of bladder dysfunction, detrusor-sphincter dyssynergia. This condition is marked by involuntary contractions of the sphincter muscles, which prevent urine from leaving the bladder. It can occur with the loss of the reciprocal relationship between detrusor muscle contraction and sphincter muscle relaxation. One hypothesis is that the condition is related to the reduced activity of the neurotransmitter nitric oxide in sphincter muscles. Nitric oxide is involved in relaxation of the sphincter. Reduced levels would therefore increase sphincter contraction (Mamas et al., 2003). Detrusor-sphincter dyssynergia can also arise from lesions to the pontine reticular nucleus and the reticular formation (Sakakibara et al., 1996).

Bowel Function Disruption

Bowel dysfunction frequently occurs after a spinal cord injury because the brain and spinal cord have major roles in stool elimination. Although the movement of feces down the length of the bowel is partly controlled by independent neurocircuits that reside within the bowel,[4] the brain and spinal cord are essential for voluntary control over defecation. Loss of bowel function is so deeply distressing and embarrassing to individuals with spinal cord injuries that it affects their social interactions and their willingness to engage in sexual activities.

The impact of a spinal cord injury on voluntary control of the bowel is known as neurogenic bowel. Neurogenic bowel comes in two types— reflexic and areflexic—depending on the location of the injury. Reflexic

---

[4]When the bowel wall is stretched, the local neurocircuits cause the muscles above the stretched area to constrict, whereas those below the stretched area are induced to relax, thus propelling feces down the bowel toward the anus.

bowel, or upper motor neuron bowel, is the result of injuries above the sacral cord. Reflexic bowel brings constipation and an inability to defecate by conscious effort. The anal sphincter muscle remains tight and can be stimulated manually to induce defecation. Areflexic bowel, or lower motor neuron bowel, results from injuries at or below the sacral cord. It also causes constipation and incontinence. The anal sphincter becomes so flaccid that it is incapable of being manually stimulated to induce defecation. Both types of neurogenic bowel carry the risk of serious complications, including bowel obstruction, colorectal distention, and a life-threatening rise in blood pressure triggered by a distended bladder or bowel.

Control of Sexual Function by the Spinal Cord and Brain

Many aspects of human sexuality are under reflexive control by various centers in the spinal cord, most frequently in the sacral and in the thoracic and lumbar regions. The site and extent of injury are thus key determinants of sexual function. Several brain regions—most notably, the limbic system and the hypothalamus—also contribute to sexual function by exerting some degree of control over neuronal centers located in the spinal cord, especially sexual drive or inhibition. A large proportion of men and women with spinal cord injuries report reduced sexual desire (Alexander et al., 1993; Sipski and Alexander, 1993) and reduced fertility (Elliot, 2002). Male infertility appears to be the result of abnormalities in semen, especially low sperm motility and viability and increased numbers of leukocytes (Randall et al., 2003).

For men, the sexual response includes three separate functions: erection, ejaculation, and orgasm. Erection has two descriptive types, both of which are controlled by distinct spinal cord reflexes. Psychogenic (or mentally induced) erection is controlled by the T11 to L2 segments of the spinal cord, whereas reflexogenic erections are mediated by the sacral cord. Ejaculation is a more complex process, with two stages mediated by the region from T10 to S4, which controls certain sympathetic, parasympathetic, and somatic nerves. A physiological component of an orgasm is rhythmic pelvic floor contractions and other smooth-muscle contractions mediated by sacral regions of the spinal cord. The experience of orgasm as pleasurable depends on processing and interpretation by the brain. Damage to the relevant spinal cord centers or disruption of connections to the brain can thus lead to various types of sexual dysfunction. Dysfunction in the urinary or the gastrointestinal system also has a bearing on ejaculation and orgasm, as does an individual's mental state, such as depression or anxiety (Elliot, 2002).

For women, the sexual response depends on arousal and orgasm. Sexual arousal involves vaginal lubrication; swelling of the clitoris; and increases in heart rate, respiratory rate, and blood pressure. Vaginal lubrication has two types, psychogenic or reflexive, which are controlled by the regions of the spinal cord from T10 to L2 and S2 to S5, respectively. Orgasm has been directly investigated in laboratory-based studies with women with spinal cord injuries. Overall, only 52 percent of women with spinal cord injuries were able to stimulate themselves to orgasm, regardless of the nature of their injury (Sipski, 2001). Women with injuries of the sacral cord were significantly less likely to reach orgasm than women with spinal cord injuries at other, higher levels. Researchers therefore postulate that an intact sacral reflex is necessary for orgasm (Sipski, 2001; Benevento and Sipski, 2002).

SUMMARY

Although much progress has been made, especially in the past 25 years, in understanding the basic biology of the nervous system and the complex pathways in the pathophysiology of spinal cord injuries that involve the immune, vascular, and nervous systems, much remains to be learned. As emphasized in the following chapters, this basic research is the underpinning of progress that will be made in developing therapeutic interventions.

Many research avenues remain to be examined to understand the biochemical mechanisms responsible for spinal cord injuries and thus the targets for the development of therapeutic interventions. Research is needed on the processes involved in cellular death and the immediate sequelae of apoptotic and necrotic cell death. The molecular mechanisms that promote and inhibit axonal regeneration need to be further explored, as do the molecular mechanisms that direct axons to their appropriate targets and regulate the formation and maintenance of appropriate and functional synaptic connections and circuitry.

Moving this research forward involves opportunities and challenges that are not isolated to spinal cord injury research. Rather, this research has far-reaching potential to both inform and be informed by many other fields of research and the efforts that are under way to examine other neurological diseases and conditions.

REFERENCES

Aguayo AJ, David S, Richardson P, Bray GM. 1982. Axonal elongation in peripheral and central nervous system transplants. *Advances in Cell Neurobiology* 3: 215-234.
Alexander CJ, Sipski ML, Findley TW. 1993. Sexual activities, desire, and satisfaction in males pre- and post-spinal cord injury. *Archives of Sexual Behavior* 22(3): 217-228.
Anderson AJ. 2002. Mechanisms and pathways of inflammatory responses in CNS trauma: Spinal cord injury. *Journal of Spinal Cord Medicine* 25(2): 70-79.

Anthes DL, Theriault E, Tator CH. 1996. Ultrastructural evidence for arteriolar vasospasm after spinal cord trauma. *Neurosurgery* 39(4): 804-814.

ASIA (American Spinal Injury Association). 2000. *International Standards for Neurological Classification of SCI.* Chicago: American Spinal Injury Association.

Bareyre FM, Schwab ME. 2003. Inflammation, degeneration and regeneration in the injured spinal cord: Insights from DNA microarrays. *Trends in Neurosciences* 26(10): 555-563.

Beattie MS, Farooqui AA, Bresnahan JC. 2000. Review of current evidence for apoptosis after spinal cord injury. *Journal of Neurotrauma* 17(10): 915-925.

Benevento BT, Sipski ML. 2002. Neurogenic bladder, neurogenic bowel, and sexual dysfunction in people with spinal cord injury. *Physical Therapy* 82(6): 601-612.

Brown TG. 1914. On the nature of fundamental activity of the nervous centers; together with an analysis of the conditioning of rhythmic activity in procession, and a theory of the evolution of function in the nervous system. *Journal of Physiology* 48: 18-46.

Bryce TN, Ragnarsson K. 2002. Pain management in persons with spinal cord disorders. In: Lin V, Cardenas DD, Cutter NC, Frost FS, Hammond MC, Lindblom LB, Perkash I, Waters R, eds. *Spinal Cord Medicine: Principles and Practice.* New York: Demos Medical Publishing. Pp. 441-460.

Bunge MB, Wood PM. 2004. Transplantation of Schwann cells and olfactory ensheathing cells to promote regeneration in the CNS. In: Selzer ME, Clarke S, Cohen LG, Dincan PW, Gage FH, eds. *Textbook of Neural Repair and Rehabilitation.* Cambridge, United Kingdom: Cambridge University Press.

Bunge RP, Puckett WR, Becerra JL, Marcillo A, Quencer RM. 1993. Observations on the pathology of human spinal cord injury. A review and classification of 22 new cases with details from a case of chronic cord compression with extensive focal demyelination. *Advances in Neurology* 59: 75-89.

Bunge RP, Puckett WR, Hiester ED. 1997. Observations on the pathology of several types of human spinal cord injury, with emphasis on the astrocyte response to penetrating injuries. *Advances in Neurology* 72: 305-315.

Burchiel KJ, Hsu FP. 2001. Pain and spasticity after spinal cord injury: Mechanisms and treatment. *Spine* 26(24 Suppl): S146-160.

Bussel B, Roby-Brami A, Neris OR, Yakovleff A. 1996. Evidence for a spinal stepping generator in man. *Paraplegia* 34(2): 91-92.

Caceci T, El-Shafey S. 2002. *Neutrophils.* [Online]. Available: http://education.vetmed.vt.edu/Curriculum/VM8054/Labs/Lab6/Examples/exneutro.htm [accessed August 18, 2004].

Cairns DM, Adkins RH, Scott MD. 1996. Pain and depression in acute traumatic spinal cord injury: Origins of chronic problematic pain? *Archives of Physical Medicine and Rehabilitation* 77(4): 329-335.

Craner MJ, Newcombe J, Black JA, Hartle C, Cuzner ML, Waxman SG. 2004. Molecular changes in neurons in multiple sclerosis: Altered axonal expression of $Na_v1.2$ and $Na_v1.6$ sodium channels and Na^+/Ca^{2+} exchanger. *Proceedings of the National Academy of Sciences (U.S.A.)* 101(21): 8168-8173.

Crowe MJ, Bresnahan JC, Shuman SL, Masters JN, Beattie MS. 1997. Apoptosis and delayed degeneration after spinal cord injury in rats and monkeys. *Nature Medicine* 3(1): 73-76.

CRPF (Christopher Reeve Paralysis Foundation). 2002. *The Spinal Cord and Muscles Working Together.* [Online]. Available: http://www.christopherreeve.org/Research/Research.cfm?ID=178&c=21 [accessed January 11, 2005].

Dammann O, Durum S, Leviton A. 2001. Do white cells matter in white matter damage? *Trends in Neurosciences* 24(6): 320-324.

de Groat WC. 1995. Mechanisms underlying the recovery of lower urinary tract function following spinal cord injury. *Paraplegia* 33(9): 493-505.

Dowling JE, 2001. *Neurons and Networks: An Introduction to Behavioral Neuroscience.* Cambridge, MA: Harvard University Press.

El Masry WS, Tsubo M, Katoh S, El Miligui YH, Khan A. 1996. Validation of the American Spinal Injury Association (ASIA) motor score and the National Acute Spinal Cord Injury Study (NASCIS) motor score. *Spine* 21(5): 614-619.

Elliot S. 2002. Sexual dysfunction and infertility in men with spinal cord disorders. In: Lin V, Cardenas DD, Cutter NC, Frost FS, Hammond MC, Lindblom LB, Perkash I, Waters R, eds. *Spinal Cord Medicine: Principles and Practice.* New York: Demos Medical Publishing. Pp. 349-368.

Emery E, Aldana P, Bunge MB, Puckett W, Srinivasan A, Keane RW, Bethea J, Levi AD. 1998. Apoptosis after traumatic human spinal cord injury. *Journal of Neurosurgery* 89(6): 911-920.

Faden AI, Simon RP. 1988. A potential role for excitotoxins in the pathophysiology of spinal cord injury. *Annals of Neurology* 23(6): 623-626.

Fawcett JW, Asher RA. 1999. The glial scar and central nervous system repair. *Brain Research Bulletin* 49(6): 377-391.

Fournier AE, GrandPre T, Gould G, Wang X, Strittmatter SM. 2002. Nogo and the Nogo-66 receptor. *Progress in Brain Research* 137: 361-369.

Fulton JA, Keller AD. 1932. *The Sign of Babinski: A Study of the Evolution of Cortical Dominance in Primates.* Springfield, IL: Charles C. Thomas.

Gensert JM, Goldman JE. 1997. Endogenous progenitors remyelinate demyelinated axons in the adult CNS. *Neuron* 19(1): 197-203.

Hains BC, Black JA, Waxman SG. 2003a. Primary cortical motor neurons undergo apoptosis after axotomizing spinal cord injury. *Journal of Comparative Neurology* 462(3): 328-341.

Hains BC, Klein JP, Saab CY, Craner MJ, Black JA, Waxman SG. 2003b. Upregulation of sodium channel $Na_v1.3$ and functional involvement in neuronal hyperexcitability associated with central neuropathic pain after spinal cord injury. *Journal of Neuroscience* 23(26): 8881-8892.

Harper GP, Banyard PJ, Sharpe PC. 1996. The International Spinal Research Trust's strategic approach to the development of treatments for the repair of spinal cord injury. *Spinal Cord* 34(8): 449-459.

Hiersemenzel LP, Curt A, Dietz V. 2000. From spinal shock to spasticity: Neuronal adaptations to a spinal cord injury. *Neurology* 54(8): 1574-1582.

Hulsebosch CE. 2002. Recent advances in pathophysiology and treatment of spinal cord injury. *Advances in Physiology Education* 26(1-4): 238-255.

Imaizumi T, Kocsis JD, Waxman SG. 1997. Anoxic injury in the rat spinal cord: Pharmacological evidence for multiple steps in Ca^{2+}-dependent injury of the dorsal columns. *Journal of Neurotrauma* 14(5): 299-311.

Jones LL, Sajed D, Tuszynski MH. 2003. Axonal regeneration through regions of chondroitin sulfate proteoglycan deposition after spinal cord injury: A balance of permissiveness and inhibition. *Journal of Neuroscience* 23(28): 9276-9288.

Kandel ER, Schwartz JH, Jessell JH, eds. 1991. *Principles of Neural Science.* New York: Elsevier.

Kaplan SA, Chancellor MB, Blaivas JG. 1991. Bladder and sphincter behavior in patients with spinal cord lesions. *Journal of Urology* 146(1): 113-117.

Kipnis J, Mizrahi T, Hauben E, Shaked I, Shevach E, Schwartz M. 2002. Neuroprotective autoimmunity: Naturally occurring $CD4^+CD25^+$ regulatory T cells suppress the ability to withstand injury to the central nervous system. *Proceedings of the National Academy of Sciences (U.S.A.)* 99(24): 15620-15625.

Koyanagi I, Tator CH, Lea PJ. 1993. Three-dimensional analysis of the vascular system in the rat spinal cord with scanning electron microscopy of vascular corrosion casts. Part 1: Normal spinal cord. *Neurosurgery* 33(2): 277-283.

Kuhn RA. 1950. Functional capacity of the isolated human spinal cord. *Brain* 73: 1-51.

Lentz TL. 1971. *Cell Fine Structure: An Atlas of Drawings of Whole-Cell Structure.* Philadelphia: W. B. Saunders Company.

Levi ADO. 2004. Approach to the patient and diagnostic evaluation. In: Winn HR, Youmans JR, eds. *Neurological Surgery: A Comprehensive Reference Guide to the Diagnosis and Management of Neurological Problems.* Vol. 4. 5th ed. Philadelphia: W. B. Saunders. Pp. 4869-4884.

Lindholm D, Castren E, Kiefer R, Zafra F, Thoenen H. 1992. Transforming growth factor-beta 1 in the rat brain: Increase after injury and inhibition of astrocyte proliferation. *Journal of Cell Biology* 117(2): 395-400.

Liu XZ, Xu XM, Hu R, Du C, Zhang SX, McDonald JW, Dong HX, Wu YJ, Fan GS, Jacquin MF, Hsu CY, Choi DW. 1997. Neuronal and glial apoptosis after traumatic spinal cord injury. *Journal of Neuroscience* 17(14): 5395-5406.

Mamas MA, Reynard JM, Brading AF. 2003. Nitric oxide and the lower urinary tract: Current concepts, future prospects. *Urology* 61(6): 1079-1085.

Maynard FM, Karunas RS, Waring WP III. 1990. Epidemiology of spasticity following traumatic spinal cord injury. *Archives of Physical Medicine and Rehabilitation* 71(8): 566-569.

Merck & Co., Inc. 2004. *Drawing of Neuron.* [Online]. Available: http://www.merck.com/ mrkshared/mmanual_home/illus/i59_3.gif [accessed April 22, 2004].

Nance PW. 1999. Rehabilitation pharmacotherapy: Preface. *Physical Medicine & Rehabilitation Clinics of North America* 10(2): xv-xvi.

Popovich PG, Jones TB. 2003. Manipulating neuroinflammatory reactions in the injured spinal cord: Back to basics. *Trends in Pharmacological Sciences* 24(1): 13-17.

Raineteau O, Schwab ME. 2001. Plasticity of motor systems after incomplete spinal cord injury. *Nature Reviews Neuroscience* 2(4): 263-273.

Randall JM, Evans DH, Bird VG, Aballa TC, Lynne CM, Brackett NL. 2003. Leukocytospermia in spinal cord injured patients is not related to histological inflammatory changes in the prostate. *Journal of Urology* 170(3): 897-900.

Ray SK, Hogan EL, Banik NL. 2003. Calpain in the pathophysiology of spinal cord injury: Neuroprotection with calpain inhibitors. *Brain Research—Brain Research Reviews* 42(2): 169-185.

Sakakibara R, Hattori T, Yasuda K, Yamanishi T. 1996. Micturitional disturbance and the pontine tegmental lesion: Urodynamic and MRI analyses of vascular cases. *Journal of the Neurological Sciences* 141(1-2): 105-110.

Schnell L, Schwab ME. 1990. Axonal regeneration in the rat spinal cord produced by an antibody against myelin-associated neurite growth inhibitors. *Nature* 343(6255): 269-272.

Schnell L, Fearn S, Klassen H, Schwab ME, Perry VH. 1999. Acute inflammatory responses to mechanical lesions in the CNS: Differences between brain and spinal cord. *European Journal of Neuroscience* 11(10): 3648-3658.

Schurch B, Wichmann W, Rossier AB. 1996. Post-traumatic syringomyelia (cystic myelopathy): A prospective study of 449 patients with spinal cord injury. *Journal of Neurology, Neurosurgery & Psychiatry* 60(1): 61-67.

Schwartz M, Kipnis J. 2001. Protective autoimmunity: Regulation and prospects for vaccination after brain and spinal cord injuries. *Trends in Molecular Medicine* 7(6): 252-258.

Sekhon LH, Fehlings MG. 2001. Epidemiology, demographics, and pathophysiology of acute spinal cord injury. *Spine* 26(24 Suppl): S2-12.

Shier D, Butler J, Lewis R. 2004. *Hole's Human Anatomy & Physiology*. 10th ed. Boston: McGraw-Hill Higher Education.

Shik ML, Severin FV, Orlovskii GN. 1966. Control of walking and running by means of electric stimulation of the midbrain. *Biofizika* 11(4): 659-666.

Shik ML, Severin FV, Orlovsky GN. 1969. Control of walking and running by means of electrical stimulation of the mesencephalon. *Electroencephalography & Clinical Neurophysiology* 26(5): 549.

Siddall PJ, McClelland JM, Rutkowski SB, Cousins MJ. 2003. A longitudinal study of the prevalence and characteristics of pain in the first 5 years following spinal cord injury. *Pain* 103(3): 249-257.

Sipski ML. 2001. Sexual response in women with spinal cord injury: Neurologic pathways and recommendations for the use of electrical stimulation. *Journal of Spinal Cord Medicine* 24(3): 155-158.

Sipski ML, Alexander CJ. 1993. Sexual activities, response and satisfaction in women pre- and post-spinal cord injury. *Archives of Physical Medicine and Rehabilitation* 74(10): 1025-1029.

Stimson D. 2001. From clear-cut endings to complex beginnings: Researchers probe the origins of Charcot-Marie-Tooth disease. *Quest* 8(1): 1-4.

Stys PK, Ransom BR, Waxman SG. 1992a. Tertiary and quaternary local anesthetics protect CNS white matter from anoxic injury at concentrations that do not block excitability. *Journal of Neurophysiology* 67(1): 236-240.

Stys PK, Waxman SG, Ransom BR. 1992b. Ionic mechanisms of anoxic injury in mammalian CNS white matter: Role of Na^+ channels and Na^+-Ca^{2+} exchanger. *Journal of Neuroscience* 12(2): 430-439.

Taber CW, Thomas CL, eds. 1997. *Taber's Cyclopedic Medical Dictionary*. Philadelphia: F.A. Davis.

Tator CH, McCormick PC, Piepmeier JM, Benzel EC, Young W. 1998. Biology of neurological recovery and functional restoration after spinal cord injury. *Neurosurgery* 42(4): 696-708.

Terre R, Valles M, Vidal J. 2000. Post-traumatic syringomyelia following complete neurological recovery. *Spinal Cord* 38(9): 567-570.

Vierck CJ Jr, Siddall P, Yezierski RP. 2000. Pain following spinal cord injury: Animal models and mechanistic studies. *Pain* 89(1): 1-5.

Vilensky JA, O'Connor BL. 1998. Stepping in nonhuman primates with a complete spinal cord transection: Old and new data, and implications for humans. *Annals of the New York Academy of Sciences* 860: 528-530.

Walsh FS, Doherty P. 1997. Neural cell adhesion molecules of the immunoglobulin superfamily: Role in axon growth and guidance. *Annual Review of Cell and Developmental Biology* 13: 425-456.

Waxman SG. 2001. Acquired channelopathies in nerve injury and MS. *Neurology* 56(12): 1621-1627.

Willson CA, Irizarry-Ramirez M, Gaskins HE, Cruz-Orengo L, Figueroa JD, Whittemore SR, Miranda JD. 2002. Upregulation of EphA receptor expression in the injured adult rat spinal cord. *Cell Transplantation* 11(3): 229-239.

Wolman L. 1965. The disturbance of circulation in traumatic paraplegia in acute and late stages: A pathological study. *Paraplegia* 59: 213-226.

Woolf CJ, Mannion RJ. 1999. Neuropathic pain: Aetiology, symptoms, mechanisms, and management. *Lancet* 353(9168): 1959-1964.

Yezierski RP. 2000. Pain following spinal cord injury: Pathophysiology and central mechanisms. *Progress in Brain Research* 129: 429-449.

Yoshimura N. 1999. Bladder afferent pathway and spinal cord injury: Possible mechanisms inducing hyperreflexia of the urinary bladder. *Progress in Neurobiology* 57(6): 583-606.

Young W. 1992. Role of calcium in central nervous system injuries. *Journal of Neurotrauma* 9 Suppl(1): S9-25.

Young W. 2002. *Spinal Cord Injury Levels & Classification.* [Online]. Available: http://www.sci-info-pages.com/levels.html [accessed September 30, 2003].

3

TOOLS FOR ASSESSING SPINAL CORD INJURY AND REPAIR

Because the spinal cord is encased in the protective armor of the vertebrae, investigation of the site of the injury or the effects of potential therapies has required the development of a diverse set of research tools. In the past 40 years the rapid progress in the technologies available to perform experiments has largely been responsible for the great strides that have been made in understanding the basic principles of neuroscience. Studies with animal models have been instrumental in the rapid development of neuroscience and understanding of the biology of the spinal cord. The advent of cell culture techniques has provided a means to isolate and grow cells. Researchers can now isolate specific molecules and proteins and examine their roles in neuronal injury and repair in laboratory animals that mimic human spinal cord injuries. Recent advances in imaging techniques and methods for investigation of the actions of genes have advanced the understanding of spinal cord injuries even further. They also provide researchers with the tools that they need to examine changes in the spinal cord at the molecular and structural levels, for example, improving knowledge of the inhibitory conditions that serve as barriers to neuronal regeneration.

This chapter describes the important genetic and in vitro tools that have been developed to advance spinal cord injury research; the key animal models that are used to mimic human spinal cord injuries and the major limitations of the existing animal models; and the outcome measures that have been developed to assess spinal cord injuries and the effectiveness of experimental therapies, including the development of imaging technologies.

MOLECULAR, GENETIC, AND IN VITRO TOOLS

Techniques have been developed that allow researchers to isolate and grow populations of neurons to investigate the effects of specific proteins and molecules on neuronal injury and repair. Neurons can be grown in isolation or with glial cells such as oligodendrocytes or Schwann cells to study the processes of axonal outgrowth and myelination. Investigators use molecular biology-based techniques, such as DNA or protein analysis, that can be used to easily visualize or analyze outcomes.

Demonstrating the power of a cell culture experiment, the simple growth-cone turning assay led to the discovery that altering various molecules inside the growing axon regulates protein and cyclic nucleotide activities, which, in turn, can convert an axon's response to a growth-inhibiting molecule from one of repulsion to one of attraction (Song et al., 1998). When this application is applied to regenerating axons in the rat spinal cord, investigators showed that the regrowth of transected neurons has the potential to be enhanced considerably (Neumann et al., 2002; Qiu et al., 2002). Furthermore, the recent elucidation of the signaling pathways responsible for this switch in response may lead to the discovery of a strategy for enhancing axon regeneration (Wen et al., 2004).

Often, in vitro assays can be used in experiments with animal models, thus allowing researchers to verify and examine the effects detected in vitro to be evaluated in a more complex system. For example, chondroitin sulfate proteoglycans were found to inhibit neurite outgrowth in in vitro experiments (Snow et al., 1990). Analysis with animal models demonstrated that the levels of these proteoglycans are enhanced, or up-regulated, during central nervous system (CNS) injury (Snow et al., 1990) and led to the development of a strategy to break down these substances and promote the regrowth of axons in the intact rat spinal cord after an injury (Bradbury et al., 2002).

Animal Models for Molecular and Genetic Studies

Models consisting of multiple-transgenic animals have been developed to investigate molecular mechanisms and to identify the molecules critical for specific processes (Table 3-1). These models provide a better understanding of the genetic and molecular basis by which spinal cord circuits, specific neuronal subtypes, and synapses are formed (Shirasaki and Pfaff, 2002; Lanuza et al., 2004). For example, by studying the development of the nervous system of the fruit fly (Drosophila melanogaster), researchers have identified numerous molecules that can regulate the growth of the axon and the formation of neuronal connections (Vaessin et al., 1991; Kidd et al., 1998; Kraut et al., 2001; Jin, 2002). This information should provide

TABLE 3-1 Animal Models Commonly Used to Identify Genes Involved in Axon Growth and Circuit Formation

Animal	Technique(s)	Primary Utility
Fruit fly	Transgenic	Identify and investigate molecular expression patterns; perform genetic experiments to identify the molecules involved in axon growth and guidance and the reformation of neuronal connections
Worm	Transgenic	Identify and investigate molecular expression patterns and perform genetic experiments
Fish	Transgenic, transection,	Examine motor control and the central pattern generator after transection of the spinal cord and investigate axonal regeneration models
Mouse	Transgenic, imaging	Identify and investigate molecular expression patterns; perform genetic experiments to identify the molecules involved in axon growth and guidance and the reformation of neuronal connections; examine cellular and molecular basis of spinal cord circuits

the insights needed to reconstruct effective circuits once axonal regeneration has been achieved.

ANIMAL MODELS OF SPINAL CORD INJURY

Animal models allow in-depth investigation of the anatomical and molecular changes that occur in response to a spinal cord injury at a level of detail that would not be possible or ethical in studies with humans. These insights are critical for the design and interpretation of the results of studies with humans. Without the knowledge gleaned from studies with animals, the spinal cord would remain the equivalent of a black box and therapies aimed at restoring function would be limited. For example, experiments with rodents demonstrated that the neurons in the spinal cord are able to regenerate after an injury (Richardson et al., 1980; Xu et al., 1995).

Researchers have developed a variety of animal models that mimic different attributes associated with spinal cord injuries. Depending on the purpose of the study and the specific aspect of the injury to be investigated, researchers determine which animal model most closely replicates the injury in humans (Tables 3-2 and 3-3). In 2000, the International Spinal Research Trust published guidelines that describe four characteristics that are required for an optimal model of spinal cord injury (Ramer et al., 2000):

- The nature and the extent of the lesion should be precisely defined. If there is doubt about the extent of a lesion or whether axons have been spared, then interpretations of regeneration can be misleading.
- A histological method should be available to detect the growth of axons through the lesion.
- A method should be available to analyze the functional synaptic transmission beyond the lesion by measuring the electrical activity that neurons use to communicate with one another.
- A behavioral measure should be available that is capable of detecting restoration of known circuits.

It is important to examine therapies in a system that best mimics the condition of the individual with a spinal cord injury. For example, therapies designed for individuals with chronic conditions should not be tested in animal models immediately after the animal has received the injury but should be tested only after the animal is in the chronic stage of the injury (Kwon et al., 2002a; Houle and Tessler, 2003; Kleitman, 2004). Further-

TABLE 3-2 Value of Animal Models for Spinal Cord Injury Research

- Allows in-depth investigation of the anatomical changes that occur in response to an injury
- Regeneration of axonal tracts between the brain and the spinal cord can be studied in detail
- Individual components of the complex neural circuitry required for sensory perception and motor control can be examined
- Factors that influence DNA and proteins can be characterized
- Provides a means to examine the effects of specific genes
- Provides a tool to identify and test the efficacies of potential therapeutic agents and targets
- Identifies clinical end points that can be used to assess the efficacies of therapeutic agents

TABLE 3-3 Criteria for Choosing an Ideal Animal Model

- Ability to match the behavioral complication to a morphology deficit
- Similarities and differences between the anatomy and cellular composition of the animal and human spinal cord
- Similarity of the whole injury process, including genetic changes and progression, to that observed in humans
- Similarities and differences between the timing of the stages of injury and life cycle in animals and humans
- Similarities and differences in the genetic backgrounds of the animal strains and species that may influence the response and recovery from a spinal cord injury
- Economics of the model, including the costs of care and feeding, and regulations

SOURCE: Croft, 2002.

more, each type of spinal cord injury (Chapter 2) is different and presents its own set of challenges; therefore, each requires its own standard animal model that reliably mimics the complications experienced by individuals with that type of spinal cord injury.

A number of animal models have been developed, including models that mimic compression, contusion, and transection (Table 3-4). Blunt contusion injuries account for 30 to 40 percent of all human spinal cord injuries (Hulsebosch, 2002); thus, the contusion model provides an important tool that researchers can use to examine the neuropathology of the injury and to test the efficacies of different therapeutic agents. In 1978, the clip compression technique was developed by researchers to simulate the continual pressure and displacement of the spinal cord common in spinal cord injuries, which is not reproduced in contusion injuries (Rivlin and Tator, 1978). This procedure has provided researchers with a great deal of information about the pathophysiology of the spinal cord during the acute stages of the injury; the timing, necessity, and effectiveness of releasing the pressure from the spinal cord; and potential therapies (Kwon et al., 2002b). To target and eliminate particular groups of neurons, methods that generate microlesions (Magavi et al., 2000) and that leave the vast majority of the nervous system intact have been developed. Using this strategy, the functional consequences that result from losing the nerve groups can be systematically examined. Researchers are determining the neuronal populations responsible for specific spinal cord injury deficits, including the root causes of chronic pain (Gorman et al., 2001).

TABLE 3-4 Commonly Used Animal Models of Spinal Cord Injury

Animal and Injury Modeled	Primary Utility and Potential Issues
Primate transection	• Test the safety and efficacies of therapies • Determine the role of the central pattern generator in bipedal animals • Ethical complications with the use of primates • High cost of animal maintenance • Limited number of animals that can be prepared for experimentation • Spatial arrangement of the tracts differs from that in humans

Cat
  contusion,
  transection
	• Examine and define spinal cord circuitry and the central pattern generator
	• Central pattern generator may have different amounts of brain regulation compared with that in humans
	• Spatial arrangement of the tracts differs from that in humans
	• Chromosomes and genes are organized differently from those in humans

Mouse
  contusion,
  compression,
  transection,
  transgenic,
  microlesion
  formation
	• Investigate molecular and anatomical changes that occur in response to injury; however, mice respond differently than humans to spinal cord injury
	• Examine specific molecular targets for potential therapeutic targets
	• Modify genes to test the effect on restoration or loss of function
	• Difficult to assess upper extremity function
	• Genetic variability in injury response, including scar formation
	• Differences in scale size of spinal cord between mice and humans
	• Spatial arrangement of the tracts differs between mice and humans
	• Chromosomes and genes are organized differently from those in humans

Rat
  contusion,
  compression,
  transection,
  microlesion
  formation
	• Investigate molecular and anatomical changes that occur in response to injury
	• Difficult to assess upper extremity function
	• Differences in scale size of spinal cord in rats versus humans
	• Chromosomes and genes are organized differently from those in humans

NOTE: Contusion refers to a bruising of the spinal cord. Transection models are used to simulate lacerations to the spinal cord. Transgenic refers to modification of the animal's genetic profile, which is done by deleting or modifying existing genes or introducing a novel gene.

Issues Regarding Animal Models

Mimicking Transection and Compression Injuries

To make certain that the results from transection experiments are correctly interpreted and to minimize the variability in results, it is important that transection methods be standardized and that control animals be prepared at the same time that the experimental animals are treated. For example, to ensure that the recovery of function is due to axonal regeneration and not spared spinal cord circuitry, researchers must precisely perform transections of the spinal cord and must be sure that the axons projecting from the neurons are completely severed. If not all of the axons are severed, sparing and sprouting from uninjured axons become issues. It is important to note that damage to the dura mater as a result of a penetrating injury (including experimental transection) provides a route for the invasion of fibroblasts into the injury site (Zhang et al., 1996, 2004). Furthermore, in mice, there is extensive invasion of fibroblasts even without damage to the dura and the fibroblasts participate in the formation of a tissue matrix that is supportive for regeneration of at least some types of CNS axons. Following penetrating injuries, the potential contribution of fibroblasts (positive or negative) must be considered in evaluating experimental interventions to promote repair and functional recovery

By virtue of the means by which compression injuries occur, there is a large amount of variability in the severities of spinal cord injuries. However, when initial compression studies are performed, it is important to be able to study a large population of animals that have the exact same initial injury characteristics before the experimental therapeutic intervention. Protocols have been developed to help minimize the variability in injury from animal to animal. Three impactors are widely accepted as standard methods for the delivery of contusion injuries to rodents: the Ohio State University (OSU) impactor, the Infinite Horizons device, and the Multicenter Animal Spinal Cord Injury Study (MASCIS) impactor (Bresnahan et al., 1987; Noyes, 1987; Kwo et al., 1989; Gruner, 1992; Young, 2002).

Genetic Variability Between and Among Species

Although it is important to test therapeutic interventions in animals before they can become established treatments in the clinic, genetic differences between animal species can potentially result in different responses to spinal cord injuries or treatments. For example, in response to injury, humans and rats develop a cavity in the spinal cord, but this does not occur in mice (although the precise cellular and molecular bases for this are not yet

---

BOX 3-1
The Story of Nogo-Knockout Mice:
Cooperation, Collaboration, and Genetic Variability

Three groups of investigators recently used the gene-knockout strategy to examine whether Nogo, a potential inhibitor of axon growth (see Chapter 2), was responsible for preventing neuronal regeneration after an injury (Steward et al., 2003). Researchers coordinated their research efforts and published their findings in papers published in the same issue of the journal. Each group removed a specific part of a mouse's chromosome that is responsible for Nogo, with the hypothesis that if Nogo is responsible for inhibiting neurons from growing, then its removal would facilitate regeneration after a spinal cord injury. However, the experiments found contradictory results. One study reported that the loss of Nogo increased the extent of neuronal regeneration, as predicted (but only in young mice), and the second study reported a more modest enhancement; however, the third group did not find any significant difference (Kim et al., 2003; Simonen et al., 2003; Zheng et al., 2003). The various results could have been due to differences in the ages and the genetic backgrounds of the mice, the strategy used to delete the Nogo gene, and the compensatory changes in other genes. In order to better understand the differences in these results, two of the groups have set up a collaboration to share their mice and perform their own analyses. This example demonstrates the value of genetic techniques, the importance of consistency in experimental design, the need to replicate experimental results, and the value of collaborative and collegial interactions between research groups.

---

well understood). In amphibians, regeneration readily occurs directly through the glial scar.

Different strains of the same animal species may respond differently to spinal cord trauma. For example, the nature and the extent of the secondary injury and wound healing vary in different strains of mice (Inman et al., 2002). Although these differences in responses between strains and species complicate comparison of the results of studies with different animal species, they may provide important insights about the specific genes that affect postinjury signaling cascades (Inman et al., 2002). Furthermore, the differences observed in experiments with the Nogo gene (Box 3-1) provide important lessons about the necessity to replicate experiments.

Scale

The human spinal cord is more than four times as long as the rat's entire CNS (brain and spinal cord). Figure 3-1 demonstrates the difference in size between the entire CNS of a rat and the caudal end of a human spinal cord. A contusion or transection trauma in humans can affect upwards of 2 to 3 centimeters of the spinal cord, which is approximately 10

(A)

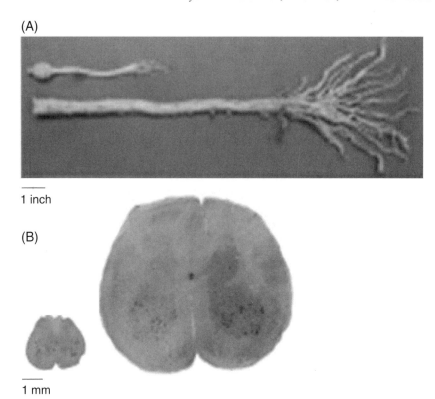

1 inch

(B)

1 mm

FIGURE 3-1 Size discrepancy between the rat and the human spinal cords.
The human spinal cord is more than four times as long as the entire CNS of the rat.
(A) A caudal segment of the human spinal cord, including the cauda equina. The
human cauda equina is approximately the same length as the entire CNS of a rat,
which includes its brain. (B) The diameter of the human spinal cord is also much
larger than that of the rat spinal cord. Twenty slices of a rat spinal cord can fit
inside one slice of a human cord.
SOURCE: Reprinted with permission, from Dobkin and Havton, 2004. Copyright
2004 from *Annual Reviews*.

times the length of the 1 to 3 millimeters often affected by contusion injuries in rats (Metz et al., 2000). Consequently, regeneration of nerve fibers
over a few vertebral segments in a rat—which can result in the restoration
of function—is equivalent to only a fraction of the distance that is needed to
restore function in humans (Dobkin and Havton, 2004). Furthermore, because neurons from both species demonstrate the same degree of spontaneous sprouting of their axons, approximately 2 millimeters (von Meyenburg
et al., 1998), there are added complexities in promoting sufficient axon

growth in humans (Dobkin and Havton, 2004). Although parts of the white matter of the human spinal cord are almost as large as the entire diameter of the rat spinal cord (Figure 3-1), there is no significant difference in the capacity for oligodendrocyte precursor cells to migrate to remyelinate axons in rats and humans.

One of the issues regarding the differences in scale between smaller laboratory animals and humans that has been discussed is the extent to which testing is needed in primate models. Depending on the treatment, it may be advisable to examine the efficacies of some cell therapies in primates. However, there are also limitations in the use of non-human primates for mimicking human responses. For example, some types of monkeys have specific antibodies that can attack and inhibit the survival of human cells. Additionally, the bioavailability and metabolism of anti-rejection drugs in non-human primates and humans differ significantly. Therefore, rodents have frequently been used as the preferred model to study the efficacies of new immunosuppressive agents because of similarities in metabolism between rodents and humans. In addition, experiments are sometimes performed in rabbits and cats, which have larger spinal cords and are also less expensive and easier to maintain than primates. Furthermore, few tests have been developed to assess changes in spinal cord recovery in nonhuman primates. The committee believes that every therapy need not necessarily be tested in primates before clinical trials are performed with humans and that tests with primates be limited to those that will answer questions that are best explored only with non-human primate models.

Next Steps

The promise accorded by the methodical testing of therapies with animal models is beginning to pay off. Scientists have identified numerous inhibitory molecules and receptors that prevent the regeneration of neurons in the spinal cord and have clarified the pathways by which the inhibitory response can be modulated.

Additional resources and tools are still needed in some areas, however. Animal models need to be developed for solid spinal cord injuries, as they account for a significant portion of human spinal cord injuries (Hulsebosch, 2002). Primate models of contusion injury are particularly needed, as well as standard animal models for cervical spinal cord injuries. Furthermore, there is no standard laboratory animal model that spinal cord injury researchers can use to examine fine motor control of the upper extremities or the loss of the sensory modality proprioception, which is responsible for limb position and immediately varying the degree of muscle contraction in response to external stimuli. When individuals with spinal cord injuries lose their proprioception, they are unable to move freely and interact comfortably with the external environment (see Box 5-1). Therefore, the development of a standard animal model that mimics the loss of proprioception will facilitate the development of therapies in a timely fashion.

It is important that researchers use standardized animal models and that they use them consistently. The National Institute of Neurological Disorders and Stroke (NINDS), in recognition of the need to train researchers who work on spinal cord injuries, collaborated with Ohio State University to design a course that emphasizes competency in the technical approaches required for standard animal care and treatment and experimental design (Ohio State University, 2004). In addition, the University of California at Irvine has developed a similar course. These courses provide researchers with the opportunity to be trained to use the same standards for animal research. By training multiple researchers to use standard techniques, consistent animal injury models can be implemented. These models will increase the extent to which research results can be compared and improve the extent to which animal models can be used to predict clinical outcomes in humans.

OUTCOME MEASURES USED TO ASSESS INJURY AND RECOVERY

Because of the variations in the severity and the nature of the outcomes that individuals with spinal cord injuries experience, it is often difficult for health care professionals and researchers to assess the success of a particular intervention. Similarly, it is difficult for preclinical researchers to consistently assess progress in laboratory animal experiments and to determine the amount of progress, if any, that results from natural recovery, drug therapy, surgical intervention, or rehabilitation.

Outcome Measures Used to Assess Spinal Cord Injury in Animal Models

Tests developed to examine the recovery of function in laboratory animals have been designed primarily to examine motor function (Table 3-5; Appendix D). However, to accelerate the translation of research in other areas, including sexual function, bladder and bowel control, and chronic pain relief, standard tests need to be developed to assess experimental therapies for each of these major complications (Widerstrom-Noga and Turk, 2003).

Researchers use a standard scale, the Basso, Beattie, and Bresnahan (BBB) scale, to assess the recovery of motor function in rats (Basso et al., 1995). The foundation of the BBB scale is the assessment of hind-limb movements in rats with spinal cord injuries. The 21-point BBB scale is sensitive enough that small gains in motor function are reflected in changes

TABLE 3-5 Tools Used to Assess Spinal Cord Injuries in Laboratory Animals

---

Functional recovery

Basso, Beattie, and Bresnahan (BBB) scale, an open-field locomotor test for rats
- Is based on 5-point Tarlov scale
- Analyzes hind-limb movements of a rat in an open field
- Is a 21-point scale used to assess locomotor coordination
- Rates parameters such as joint movements, the ability for weight support, limb coordination, foot placement, and gait stability
- Small changes in tissue correlate to large changes on the scale
- Assesses walking, not other movements requiring coordinated spinal cord activity
- Does not assess pain, bowel, bladder, or sexual function

Basso Mouse Scale (BMS), an open-field locomotor test for mice
- Is an adaptation of rat BBB scale to examine the recovery of hind-limb locomotor function
- Assesses walking, not other movements requiring coordinated spinal cord activity
- Does not assess pain, bowel, bladder, or sexual function

Neuronal activity assessment by electrophysiology
- Assesses MEPs or SSEP
- Stimulates corresponding cortical areas of the brain and records response in target nerves to see if connections are still functional
- Correlates to impairment of locomotor activity
- Is noninvasive
- Neuronal activity may not correlate with functional changes
- Hard to assess subtle but critical improvements to circuitry
- Does not directly assess pain, bowel, bladder, or sexual function

Forepaw withdrawal
- Investigates recovery of heat perception
- The forepaw is placed on a heat block and the time that it takes for the animal to withdraw it is measured
- Forepaw withdrawal requires motor function
- Does not assess pain, bowel, bladder, or sexual function

Directed forepaw reaching
- Looks at coordinated limb and muscle movement
- Requires rats to reach under a barrier and pick up food with forepaws
- Limited scale for assessment
- Does not assess pain, bowel, bladder, or sexual function

Morphological assessment of recovery

Histology
- Is used to look at the morphology of axons and assess the degree of tissue sparing, injury, and recovery

Continued

TABLE 3-5 Continued

- Is used for anterograde and retrograde tracing of axons: a substance is injected above or below the location of the injury to determine if the neuron transports it up past the injury location
- Uses electron microscopy to look at the morphology of the spinal cord at very high resolution
- Uses antibody staining to determine the protein distribution in cells
- Assessments cannot be made in real time
- Cannot be performed with living animals

Real-time imaging of the spinal cord
- Uses MRI, CT, and PET, which are safe, noninvasive methods that provide detailed images of hard-to-view areas of the spine
- Resolution is not high enough to detect changes to individual cells

Genetically encoded reporter molecules
- Axon regrowth and formation of functional connections are visualized by use of genetically encoded reporter molecules in intact animal models or in isolated spinal cord preparations
- Requires a correlation to improvements in physiological function

NOTE: Abbreviations: BBB = Basso, Beattie, and Bresnahan; BMS = Basso Mouse Scale; CT = computed tomography; MEPs = motor evoked potential; MRI = magnetic resonance imaging; PET = positron emission tomography; SSEP = somatosensory evoked potential.

in the outcome score. However, the scale has several limitations as it assesses only the functional recovery of the hind limbs and not other elements of fine motor control that are required for coordinated activity regulated by the spinal cord; does not examine the recovery of sensory modalities, including pain and temperature sensations; does not assess other complications that arise as a result of spinal cord injuries, including bowel and bladder function, pain, or sexual capacity; and is not linear.

Outcome Measures Used to Assess Spinal Cord Injury in Humans

Clinicians have available more than 30 assessment tests and surveys that they can use to examine individuals with spinal cord injuries (see Appendix D), including the American Spinal Injury Association (ASIA) scale and measures that assess all the major complications associated with spinal cord injuries. As discussed in further detail in Chapter 5, each of these measures assesses a specific aspect of recovery from spinal cord injury or evaluates the individual's quality of life and is not designed to examine all the major complications that arise because of a spinal cord injury.

MONITORING REAL-TIME PROGRESSION OF
SPINAL CORD INJURIES

Biomarkers

It is hoped that in the near future biomarkers will be available for diagnosis or prediction of the clinical course of an individual after a spinal cord injury; however, no biomarkers are currently available to identify the changes occurring in the cells in the living spinal cord, such as neurite outgrowth, cell death, or changes in gene expression. Researchers have identified a large number of potential biomarkers (Table 3-6) and are developing practical methods to assess changes to those markers that could be used in the clinical setting. Once biomarkers are available and validated, they could be used to aid researchers and clinicians with making a diagnosis and establishing a prognosis, monitoring changes over time, and evaluating therapeutic interventions.

Trauma to the spinal cord affects a large number of biochemical cascades and reactions, but specific details about the genes involved in these processes are not well understood. Most of these changes are reflected by changes in mRNA and protein levels (Table 3-7). Since mRNA is copied, or transcribed, from DNA and provides the transcript that the cell uses to synthesize new proteins, analysis of mRNA or protein levels could reveal information about changes in cellular events. Advances in microarray technologies over the last decade have made it possible for researchers to examine the expression patterns of hundreds, if not thousands, of genes at the same time by comparing changes in gene activity in spinal cord samples from healthy and injured individuals. Using biomarkers, microarrays, and other tools, investigators have started to assess the complexity of the biological response to spinal cord injury. The full potential uses of biomarkers for spinal cord injury research include the following:

• *Diagnosis and prognosis.* The expression profile of a biomarker, especially proteins, could provide clinicians with information that aids in establishment of a diagnosis and a prognosis of a patient's injury. For instance, the progression of multiple sclerosis (MS) can be determined by examining the levels of a major myelin component, myelin basic protein, whose concentration increases in the cerebrospinal fluid in response to a demyelinating episode. Experiments with laboratory animals have identified similar gene expression fluctuations in response to spinal cord injuries. For example, the onset of the acute immune response is characterized by increases in the levels of the interleukin-6 protein (Segal et al., 1997; Carmel et al., 2001; Song et al., 2001; Nesic et al., 2002), whereas apoptosis, or the controlled death of cells that begins in the secondary stage of the injury, is regulated, in part, by changes in the levels of the Fas protein (Li et al., 2000;

TABLE 3-6 Criteria for Determining and Validating a Biomarker Used to Monitor Spinal Cord Injury Progression and Recovery of Function

Necessary properties of a progression marker	• Describe a biological process that changes with the progression of the disease or recovery • Correlate with clinical deterioration
Necessary properties of a biomarker measure used as a progression indicator	• Objective (i.e., it should be amenable to a blinded or a centralized assessment) • Reproducible (i.e., repeat measurements of the progression indicator for the same patient should be highly correlated) • Specific to changes in progression indicator; otherwise, the effects of other changes in the biomarker (e.g., compensatory changes related to drugs used to treat the injury or to agent under study in a clinical trial) should be known so that suitable adjustments in the analysis of clinical trial data can be made • Low signal-to-noise ratio for the biomarker measure • Safe and tolerable and should not require maneuvers that could unblind the study
Other desirable properties of a biomarker measure used as a progression indicator	• Relatively inexpensive and easy to use • Capable of being used in repeated studies with a particular individual with a spinal cord injury
Data needed to support the use of progression indicator or biomarker measurement for application to a clinical trial for study of spinal cord injury progression	• Data from longitudinal studies should be available for a sufficient number of individuals with spinal cord injuries to allow an informative assessment of the distributional properties (e.g., mean and variance) of the progression measure over periods of time pertinent to future clinical trials; such data are needed to allow calculation of the sample size and power for trials to evaluate the effects of specific treatments on spinal cord injury progression

NOTE: This table is based on recommendations for the development of biomarkers for use in monitoring the progression of Parkinson's disease.
SOURCE: Adapted from Brooks et al., 2003.

Casha et al., 2001). Thus, identification of specific fluctuations in the levels of proteins like interleukin-6 and Fas could inform clinicians about changes in an individual's level of injury.

• *Treatment guidance.* Analysis of gene expression during the course of the injury and recovery could provide clinicians with detailed information about the molecular events that are responsible for changes in spinal cord reorganization that occur over time. With this knowledge, physicians might be able to avoid preventable complications and specifically target ongoing events when they treat spinal cord injuries.

• *Outcomes assessment.* Biological expression data that are correlated to functional improvement, such as increased locomotion, improved bowel function, or reduced spasticity, may provide helpful means of assessing beneficial or harmful changes to the spinal cord that may be missed when the primary clinical end points are behavioral. The development of biomarkers that are specific for neuronal cell death, myelination, or nerve regeneration would be beneficial to both basic researchers and clinicians.

• *Potential therapeutic targets.* The analysis of changes in specific gene products that are up- and down-regulated in response to a spinal cord injury could also provide researchers with a tool to identify specific targets that could be used for future drug development. Understanding of the molecular and cellular mechanisms involved in spinal cord injuries may permit identification of specific targets for therapeutic benefit.

Traditionally, biomarkers were identified by examining candidate genes involved in cellular events that occur as a result of a spinal cord injury and looking for other genes that were associated with the function of the candidate gene. This strategy led to the identification of many candidate genes, such as the Nogo gene and several of the interleukin genes, which have helped define the biological processes affected by a spinal cord injury. Although the individual process of identifying genes involved in a spinal cord injury has been critical for advancing the research, the process is also intrinsically biased and limited in its scope because of its dependence on previous detailed knowledge about the biological system under study. Another limitation is that changes in individual biomarkers may be induced by events other than spinal cord injuries. For example, the activities of the immediate-early genes c-fos and c-jun have been correlated to neurite outgrowth, but they are also involved in many other processes, including cancer metastasis. Therefore, for a single biomarker to provide sufficient predictive value, it must be specific to spinal cord injuries and provide a sensitive measure for the assessment of the process being examined. Consequently, changes in multiple genes will need to be assessed to understand gene responses specifically related to spinal cord injuries as is true in assessing breast cancer (Hollon, 2002).

Protein Expression Profiles of Spinal Cord Injury

Because the body contains more than 1 million proteins that regulate metabolism and disease (Watkins, 2001), proteomic techniques that ana-

TABLE 3-7 Changes in Gene Expression After Spinal Cord Injury, by Stage of Injury

Gene Function	Primary Stage	Secondary Stage	Chronic Stage
Apoptosis	Caspases, c-jun, p53, Fas, FasL, CD95, rho	Caspases, c-jun, NF-κB, HSP70	None
Growth and differentiation	Vimentin, TGFβ, ANIA-6	Vimentin, TGF, VGF, BDNF, TrkB (–)	Vimentin, TrkB, BMPs
Inflammation	IL-6, IL-1β, IGFs, SOCS, MCP-1 (IESR-JE), ICAM-1, iNOS, GFAP, IL-4r, COX-2, IL-2Rα, HSP27	IL-6, IL-1, IGFs, SOCS, MCP-1 (IESR-JE), ICAM-1, iNOS, GFAP, TNF receptor, COX-3 (–), HSP27	IL-6, IL-1β, IGFs, HSP27
Regulation of ion transport	Ca^{2+} ATPase (–)	Ca^{2+} ATPase (–), K^+ channels, Na^+ channels (–), Na^+/K^+ ATPase (–)	Ca^{2+} ATPase (–)
Protection of neurons	None	Metallothionein I and II, survival motoneuron	Metallothionein I and II
Communication between neurons	SNAP-25 (–), syntaxins (–), glutamate receptors	SNAP-25 (–), syntaxins (–), synapsins (–), somatostatin (–), GABA transporters (–), glutamate receptors, GABA receptors (–), glutamate transporter	GABA receptors

lyze changes to individual or multiple proteins have the potential to provide investigators with information about cellular responses to spinal cord injuries. For example, Western blotting and immunohistochemistry allow investigators to examine modifications to a protein's structure that may change its activity and cellular distribution.

Protein arrays, like DNA arrays, allow researchers to screen simultaneously many proteins for changes in expression levels that result from the onset of a disease or a therapeutic approach. However, protein arrays are not as encompassing as DNA arrays. Current protein array technology only allows about 10 percent of a cell's total proteome to be represented on an array (2,000 to 3,000 proteins can be represented on a protein array,

TABLE 3-7 Continued

Gene Function	Primary Stage	Secondary Stage	Chronic Stage
Repair and regeneration of neurons and glia	Nestin, JAK, STAT, c-fos	Nestin, vimentin, dynamin (–), c-fos	Semaphorin, GAS-7, epithelins 1 and 2, platelet factor 4
Proteins that relay exterior information to the nucleus	PDE, CaM kinases (–)	PDE, MAP kinases, CaM kinases (–)	None
Proteins that generate and maintain cellular structure	None	MOG (–), neurofilaments, LAMP (–), MAP-2, tau (–)	None
Regulation of DNA synthesis	Fra-1, NGFI-A	Fra-1, NGFI-A	None

NOTE: Analysis of proteomic and DNA gene array studies identified significant changes in gene expression in response to a spinal cord injury. Classification of these genes into specific functions provides further insight into the processes that are changing. All genes are up-regulated unless a "(–)" notation is presented, in which case the gene is down-regulated.
SOURCES: Bregman et al., 1997; Segal et al., 1997; Li et al., 2000; Saito et al., 2000; Carmel et al., 2001; Casha et al., 2001; Fan et al., 2001; Song et al., 2001; Zurita et al., 2001; Bareyre et al., 2002; Nesic et al., 2002; Shibuya et al., 2002; Tachibana et al., 2002; Bareyre and Schwab, 2003; Di Giovanni et al., 2003; Dubreuil et al., 2003; Liu et al., 2003; Haberkorn et al., 2004.

whereas 47,000 genes can be represented on a DNA array). Such arrays could be tailored to the specific aspect of spinal cord injury being studied. In addition, advances in mass spectrometry now make it possible to characterize the levels and even the phosphorylation state of many hundreds of proteins, allowing greater insights into the specific activities of proteins.

Issues in Developing Biomarkers for Spinal Cord Injury

It is extremely difficult to obtain samples of mRNA or protein directly from spinal cord tissue without inducing further complications. The most practical sources of mRNA and protein are serum and cerebrospinal fluid.

However, a spinal tap—an invasive procedure, which requires the insertion of a special needle through the lumbar vertebral spine into the fluid space that surrounds the spinal cord—must be performed to obtain cerebrospinal fluid. Although serum is easier to collect by drawing blood samples, its analysis is complicated by the high concentration of several proteins (e.g., albumin, immunoglobulin G, and transferrin) that constitute approximately 80 percent of total serum proteins. These high background levels make it difficult to sieve through and detect changes in the levels of proteins that are present at low concentrations. Once a sample is obtained, issues about the usefulness of the contents remain. The mRNA derived from neurons and glia is not very abundant and degrades rapidly. Also, because serum and cerebrospinal fluid are indirect sources of spinal cord mRNA and proteins, the overall numbers of genes that are associated with spinal cord injuries are not well represented. Furthermore, the proteins that are present are typically restricted to those found on the exteriors of cells and the small intracellular concentrations of mRNA and proteins that are released when a cell dies, which further limits the pool of biomarkers that can be analyzed. Efforts are thus needed to improve the processes for detecting potential biomarkers.

Next Steps in Biomarker Development

Experimental therapies developed in the laboratory take as long as 7 to 15 years to enter into the clinic (Lakhani and Ashworth, 2001). To expedite this transition, spinal cord injury researchers should use strategies developed in other fields, including MS, Alzheimer's disease, and cancer biology. For example, clinical studies for MS and brain metastasis have been established to analyze changes in protein levels in the serum and cerebrospinal fluid. These trials could provide the framework for biomarker studies involving individuals with spinal cord injuries.

In 2000, the National Cancer Institute established the Early Detection Research Network (EDRN) to guide the process of biomarker discovery in an effort to produce a useful population-screening tool (Kutkat and Srivastava, 2001). This network consists of three laboratory components: biomarker discovery laboratories, biomarker validation laboratories, and clinical epidemiological centers. EDRN also helped to establish standards for the development and evaluation of biomarkers and guide the process of biomarker discovery related to cancer biology. Using EDRN as a model, the spinal cord injury community can transfer many of the recommendations and strategies developed to facilitate progress on cancer research for spinal cord injury research. In 2001 and 2004 NINDS issued two program announcements that focused on advancing proteome arrays and identifying clinical biomarkers (NINDS, 2001a, 2004); these are not specifically focused on spinal cord injuries but do offer potential for advances in this area. Additionally, NINDS put out a request for proposals (NINDS, 2001b) for studies designed to define gene expression profiles following traumatic spinal cord injuries.

Because the technologies used to identify biological markers can detect small but significant changes in gene expression, they are sensitive to slight variations in protocol. In fact, the gene profiles obtained from experimental studies are affected by differences in the instruments used to analyze the samples and by small changes in the ways in which samples are collected (e.g., the relative time after injury that tissue is collected, the location of the injury, and the quantity of the specimen) (Bareyre and Schwab, 2003). A standard set of methods is needed to minimize variability and maximize reproducibility (Bareyre and Schwab, 2003).

Visualizing the Living Spinal Cord

The spinal cord is embedded in bone and is surrounded by cerebrospinal fluid, which precludes direct visualization. The advent of neuroimaging techniques has allowed investigators to visualize the spinal cord so that they can begin to study the progression of spinal cord injuries. Magnetic resonance imaging (MRI) and computed tomography (CT) provide real-time information about the state of the injury and recovery. Moreover, imaging is noninvasive and the same region of the spinal cord can be repeatedly visualized to identify changes occurring over time. Imaging technologies, biomarkers, and molecular genetic technologies are being combined to provide researchers with powerful tools to monitor the progression of the injury and recovery through the visualization of specific molecular markers that define cellular events and functional changes.

MRI is a safe and noninvasive method of evaluating the spinal cord that provides detailed pictures of hard-to-view areas of the spine, including the spinal canal, vertebra, and soft tissue (Levitski et al., 1999). Clinicians use MRI after an individual has an acute spinal cord trauma to visualize the location and the extent of the spinal cord trauma and compressive lesions (e.g., blood clots) (AANS/CNS, 2002). It is superior to positron emission tomography (PET), CT, and other imaging technologies for the detection of abscesses or other masses near the spinal cord and is used to monitor patients with chronic compression injuries. However, imaging technologies have practical limits in the setting of acute spinal cord traumas, as a patient may not be stable enough to enter an MRI machine or may have other medical priorities that take precedence over receiving a detailed image of the spinal cord.

Functional MRI (fMRI) can provide second-by-second images of the brain to reveal changes in neuronal activity in response to different sensory stimuli and mental tasks. It allows researchers and clinicians to study the changes in injured neuronal circuits. However, fMRI relies on the metabolic changes that occur in response to neural activity and the images obtained by fMRI are not a direct measure of neural activity. Therefore, caution should be placed on interpretation of the accuracies of the spatial maps generated by fMRI (Ugurbil et al., 2003). The National Institutes of Health has recommended that fMRI techniques be developed to assess the degree of loss and recovery of sensation in rodents with contusion injuries to their spinal cords (Hofstetter et al., 2003; NINDS, 2004).

Radiologists use CT scans as a standard procedure to clarify areas of clinical concern (Youmans, 1996; AANS/CNS, 2002). Although MRI is better suited for analyzing the soft tissue of the spinal cord, the strength of using CT scans is in investigating the bone structure and detecting fractures of the vertebrae (Figure 3-2). Helical CT scans offer advantages over traditional radiology X-rays due to their speed in accruing the images and increased accuracy (4.5 minutes and 98.5 percent, respectively, for helical CT compared with 25 minutes and 43 percent, respectively, for X-rays). Therefore, in conjunction with MRI, CT scans provide useful tools for emergency clinicians (Nunez et al., 1994).

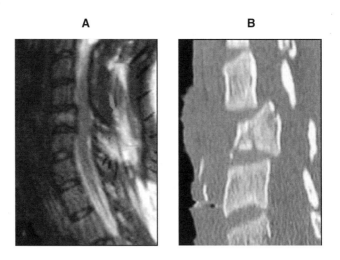

FIGURE 3-2 MRI (A) and CT (B) of an injured spinal cord. Imaging of a spinal cord contusion injury by MRI and CT helps to reveal different aspects of the injury. The MRI image on the left reveals the soft spinal cord and bone, whereas the CT scan image on the right clearly delineates bone structures.
SOURCE: Reprinted with permission, from AANS, 1999. Copyright 1999 from AANS.

Unlike MRI, fMRI, and CT scans, PET scans detect and localize specific naturally occurring proteins; molecules, such as sugars and water; and other substances, such as neurotransmitters, which have been modified to emit radioactive energy.

At present, PET scans are not commonly used in the clinic to assess spinal cord injuries. However, as discussed below, the technology has much potential to provide researchers and clinicians with a means by which to visualize changes in gene expression in the spinal cord.

Next Steps: Future Imaging Technologies

Imaging technologies provide clinicians with important tools to gauge the responses of patients to different therapies (Jacobs et al., 2003). The creation of sensitive assays that merge image-based technologies with biomarker research will allow investigators and clinicians to use specific tracers to localize molecular, genetic, and cellular processes in real time, thus providing further insight into the biological processes that affect the progression of the injury (Blasberg and Gelovani, 2002).

As of January 2005, no clinical studies in the United States were specifically examining the use of imaging marker technologies for the study of spinal cord injuries. In comparison, markers are used to assess the state of MS and Alzheimer's disease and imaging techniques are used to monitor the effects of different treatments for these conditions. For example, imaging assays are being developed to visualize specific neurotransmitter levels and to determine if they are involved in memory loss (Brown et al., 2003).

The Future of Magnetic Resonance Technology

In animals with syringomyelia, diffusion-weighted MRI, which is sensitive to the diffusion or random motion of water molecules in tissue, can detect cystic lesions in the gray matter of the spinal cord (Schwartz et al., 1999). The increased sensitivity offered by diffusion-weighted MRI will enable physicians to detect specific complications of spinal cord injuries sooner, thus increasing the potential for treatment.

Magnetic resonance technology can be adapted to provide more than diagnostic information about the structural changes occurring in response to a spinal cord injury. In 2001, Bulte and colleagues used magnetic resonance to track oligodendrocyte stem cells that were prelabeled with super paramagnetic iron oxide nanocomposites, which are small beads invisible to the naked eye that can be detected by MR technology (Bulte et al., 1999, 2001). Using this approach, the investigators were able to track the real-time migration and integration of these oligodendrocyte stem cells for up to 6 weeks in the same animal, which is important for distinguishing the efficacies of endogenous cells versus those of the exogenous transplanted stem cells.

The Future of PET Scans

PET scan technology is being developed to inform clinicians about whether drugs can bind to the appropriate targets. For example, clinicians are using PET scans to determine if treatments are effective by looking at the uptake of glucose, which tumors need to nourish their growth (Van den Abbeele and Badawi, 2002; Pollack, 2004). These effects can be observed before structural changes in the tumor can be detected.

Two caveats about the use of PET scans must be kept in mind. First, current technology does not have enough resolution to allow complete visualization through the entire diameter of the spinal cord. Furthermore, the current spatial resolution of commercial PET scanners is 4 mm but 2.5 mm resolution has been achieved in research instruments that use motion compensation. Second, information obtained from PET scans is based on metabolic events that correlate to neural activity and may not directly correspond to the location where the changes in activity are occurring. Therefore, the images generated by PET scans could be misleading because they may not accurately represent the spatial specificities of the changes (Ugurbil et al., 2003). However, refinements to PET scans could provide important information about the cellular states of the injury, such as gene activation or suppression in response to the injury; this would provide physicians with the ability to quantify responses to different spinal cord injury treatments (Brooks et al., 2003) and to identify functional changes before the onset of structural changes identifiable by MRI (National PET Scan Management, LLC, 2004). PET ligands have been developed that can detect glucose metabolism, inflammation, and receptor abundance, including agents that track the N-methyl-D-aspartate (NMDA) receptor activity and proteases. PET measures very different process than does MRI whose spatial resolution is superior. However, PET contrast resolution for identification of proteins can be hundreds of times greater than MRI depending on the target. The potentials of PET for assessing the severity of injury and the responses to therapy await application of high resolution systems with recently developed radiopharmaceuticals.

Tracking Recovery with PET and Magnetic Resonance

Improvements to PET and MR technologies enable investigators to visualize the molecular signatures of damage and repair to the CNS. In an attempt to examine the activities of specific neuronal circuits, imaging markers that mimic neurotransmitters and receptors that are nonradioactive are being created, including the iron analog annexin V (Schellenberger et al., 2002), the fluorescent marker Cy5.5 (Petrovsky et al., 2003), and markers that do not become active until they reach their target. Future modification and adaptation of these technologies could be used to examine specific stages of regeneration, including those designed to detect neurite outgrowth, astrocyte scarring, oligodendrocyte myelination, and immunological response.

Transgenic Animals: Following the Labeled Cell

At present it is difficult to follow the path of cell transplants (such as stem cells, Schwann cells, and olfactory ensheathing cells) in the living spinal cord; therefore, it is difficult to draw conclusions about the efficacy of an experiment with such cells. Continued advancement of imaging techniques will provide a mechanism by which investigators and clinicians can assess the integration of grafted tissue or cells into the preexisting neuronal network or monitor the response to gene therapy by tracking the transgene location. Transgenic animal models have thus been developed. Specific populations of cells in these animals are genetically engineered to be fluorescent or to emit a fluorescent signal when they are functionally activated. Such approaches, which use two-photon confocal imaging to detect the signal, can be directly applied to spinal cord preparations in vitro and administered to intact mice and rats. With improvements in the current technology, the use and improvement of near-infrared markers might also provide researchers with a means to monitor the progression of a spinal cord injury and recovery in laboratory animals.

Multidisciplinary Research and Bringing Molecular Imaging to the Clinic

The promise of molecular imaging technologies can be realized only if the technologies can be successfully transferred to the clinical setting. The transfer of these technologies will require cross-disciplinary collaborations and multidisciplinary research efforts among molecular and cellular biologists, imaging scientists, nanotechnologists, and clinicians. A review article by Massoud and Gambhir (2003) identified the following goals for the transfer of molecular imaging technologies from the research laboratory to the clinic:

- develop noninvasive in vivo imaging methods that detect specific cellular and molecular processes, such as gene expression and protein-protein interactions;
- monitor multiple molecular events in concert;
- monitor the trafficking and targeting of cells;

- optimize drug and gene therapies;
- image drug effects at the molecular and cellular levels; and
- assess the molecular pathology of disease progression.

Achieving these goals and translating those achievements into reliable clinical technologies will be critical steps toward the treatment and diagnosis of spinal cord injuries at the molecular level. To achieve these objectives, continued advances need to be made to overcome the challenges of biocompatibility, probe delivery, and high-resolution signal detection (Mahmood and Weissleder, 2002).

Cross-disciplinary collaboration and multidisciplinary research is needed to bring together molecular and cellular biologists, imaging scientists, nanotechnologists, and clinicians to reach these goals (Blasberg and Gelovani, 2002). Many of the imaging techniques used to examine the CNS were designed to visualize brain tumors or to assess Alzheimer's disease, Parkinson's disease, and MS. These resources and technologies can be applied or can provide models for spinal cord injury research. For instance, investigators are examining the utility of using multiphoton imaging techniques to monitor the progression of senile plaques in mice that model Alzheimer's disease (Christie et al., 2001). This technology could also be modified to assess and monitor the progression of the glial scar formation that results from spinal cord injuries.

The cancer research field not only has led the way in developing technologies but also has helped to establish research centers that have been critical in creating a means for translating imaging technologies into the clinic. In particular, the National Cancer Institute has developed two programs: the Small Animal Imaging Resources Program (SAIRP) and the In Vivo Cellular and Molecular Imaging Centers (ICMIC) Program. These programs, along with support mechanisms sponsored by the National Institute of Biomedical Imaging and Engineering, provide mechanisms and model systems that can be used to promote the cooperative development of new imaging systems for spinal cord injury research and treatment.

RECOMMENDATIONS

Recommendation 3.1: *Increase Training Efforts on Standardized Research Tools and Techniques*
Spinal cord injury researchers should receive training in the use of standardized animal models and evaluation techniques. Pre- and postdoctoral fellowship training programs focused on spinal cord injury research should require participation in courses designed to train investigators on the appropriate use of the available tools and techniques.

Recommendation 3.2: *Improve and Standardize Research Tools and Assessment Techniques*
Preclinical research tools and animal models should be developed and refined to examine spinal cord injury progression and repair and assess the effectiveness of therapeutic interventions. These preclinical tools and assessment protocols should be standardized for each type and each stage of spinal cord injury. Particular emphasis should be placed on:

- improving imaging technologies to allow real-time assessment of the current state and progression of the injury;
- identifying biomarkers that can be used to monitor the progression of the injury and recovery;
- developing additional animal models to explore the progression of spinal cord injury and repair;
- establishing standardized sets of functional outcome measures for the evaluation of experimental therapies for each type and each stage of spinal cord injury in animal models; and
- enhancing functional assessment techniques to examine motor function as well as secondary complications, including pain and depression of the immune system.

REFERENCES

AANS (American Association of Neurological Surgeons). 1999. *Spinal Cord*. [Online]. Available: http://www.neurosurgerytoday.org/what/patient_e/spinal.asp [accessed January 25, 2005].

AANS/CNS (American Association of Neurological Surgeons/Congress of Neurological Surgeons). 2002. Radiographic assessment of the cervical spine in symptomatic trauma patients. *Neurosurgery* 50(3 Suppl): S36-43.

Bareyre FM, Schwab ME. 2003. Inflammation, degeneration and regeneration in the injured spinal cord: Insights from DNA microarrays. *Trends in Neurosciences* 26(10): 555-563.

Bareyre FM, Haudenschild B, Schwab ME. 2002. Long-lasting sprouting and gene expression changes induced by the monoclonal antibody IN-1 in the adult spinal cord. *Journal of Neuroscience* 22(16): 7097-7110.

Basso DM, Beattie MS, Bresnahan JC. 1995. A sensitive and reliable locomotor rating scale for open field testing in rats. *Journal of Neurotrauma* 12(1): 1-21.

Blasberg RG, Gelovani J. 2002. Molecular-genetic imaging: A nuclear medicine-based perspective. *Molecular Imaging: Official Journal of the Society for Molecular Imaging* 1(3): 280-300.

Bradbury EJ, Moon LD, Popat RJ, King VR, Bennett GS, Patel PN, Fawcett JW, McMahon SB. 2002. Chondroitinase ABC promotes functional recovery after spinal cord injury. *Nature* 416(6881): 636-640.

Bregman BS, McAtee M, Dai HN, Kuhn PL. 1997. Neurotrophic factors increase axonal growth after spinal cord injury and transplantation in the adult rat. *Experimental Neurology* 148(2): 475-494.

Bresnahan JC, Beattie MS, Todd FD III, Noyes DH. 1987. A behavioral and anatomical analysis of spinal cord injury produced by a feedback-controlled impaction device. *Experimental Neurology* 95(3): 548-570.

Brooks DJ, Frey KA, Marek KL, Oakes D, Paty D, Prentice R, Shults CW, Stoessl AJ. 2003. Assessment of neuroimaging techniques as biomarkers of the progression of Parkinson's disease. *Experimental Neurology* 184(Suppl 1): S68-79.

Brown D, Chisholm JA, Owens J, Pimlott S, Patterson J, Wyper D. 2003. Acetylcholine muscarinic receptors and response to anti-cholinesterase therapy in patients with Alzheimer's disease. *European Journal of Nuclear Medicine & Molecular Imaging* 30(2): 296-300.

Bulte JW, Zhang S, van Gelderen P, Herynek V, Jordan EK, Duncan ID, Frank JA. 1999. Neurotransplantation of magnetically labeled oligodendrocyte progenitors: Magnetic resonance tracking of cell migration and myelination. *Proceedings of the National Academy of Sciences (U.S.A.)* 96(26): 15256-15261.

Bulte JW, Douglas T, Witwer B, Zhang SC, Strable E, Lewis BK, Zywicke H, Miller B, van Gelderen P, Moskowitz BM, Duncan ID, Frank JA. 2001. Magnetodendrimers allow endosomal magnetic labeling and in vivo tracking of stem cells. *Nature Biotechnology* 19(12): 1141-1147.

Carmel JB, Galante A, Soteropoulos P, Tolias P, Recce M, Young W, Hart RP. 2001. Gene expression profiling of acute spinal cord injury reveals spreading inflammatory signals and neuron loss. *Physiological Genomics* 7(2): 201-213.

Casha S, Yu WR, Fehlings MG. 2001. Oligodendroglial apoptosis occurs along degenerating axons and is associated with FAS and p75 expression following spinal cord injury in the rat. *Neuroscience* 103(1): 203-218.

Christie RH, Bacskai BJ, Zipfel WR, Williams RM, Kajdasz ST, Webb WW, Hyman BT. 2001. Growth arrest of individual senile plaques in a model of Alzheimer's disease observed by in vivo multiphoton microscopy. *Journal of Neuroscience* 21(3): 858-864.

Croft BY. 2002. Animal models for imaging. *Disease Markers* 18(5-6): 365-374.

Di Giovanni S, Knoblach SM, Brandoli C, Aden SA, Hoffman EP, Faden AI. 2003. Gene profiling in spinal cord injury shows role of cell cycle in neuronal death. *Annals of Neurology* 53(4): 454-468.

Dobkin BH, Havton LA. 2004. Basic advances and new avenues in therapy of spinal cord injury. *Annual Review of Medicine* 55: 255-282.

Dubreuil CI, Winton MJ, McKerracher L. 2003. Rho activation patterns after spinal cord injury and the role of activated Rho in apoptosis in the central nervous system. *Journal of Cell Biology* 162(2): 233-243.

Fan M, Mi R, Yew DT, Chan WY. 2001. Analysis of gene expression following sciatic nerve crush and spinal cord hemisection in the mouse by microarray expression profiling. *Cellular and Molecular Neurobiology* 21(5): 497-508.

Gorman AL, Yu CG, Ruenes GR, Daniels L, Yezierski RP. 2001. Conditions affecting the onset, severity, and progression of a spontaneous pain-like behavior after excitotoxic spinal cord injury. *Journal of Pain* 2(4): 229-240.

Gruner JA. 1992. A monitored contusion model of spinal cord injury in the rat. *Journal of Neurotrauma* 9(2): 123-126.

Haberkorn U, Altmann A, Mier W, Eisenhut M. 2004. Impact of functional genomics and proteomics on radionuclide imaging. *Seminars in Nuclear Medicine* 34(1): 4-22.

Hofstetter CP, Schweinhardt P, Klason T, Olson L, Spenger C. 2003. Numb rats walk—A behavioural and fMRI comparison of mild and moderate spinal cord injury. *European Journal of Neuroscience* 18(11): 3061-3068.

Hollon T. 2002. Classifying breast cancer models. *The Scientist* 16(17): 20-24.

Houle JD, Tessler A. 2003. Repair of chronic spinal cord injury. *Experimental Neurology* 182(2): 247-260.

Hulsebosch CE. 2002. Recent advances in pathophysiology and treatment of spinal cord injury. *Advances in Physiology Education* 26(1-4): 238-255.

Inman D, Guth L, Steward O. 2002. Genetic influences on secondary degeneration and wound healing following spinal cord injury in various strains of mice. *Journal of Comparative Neurology* 451(3): 225-235.

Jacobs AH, Li H, Winkeler A, Hilker R, Knoess C, Ruger A, Galldiks N, Schaller B, Sobesky J, Kracht L, Monfared P, Klein M, Vollmar S, Bauer B, Wagner R, Graf R, Wienhard K, Herholz K, Heiss WD. 2003. PET-based molecular imaging in neuroscience. *European Journal of Nuclear Medicine & Molecular Imaging* 30(7): 1051-1065.

Jin Y. 2002. Synaptogenesis: Insights from worm and fly. *Current Opinion in Neurobiology* 12(1): 71-79.

Kidd T, Brose K, Mitchell KJ, Fetter RD, Tessier-Lavigne M, Goodman CS, Tear G. 1998. Roundabout controls axon crossing of the CNS midline and defines a novel subfamily of evolutionarily conserved guidance receptors. *Cell* 92(2): 205-215.

Kim JE, Li S, GrandPre T, Qiu D, Strittmatter SM. 2003. Axon regeneration in young adult mice lacking Nogo-a/B. *Neuron* 38(2): 187-199.

Kleitman N. 2004. Keeping promises: Translating basic research into new spinal cord injury therapies. *Journal of Spinal Cord Medicine* 27(4): 311-318.

Kraut R, Menon K, Zinn K. 2001. A gain-of-function screen for genes controlling motor axon guidance and synaptogenesis in *Drosophila*. *Current Biology* 11(6): 417-430.

Kutkat L, Srivastava S. 2001. The early detection research network: A platform for communication and collaboration. *Disease Markers* 17(1): 3-4.

Kwo S, Young W, Decrescito V. 1989. Spinal cord sodium, potassium, calcium, and water concentration changes in rats after graded contusion injury. *Journal of Neurotrauma* 6(1): 13-24.

Kwon BK, Liu J, Messerer C, Kobayashi NR, McGraw J, Oschipok L, Tetzlaff W. 2002a. Survival and regeneration of rubrospinal neurons 1 year after spinal cord injury. *Proceedings of the National Academy of Sciences (U.S.A.)* 99(5): 3246-3251.

Kwon BK, Oxland TR, Tetzlaff W. 2002b. Animal models used in spinal cord regeneration research. *Spine* 27(14): 1504-1510.

Lakhani SR, Ashworth A. 2001. Microarray and histopathological analysis of tumours: The future and the past?. *Nature Reviews—Cancer* 1(2): 151-157.

Lanuza GM, Gosgnach S, Pierani A, Jessell TM, Goulding M. 2004. Genetic identification of spinal interneurons that coordinate left-right locomotor activity necessary for walking movements. *Neuron* 42(3): 375-386.

Levitski RE, Lipsitz D, Chauvet AE. 1999. Magnetic resonance imaging of the cervical spine in 27 dogs. *Veterinary Radiology & Ultrasound* 40(4): 332-341.

Li GL, Farooque M, Olsson Y. 2000. Changes of Fas and Fas ligand immunoreactivity after compression trauma to rat spinal cord. *Acta Neuropathologica* 100(1): 75-81.

Liu CL, Jin AM, Tong BH. 2003. Detection of gene expression pattern in the early stage after spinal cord injury by gene chip. *Chinese Journal of Traumatology* 6(1): 18-22.

Magavi SS, Leavitt BR, Macklis JD. 2000. Induction of neurogenesis in the neocortex of adult mice. *Nature* 405(6789): 951-955.

Mahmood U, Weissleder R. 2002. Some tools for molecular imaging. *Academic Radiology* 9(6): 629-631.

Massoud TF, Gambhir SS. 2003. Molecular imaging in living subjects: Seeing fundamental biological processes in a new light. *Genes & Development* 17(5): 545-580.

Metz GA, Curt A, van de Meent H, Klusman I, Schwab ME, Dietz V. 2000. Validation of the weight-drop contusion model in rats: A comparative study of human spinal cord injury. *Journal of Neurotrauma* 17(1): 1-17.

National PET Scan Management, LLC. 2004. *How Does PET Compare with Other Imaging Modalities?* [Online]. Available: http://www.nationalpetscan.com/petovew.htm [accessed November 11, 2004].

Nesic O, Svrakic NM, Xu GY, McAdoo D, Westlund KN, Hulsebosch CE, Ye Z, Galante A, Soteropoulos P, Tolias P, Young W, Hart RP, Perez-Polo JR. 2002. DNA microarray analysis of the contused spinal cord: Effect of NMDA receptor inhibition. *Journal of Neuroscience Research* 68(4): 406-423.

Neumann S, Bradke F, Tessier-Lavigne M, Basbaum AI. 2002. Regeneration of sensory axons within the injured spinal cord induced by intraganglionic cAMP elevation. *Neuron* 34(6): 885-893.

NINDS (National Institute of Neurological Disorders and Stroke). 2001a. *Biomarkers and Clinical Endpoints in Pediatric Clinical Trials.* [Online]. Available: http://grants.nih.gov/grants/guide/pa-files/PA-01-043.html [accessed November 11, 2004].

NINDS. 2001b. *Gene Expression Profiling in the Nervous System Following Traumatic Spinal Cord Injury.* [Online]. Available: http://www.ninds.nih.gov/funding/2rfp_01_03.pdf [accessed October 4, 2004].

NINDS. 2004. *Functional and Dysfunctional Spinal Circuitry: Role for Rehabilitation and Neural Prostheses.* [Online]. Available: http://www.ninds.nih.gov/news_and_events/proceedings/spinalcircuitrywkshp_pr.htm [accessed November 11, 2004].

Noyes DH. 1987. Correlation between parameters of spinal cord impact and resultant injury. *Experimental Neurology* 95(3): 535-557.

Nunez DB, Ahmed AA, Coin C, et al. 1994. Clearing the cervical spine in multiple trauma victims: A time-effective protocol using helical computed tomography. *Emergency Radiology* 1(6): 273-278.

Ohio State University. 2004. *Spinal Cord Injury: A Comprehensive Course.* [Online]. Available: http://medicine.osu.edu/sci/Main.htm [accessed November 11, 2004].

Petrovsky A, Schellenberger E, Josephson L, Weissleder R, Bogdanov A Jr. 2003. Near-infrared fluorescent imaging of tumor apoptosis. *Cancer Research* 63(8): 1936-1942.

Pollack A. 2004, August 4. In drug research, some guinea pigs are now human. *The New York Times.* p. A2.

Qiu J, Cai D, Filbin MT. 2002. A role for cAMP in regeneration during development and after injury. *Progress in Brain Research* 137: 381-387.

Ramer MS, Harper GP, Bradbury EJ. 2000. Progress in spinal cord research: A refined strategy for the International Spinal Research Trust. *Spinal Cord* 38(8): 449-472.

Richardson PM, McGuinness UM, Aguayo AJ. 1980. Axons from CNS neurons regenerate into PNS grafts. *Nature* 284(5753): 264-265.

Rivlin AS, Tator CH. 1978. Effect of duration of acute spinal cord compression in a new acute cord injury model in the rat. *Surgical Neurology* 10(1): 38-43.

Saito N, Yamamoto T, Watanabe T, Abe Y, Kumagai T. 2000. Implications of p53 protein expression in experimental spinal cord injury. *Journal of Neurotrauma* 17(2): 173-182.

Schellenberger EA, Hogemann D, Josephson L, Weissleder R. 2002. Annexin V-Clio: A nanoparticle for detecting apoptosis by MRI. *Academic Radiology* 9(Suppl 2): S310-311.

Schwartz ED, Yezierski RP, Pattany PM, Quencer RM, Weaver RG. 1999. Diffusion-weighted MR imaging in a rat model of syringomyelia after excitotoxic spinal cord injury. *American Journal of Neuroradiology* 20(8): 1422-1428.

Segal JL, Gonzales E, Yousefi S, Jamshidipour L, Brunnemann SR. 1997. Circulating levels of IL-2R, ICAM-1, and IL-6 in spinal cord injuries. *Archives of Physical Medicine and Rehabilitation* 78(1): 44-47.

Shibuya S, Miyamoto O, Auer RN, Itano T, Mori S, Norimatsu H. 2002. Embryonic interme-diate filament, nestin, expression following traumatic spinal cord injury in adult rats. *Neuroscience* 114(4): 905-916.

Shirasaki R, Pfaff SL. 2002. Transcriptional codes and the control of neuronal identity. *Annual Review of Neuroscience* 25: 251-281.

Simonen M, Pedersen V, Weinmann O, Schnell L, Buss A, Ledermann B, Christ F, Sansig G, van der Putten H, Schwab ME. 2003. Systemic deletion of the myelin-associated out-growth inhibitor Nogo-A improves regenerative and plastic responses after spinal cord injury. *Neuron* 38(2): 201-211.

Snow DM, Lemmon V, Carrino DA, Caplan AI, Silver J. 1990. Sulfated proteoglycans in astroglial barriers inhibit neurite outgrowth in vitro. *Experimental Neurology* 109(1): 111-130.

Song G, Cechvala C, Resnick DK, Dempsey RJ, Rao VL. 2001. GeneChip analysis after acute spinal cord injury in rat. *Journal of Neurochemistry* 79(4): 804-815.

Song H, Ming G, He Z, Lehmann M, McKerracher L, Tessier-Lavigne M, Poo M. 1998. Conversion of neuronal growth cone responses from repulsion to attraction by cyclic nucleotides. *Science* 281(5382): 1515-1518.

Steward O, Zheng B, Tessier-Lavigne M. 2003. False resurrections: Distinguishing regener-ated from spared axons in the injured central nervous system. *Journal of Comparative Neurology* 459(1): 1-8.

Tachibana T, Noguchi K, Ruda MA. 2002. Analysis of gene expression following spinal cord injury in rat using complementary DNA microarray. *Neuroscience Letters* 327(2): 133-137.

Ugurbil K, Toth L, Kim DS. 2003. How accurate is magnetic resonance imaging of brain function? *Trends in Neurosciences* 26(2): 108-114.

Vaessin H, Grell E, Wolff E, Bier E, Jan LY, Jan YN. 1991. Prospero is expressed in neuronal precursors and encodes a nuclear protein that is involved in the control of axonal out-growth in *Drosophila*. *Cell* 67(5): 941-953.

Van den Abbeele AD, Badawi RD. 2002. Use of positron emission tomography in oncology and its potential role to assess response to imatinib mesylate therapy in gastrointestinal stromal tumors (GISTs). *European Journal of Cancer* 38(Suppl 5): S60-65.

von Meyenburg J, Brosamle C, Metz GA, Schwab ME. 1998. Regeneration and sprouting of chronically injured corticospinal tract fibers in adult rats promoted by NT-3 and the mAb IN-1, which neutralizes myelin-associated neurite growth inhibitors. *Experimental Neurology* 154(2): 583-594.

Watkins K. 2001. Making sense of information mined from the human genome is a massive undertaking for the fledgling industry. *Chemical & Engineering News* 79(8): 26-45.

Wen Z, Guirland C, Ming GL, Zheng JQ. 2004. A CaMKII/calcineurin switch controls the direction of Ca^{2+}-dependent growth cone guidance. *Neuron* 43(6): 835-846.

Widerstrom-Noga EG, Turk DC. 2003. Types and effectiveness of treatments used by people with chronic pain associated with spinal cord injuries: Influence of pain and psychoso-cial characteristics. *Spinal Cord* 41(11): 600-609.

Xu XM, Guenard V, Kleitman N, Bunge MB. 1995. Axonal regeneration into Schwann cell-seeded guidance channels grafted into transected adult rat spinal cord. *Journal of Com-parative Neurology* 351(1): 145-160.

Youmans JR, ed. 1996. *Neurological Surgery: A Comprehensive Reference Guide to the Diagnosis and Management of Neurological Problems*. Philadelphia: W. B. Saunders.

Young W. 2002. Spinal cord contusion models. *Progress in Brain Research* 137: 231-255.

Zhang YP, Iannotti C, Shields LB, Han Y, Burke DA, Xu XM, Shields CB. 2004. Dural closure, cord approximation, and clot removal: Enhancement of tissue sparing in a novel laceration spinal cord injury model. *Journal of Neurosurgery: Spine* 100(4): 343-352.

Zhang Z, Fujiki M, Guth L, Steward O. 1996. Genetic influences on cellular reactions to spinal cord injury: A wound-healing response present in normal mice is impaired in mice carrying a mutation (Wld(s)) that causes delayed Wallerian degeneration. *Journal of Comparative Neurology* 371(3): 485-495.

Zheng B, Ho C, Li S, Keirstead H, Steward O, Tessier-Lavigne M. 2003. Lack of enhanced spinal regeneration in Nogo-deficient mice. *Neuron* 38(2): 213-224.

Zurita M, Vaquero J, Zurita I. 2001. Presence and significance of CD-95 (Fas/APO1) expression after spinal cord injury. *Journal of Neurosurgery* 94(2 Suppl): 257-264.

4

CURRENT THERAPEUTIC INTERVENTIONS

As a result of recent advances in science and technology, individuals with a spinal cord injury have improved survival rates, increased opportunities for independent living, and longer life spans—all difficult to imagine possible even a few decades ago. Beginning at the accident scene, immobilization of the spine prevents or reduces the severity of a spinal cord injury, and advances in emergency response have improved the medical care for other urgent and life-threatening problems often associated with spinal cord injuries, including significant blood loss, blocked respiratory pathways, major head or body system trauma, and a dramatic drop in blood pressure. Improvements in rehabilitative care and treatment options have also provided significant functional enhancement and improved daily function.

Organized according to the stage of the injury and the targets for therapeutic intervention, this chapter describes the current standards of care and the treatment options for reducing the sequelae and secondary complications associated with spinal cord injuries, including improving sexual, bowel, and bladder functions; minimizing pulmonary embolisms, depression, and spasticity; alleviating pain; and enhancing function. The following chapter provides details of the progress that is being made in neuronal repair and regeneration and discusses the committee's recommendations for moving forward in developing therapeutic interventions.

CURRENT STANDARDS OF CARE

Clinical practice guidelines are used in all areas of medicine to promote the best available treatments backed by scientific evidence. Given the complexity of spinal cord injuries, only a limited number of guidelines have been developed or are under development. Clinical practice guidelines for spinal cord injuries have come largely from two professional groups, both of which rated the evidence by similar criteria to arrive at formal treatment recommendations. Guidelines from the American Association of Neurological Surgeons and the Congress of Neurological Surgeons (AANS/CNS) deal with acute care, and those developed by the Consortium for Spinal Cord Medicine deal with acute and chronic care (Table 4-1) (PVA, 2002). Other groups have developed additional evidence-based clinical guidelines (AHRQ, 1998). Panels accord the greatest weight to evidence from randomized, prospective, controlled clinical trials and the least weight to evidence from case reports describing one or more patients who improved with treatment. A lack of clinical guidelines for a particular treatment does

TABLE 4-1 Clinical Practice Guidelines for Treatment of Spinal Cord Injury

Current Guidelines

    Acute Care

- Acute management of autonomic dysreflexia: Individuals with spinal cord injury presenting to health care facilities (1997, 2001)[a]
- Pressure ulcer prevention and treatment following spinal cord injury: A clinical practice guideline for health-care professionals (2000)[a]
- Diagnosis of occipital condyle fractures by computed tomography (CT) imaging[b]
- Isolated fractures of the axis in adults[b]
- Management of pediatric cervical spinal injuries[b]

    Chronic Care

- Neurogenic bowel management in adults with spinal cord injury (1998)[a]
- Depression following spinal cord injury: A clinical practice guideline for primary care physicians (1998)[a]
- Outcomes following traumatic spinal cord injury: Clinical practice guidelines for health-care professionals (1999)[a]
- Prevention of thromboembolism in spinal cord injury (1997[a], 2002[b])

Guidelines Under Development

- Respiratory management[a]
- Preservation of the upper extremity function[a]
- Bladder management[a]
- Acute management of spinal cord injury[a]
- Sexuality and reproductive health[a]
- Treatment of spasticity[a]

[a]Consortium for Spinal Cord Medicine.
[b]American Association of Neurological Surgeons and the Congress of Neurological Surgeons.
SOURCES: Apuzzo, 2002; PVA, 1998, 2000, 2001, 2002.

not mean that the treatment is ineffective; rather, some treatments have not been entered into clinical trials to examine efficacy.

THERAPIES FOR ACUTE INJURIES

Acute care begins at the scene of an injury, continues through transport of the patient, and ends with early evaluation and care at a trauma center. The complex medical challenges faced in treating patients who suffer a spinal cord injury begin at the injury scene where often the patient not only needs to be immobilized because of concerns about a spinal cord injury but also requires immediate attention for other urgent and life-threatening problems: significant blood loss, blocked respiratory pathways, major head or body system trauma, or a dramatic drop in blood pressure. One indicator of the progress that has been made in acute care is that patients increasingly arrive at the emergency department with less severe injuries. Most patients (55 percent) in the 1970s came to regional centers with complete spinal cord injuries, whereas today approximately 39 percent arrive with complete injuries (AANS/CNS, 2002a). The transformation to less severe injury is most likely the result of improved emergency medical services (EMS) at the accident scene and more careful handling and patient care during transport (Garfin et al., 1989). Apart from immobilization at the accident scene, few therapies for acute spinal cord injuries have been proven to be effective and safe.

Immobilization at the Scene and Transport to Acute Care

At the scene of the injury, the primary considerations related to the spinal cord injury are to stabilize the spine and to ensure rapid transport to the nearest acute-care facility. These goals are vital to preventing further injury, considering that it has been estimated that in the past between 3 and 25 percent of spinal cord injuries took place after the initial trauma, either during transport or early in the course of patient evaluation (Hachen, 1974). In the United States, the practice of immobilizing the neck and spine of all trauma patients at the scene has become nearly universal. Immobilization at the scene is supported by clinical experience and by biomechanical evidence that it reduces the pathological motion of the spinal column.

A major improvement in EMS arrival and transport times has led in recent decades to striking decreases in rates of mortality, injury severity, complications, and lengths of hospital stays (Hachen, 1974; Tator et al., 1993). In the mid-1990s, a large clinical trial conducted in multiple states noted the rapid times of EMS arrival at the scene (e.g., 4 minutes for 25 percent of cases) and arrival to the first emergency department in about 1 hour (Geisler et al., 2001). The elapsed time from the injury to the arrival at a specialized trauma center averaged 6.2 hours. Also, the quality of the care administered during transport has improved. Before 1968, many deaths took place in transit as a result of inadequate respiratory or cardiovascular support. Current treatment guidelines call for rapid transport to the closest facility with the capacity to evaluate and treat spinal cord injuries (AANS/CNS, 2002c).

Despite the progress in care at the scene of the injury, there are as yet no demonstrably effective pharmacological therapies that can be administered at the scene or during transport. Further attention needs to be given to the development of acute-care therapeutic interventions and to evaluation of other emergency response efforts that might improve patient outcomes, such as methods to relieve compression of the spinal cord and prevent further cell death, edema, and ischemia.

Decompression of the Spinal Cord

Decompression of the spinal cord, if it is performed during the appropriate time window, may provide a benefit to individuals with spinal cord injuries. In many patients, surgery is performed soon after the injury to remove the tissue debris, bone, disc, and fluid that compress the spinal cord. The goal is to alleviate pressure and to improve the circulation of blood and cerebrospinal fluid, particularly for those with central cervical spinal cord injuries (Dobkin and Havton, 2004). Yet there are many unknowns about the value and timing of this procedure. Studies of decompression in rodents after a spinal cord injury demonstrate that the longer compression of the spinal cord exists, the worse the prognosis for neurological recovery (Dimar et al., 1999).

A meta-analysis found that although decompression clearly improves neurological recovery in animal models, the findings for humans are less impressive (Fehlings et al., 2001). Studies favoring decompression have mostly been case studies, which are less robust types of analyses than randomized controlled trials. No prospective clinical trials of the benefits and risks of decompression have been conducted. Furthermore, in the studies that have already been completed, the timing of surgery was not uniform, so the optimal timing remains unknown. Nevertheless, the best indication about timing comes from a large case series that found that the greatest benefits were obtained when decompression was performed within 6 hours of the injury (Aebi et al., 1986). Some evidence, on the other hand, indicates that decompression of the spinal cord may be harmful and is best avoided, as long as the individuals are provided with nonsurgical therapies (Fehlings et al., 2001). Weighing the evidence as a whole, two professional groups adopted the position that decompression does not constitute the standard of care but should remain an option (Silber and Vaccaro, 2001;

AANS/CNS, 2002c). The Christopher Reeve Paralysis Foundation is in the process of developing an international clinical trials network (see Chapter 6) and is examining the feasibility of performing a clinical trial to examine the optimal timing for spinal cord decompression.

Neuroprotection

Several human clinical trials of potential neuroprotective therapies after spinal cord injury were conducted in the 1980s and 1990s (Mirza and Chapman, 2001); however, none of these conclusively demonstrated a benefit for increasing function after a spinal cord injury. The most high profile clinical trials were of the medications methylprednisolone and the ganglioside GM-1. After careful review of the results by two separate panels, neither of the two medications received endorsement as a standard of care (Fehlings and Spine Focus Panel, 2001; AANS/CNS, 2002c).

The three clinical trials of methylprednisolone, a corticosteroid, were sponsored by the National Acute Spinal Cord Injury Study (NASCIS) (Bracken et al., 1984, 1990, 1997). The trials were launched after it was reported that methylprednisolone preserved neurological function in animal models by inhibiting ischemia, axon degeneration, and inflammation, among other effects. The first human clinical trial in the early 1980s compared high- versus low-dose methylprednisolone (Bracken et al., 1984); the second clinical trial compared the effects of methylprednisolone with those of another agent and a placebo (Bracken et al., 1990); and the third clinical trial compared the timing of methylprednisolone treatment (Bracken et al., 1997). Concerns have been raised about the robustness of the statistical analyses and the heterogeneity of the populations with spinal cord injuries used in the studies, which made it difficult to compare due to differences in the baseline characteristics of the study populations (Bracken and Holford, 2002) (see Chapter 6 and Appendix E). Consequently, it has been stated that the data describing improved recovery from methylprednisolone treatment are weak and that the improvements observed may represent random events (Hurlbert, 2000). In some cases the trials documented serious side effects, the most prominent of which were higher infection rates, respiratory complications, and gastrointestinal hemorrhage.

Another pharmacological therapy, the ganglioside GM-1, a lipid that is abundant in mammalian central nervous system membranes, was also reported to show improvement in animal models but has not been found to be useful in humans. Its potential therapeutic value was suggested by its ability to prevent apoptosis and to induce neuronal sprouting in animal models. However, the findings from a large-scale clinical trial were negative when the results for the treated group were compared with individuals who received placebo (AANS/CNS, 2002c).

Similarly, experiments with rodents (Behrmann et al., 1994) and cats (Faden et al., 1981) have demonstrated that thyrotropin-releasing hormone (TRH) can significantly improve long-term motor recovery after a spinal cord injury. However, a large-scale randomized clinical trial designed to examine the effects of TRH analogs in individuals with acute spinal cord injuries was not fully completed (Pitts et al., 1995), and such an evaluation has not been revisited.

TREATING COMPLICATIONS OF SPINAL CORD INJURIES

Prevention or Elimination of Chronic Pain

Chronic pain, one of the most common sequelae of spinal cord injuries, is not adequately controlled by currently available treatments. Inadequately controlled pain not only erodes quality of life, functioning, and mood but also can lead to depression and, most tragically, suicide (Hulsebosch, 2003; Finnerup and Jensen, 2004). Some clinicians have been slow to recognize that chronic pain is real, has serious consequences, and should not be dismissed as grounds for psychiatric referral (Hulsebosch, 2003).

To assist with the development of treatments for the chronic pain associated with spinal cord injuries, an International Association for the Study of Pain task force was formed to define distinct categories and sources of pain (Vierck et al., 2000). Two categories were defined: at-level neuropathic pain and below-level neuropathic pain. At-level neuropathic pain is correlated to the amount of damage to the gray matter above and below the primary injury site (Yezierski, 2000) and the amount of secondary cellular damage caused by the release of neurotransmitters (glutamate and N-methyl-D-aspartate [NMDA]) (Tator and Fehlings, 1991) and inflammatory cytokines (Bethea et al., 1998; Vierck et al., 2000). Below-level neuropathic pain is associated with axonal disruption, loss, or damage along the spinothalamic tract (Bowsher, 1996).

Experts in spinal cord injury-associated pain consider the development of pain therapies to be a major and feasible research priority, considering the body of research that has been amassed over the past 10 years about pain mechanisms in individuals with spinal cord injuries, as well as related research on other forms of neuropathic pain. Neuropathic pain, as explained in Chapter 2, results from direct damage to neural tissue, whereas nociceptive pain is caused by damage to nonneural tissues (bone, muscles, and ligaments). Nociceptive pain is what most healthy people are familiar with, and it is more treatable and controllable with standard pain therapies like anti-inflammatory agents and analgesics. Neuropathic pain is often treated with antidepressants and anticonvulsants, but their efficacies specifically for the treatment of spinal cord injury-associated pain are weak (Finnerup and Jensen, 2004).

Few randomized controlled clinical trials of pain therapies for individuals with spinal cord injuries have been published in the medical literature, and none of the trials that have been conducted found commonly used pain therapies to be highly effective (Table 4-2) (Finnerup and Jensen, 2004). Explicit guidelines for the treatment of both pain and spasticity (see the next section) for clinicians and caregivers are lacking. However, evidence is accumulating that opioid agents given in combination with other agents may have therapeutic value (Mao et al., 1995; Wiesenfeld-Hallin et al., 1997; von Heijne et al., 2000).

The use of some therapies that encourage axonal elongation may be inadvisable because they could also cause chronic pain. For example, in addition to promoting axon regrowth, brain-derived neurotrophic factor has been found to elicit pain (Kerr et al., 1999), likely by enhancing synaptic input into the superficial dorsal horn, where nociceptive pain processing

TABLE 4-2 Randomized Controlled Trials of Pharmacological Treatments for Pain in Individuals with Spinal Cord Injuries

Active Drug	Number of Patients Tested	Outcome	Reference
Valproate	20	No effect	Drewes et al., 1994
Gabapentin	7	No effect	Tai et al., 2002
Lamotrigine	22	No effect	Finnerup et al., 2002
Amitriptyline	84	No effect	Cardenas et al., 2002
Trazodone hydrochloride	18	No effect	Davidoff et al., 1987
Lidocaine	21	Better than placebo	Loubser and Donovan, 1991
Lidocaine	10	Better than placebo	Attal et al., 2000
Mexiletine	11	No effect	Chiou-Tan et al., 1999
Morphine	9	No effect	Attal et al., 2002
Morphine	15	No effect	Sidall et al., 2000
Clonidine	15	No effect	Sidall et al., 2000
Morphine and clonidine	15	Better than placebo	Sidall et al., 2000
Ketamine	9	Better than placebo	Eide et al., 1995
Alfentanil	9	Better than placebo	Eide et al., 1995
Propofol	8	Better than placebo	Canavero et al., 1995
Baclofen	7	Better than placebo	Herman et al., 1992

SOURCE: Adapted from Finnerup and Jensen, 2004.

takes place (Garraway et al., 2003). Primary sensory neurons (also known as primary afferents) in the spinal cord convey pain information from the primary sensory neuron to the brain. After a spinal cord injury, these neurons become hyperexcitable; namely, they fire more readily than before the injury. To explain hyperexcitability, a recent study with animals revealed that projection neurons possess more sodium channels of a particular type ($Na_v1.3$) (Hains et al., 2003). Strategies to reduce the formation of this sodium channel may reduce hyperexcitability and pain. Furthermore, suppression of the activation of a key enzyme, known as MAP kinase, which aids the transmission of signals from the projection neuron's membrane to its nucleus (Kawasaki et al., 2004), may prevent the onset of pain.

Relief of Spasticity

Spasticity refers to the debilitating muscle spasms and other types of increased muscle tone that occur after a spinal cord injury. Spasticity is similar to pain in that both are highly common after spinal cord injuries and have multiple possible mechanisms that might account for their onset (see Chapter 2). The key difference between them is that spasticity results from the heightened activity of reflex pathways (proprioceptive sensory neurons and motor neurons), whereas pain reflects the heightened activities of pain pathways.

Spasticity affects, to various degrees, the vast majority of people with spinal cord injury (Kaplan et al., 1991). Treatment begins with stretching and other rehabilitation techniques. If it remains uncontrolled, drug interventions are used, and if it is severe, the treatment is surgery and administration of the drug baclofen by implanted pumps (Kirshblum, 1999). Baclofen and tizanidine have inhibitory effects on motor neurons because their actions mimic that of the inhibitory neurotransmitter γ-aminobutyric acid (GABA). No treatment for spasticity is uniformly successful or provides a complete cure, most likely because of spasticity's multiple underlying causes, but it can be controlled in many individuals (Burchiel and Hsu, 2001). The drug fampridine, a potassium channel blocker, appears to alleviate some degree of spasticity and is being evaluated in clinical trials. One of the issues in the development of drugs used to control spasticity is that they may have the undesirable effect of inhibiting spontaneous activity that might be necessary for axon regrowth (McDonald and Becker, 2003) and may deprive patients of useful muscle contraction.

Thromboembolism

Thromboembolism is a potentially life-threatening condition frequently encountered in the early weeks after a spinal cord injury. Deep vein thromboses (DVTs) are blood clots that form deep within the veins, usually in the legs and thighs, and result from slowed or halted blood flow (venous stasis) in immobilized individuals with spinal cord injuries. The most feared complication of DVT is pulmonary embolism, which can bring sudden death. Pulmonary embolism occurs when a blood clot within a deep vein dislodges and travels to the pulmonary artery, where it obstructs the passage of oxygenated blood to the rest of the body. Widespread adoption of preventive regimens in the early 1990s decreased the incidence of DVT in individuals with spinal cord injuries in acute care or rehabilitation from 14 to 9.8 percent and the incidence of pulmonary embolism from nearly 4 to 2.6 percent (Chen et al., 1999).

Today, the incidences of both DVTs and pulmonary embolism have declined because of greater awareness of the conditions and several controlled clinical trials that found that combination strategies are effective in preventing DVT and pulmonary embolism. A panel rating the quality of evidence found several treatment modalities that warranted designation as a standard of care because they had been found to be effective in controlled clinical trials (AANS/CNS, 2002b). The standards for preventing DVT call for prophylactic treatment with low-molecular-weight heparins (an anticoagulant) or adjusted-dose heparin, the use of rotating beds, or a combination of these modalities. Low-dose heparin, in combination with compression stockings or electrical stimulation, is also recommended as a standard of care. High doses of heparin have been found to lead to higher incidence of bleeding. Several other preventive treatments were also listed as options for care (AANS/CNS, 2002c).

Bladder Dysfunction

Bladder dysfunction affects virtually all individuals with spinal cord injuries (see Chapter 2). Its treatment depends on the site and the type of injury, including the extent of sacral injury. Three types of bladder problems are common after a spinal cord injury. The first, flaccid bladder, results from injury to the sacral cord, which controls reflexive contraction of the bladder. The injury leaves the bladder's detrusor muscle incapable of being contracted and thus causes urine to back up in the kidneys. The treatment is intermittent catheterization, in which a tube is inserted into the bladder to permit passive drainage at regularly scheduled intervals to prevent urine from overfilling the bladder. Bladder overfill causes damage to the bladder wall and heightens the risk of infection (Burns et al., 2001). In order to reduce the incidence of urinary tract infections, intermittent catheterization should be performed by the patient (Cardenas and Mayo, 1987).

The other two types of dysfunction are detrusor hyperreflexia and detrusor-sphincter dyssynergia. The goal of treating detrusor hyperreflexia is to prevent incontinence. Treatment of detrusor-sphincter dyssynergia is aimed at ensuring adequate drainage, low-pressure storage, and low-pressure voiding. Both of these bladder conditions can be treated with anticholinergic or other types of medications that suppress contraction of the detrusor muscles. However, in many cases these medications do not suppress contractions. Bladder augmentation (augmentation cystoplasty) is often recommended for patients who have destrusor hyperreflexia or reduced compliance that fails to respond to anticholinergics (Sidi et al., 1990). New treatments have been introduced for these conditions, including pharmacological therapies to reduce the hyperactivity of the detrusor muscle (such as botulinum toxin or capsaicin) and functional electrical stimulation (see below). For example, a Food and Drug Administration (FDA)-approved device, known as the Vocare bladder system, uses surgically implanted electrodes to stimulate the sacral nerves controlling bladder function. The patient manually controls the stimulator using an external transmitting device. The benefits of these therapies have yet to be fully investigated (Burns et al., 2001). In another strategy, male patients may undergo sphincterotomy or stent placement to use the hyperreflexia to empty the bladder. The Consortium for Spinal Cord Medicine will soon be describing the strength of the evidence in a clinical practice guideline under development.

Neurogenic Bowel Treatment

Neurogenic bowel, the absence of voluntary control over stool elimination, affects the vast majority of individuals with spinal cord injuries. Some studies have found that as many as 95 percent of individuals with spinal cord injuries require at least one therapeutic procedure so that they can defecate (Glickman and Kamm, 1996). The majority of individuals with spinal cord injuries rate bowel dysfunction as a major life-limiting problem (Kirk et al., 1997). Before they leave the hospital, most patients are taught how to care for neurogenic bowel. Care is designed to regularize bowel movements and prevent constipation, incontinence, other gastrointestinal symptoms, and serious complications from impacted bowels (see the section on autonomic dysreflexia below). It consists of a program with several components that are individualized to patients with one of two types of neurogenic bowel: reflexic bowel and areflexic bowel. Both types require dietary fiber and fluid intake, oral medications, and rectal suppositories. Treatments help to stimulate the transport of stool through the bowels and hold moisture within the stool. Key differences in treating reflexive bowel versus areflexic bowel include the type of rectal stimulant, the consistency of the stool, and the frequency of bowel care. Clinical practice guidelines for the management of neurogenic bowel were developed in 1998 (Spinal Cord Medicine Consortium, 1998).

Autonomic Dysreflexia

Autonomic dysreflexia is a potentially lethal complication of a spinal cord injury that affects people with injuries at or above the thoracic level (usually T6 or above). The condition is manifest by severe headache (caused by an abrupt elevation of blood pressure), hypertension, profuse sweating, and activation of other autonomic reflexes. Symptoms come from overactivity of the autonomic (involuntary) nervous system cells in the spinal cord because of the blocked nerve impulses from the brain that normally keep these cells under restraint. The most frequent triggers of autonomic dysreflexia are an impacted bowel or an overfull bladder. The overactive sympathetic nerve and its branches cause a narrowing of the blood vessels, which, in turn, dramatically elevates blood pressure. Death from seizures, stroke, and abnormal heart beat rhythm can ensue if autonomic dysreflexia is not urgently treated.

Because autonomic dysreflexia is most often set off by bladder distention or bowel impaction, many individuals with spinal cord injuries have learned means of self-care to avoid emergency treatment by sitting upright to check urinary drainage or empty their bowel. An array of nonpharmacological and pharmacological agents are also available for emergency medical treatment (PVA, 2001).

Pressure Ulcers

Pressure ulcers are a highly frequent and serious complication of a spinal cord injury that affect physical, psychological, and social functioning. Ulcers are lesions caused by unrelieved pressure (if the force is perpendicular) or shear (if the force is tangential) to the tissue surface. The constant pressure can also interfere with the pressure in the capillaries and can therefore affect the exchange and elimination of nutrients and metabolites. Prolonged circulatory interference ultimately leads to cell death. In severe cases, individuals can develop a severe internal infection (septic shock), which can lead to organ failure. Stage I lesions are marked by discoloration and changes in tissue consistency on the skin surface, whereas the most serious lesions, stage IV lesions, are marked by extensive tissue necrosis and damage to muscle, bone, or supporting structures. About 32 percent of individuals with spinal cord injuries admitted to specialized care centers have been reported to develop pressure ulcers during the acute care stage, and at 2 years of follow-up the prevalence of pressure ulcers was 8.9 percent (Yarkony and Heinemann, 1995). The Consortium for Spinal Cord Medicine's clinical practice guideline advocates a range of prevention strategies, including the avoidance of prolonged positional immobilization, use of support devices on beds and wheelchairs, and dietary changes. Treatments include a range of cleansing strategies, debridement, and surgery for deep stage III or stage IV ulcers. The use of electrical stimulation to enhance healing of stage III or stage IV pressure ulcers is also recommended, on the basis of data from three randomized controlled clinical trials (PVA, 2000).

Treatment of Sexual Dysfunction and Fertility

Male Sexual Dysfunction and Fertility

Treatment research has largely focused on erectile dysfunction rather than the other two components of male sexual function, ejaculation and orgasm. The greatest strides have been with oral medications for erectile dysfunction. Although most men with spinal cord injuries have erections, their quality is often not sufficient to sustain intercourse. Sildenafil (Viagra), which has been available since 1998, has been shown to have a high degree of efficacy, with up to 94 percent of men with spinal cord injuries in one study reporting improved erections and intercourse (Derry et al., 2002). Other new drugs with pharmacological and side effect profiles somewhat different from those of sildenafil have also become available (Anderson et al., 2004). Oral medications are now considered the first line of therapy and have largely supplanted less safe, more cumbersome, and costly treatments, such as penile prostheses (Benevento and Sipski, 2002). Local erectogenic neurotransmitters administered by injection, topical, or urethal forms are in development (Elliot, 2002).

Fertility problems, which are common in men with spinal cord injuries, result from poor sperm quality or ejaculatory dysfunction. Much progress has been made in enhancing male fertility through the development of penile vibratory stimulation, which has become routine for men with spinal cord injuries who wish to have children (Benevento and Sipski, 2002). Vibratory stimulation is considered preferable to another treatment, electroejaculation, because it is less invasive and may be performed at home or in a clinic setting. Studies have shown that nearly all men given one of these two treatments successfully ejaculate, after which approximately one-third of the couples achieved pregnancies (Sonksen et al., 1997). However, this success rate is still largely dependent on overcoming the low sperm quality in men with spinal cord injuries, which often requires very invasive forms of assisted reproduction, ranging from artificial insemination to in vitro fertilization and intracytoplasmic sperm injection.

Female Sexual Dysfunction and Fertility

Sexual dysfunction in women with spinal cord injuries received scant attention until the 1990s. The problems include insufficient vaginal secretions and failure to reach orgasm (especially in women with sacral injuries) (Benevento and Sipski, 2002). Women with spinal cord injuries benefit from sildenafil, which promotes increased subjective arousal (Sipski et al., 2000). In the trial, the drug worked most effectively when it was combined with manual or visual stimulation, and there were few adverse effects.

Fertility is generally preserved in women with spinal cord injuries (Charlifue et al., 1992), primarily because it does not rely on spinal circuits. Rather, fertility is controlled by the hypothalamic release of hormones that stimulate the ovaries. Pregnant women with spinal cord injuries tend to have babies with lower birth weights and tend to have more complications during pregnancy and delivery, including bladder and bowel problems, autonomic hyperreflexia, decubitus ulcers, urinary tract infections, edema, anemia, spotting, fatigue, cardiac irregularity, and preeclampsia (Charlifue et al., 1992; Jackson and Wadley, 1999).

Treatment of Bone Disorders

The reduced mobility and other pathological changes that occur in individuals with spinal cord injuries often lead to decreases in bone density (hence, a greater risk of bone fractures) and heterotopic ossification. The latter refers to the formation of bone in soft tissues near paralyzed joints. Bone density loss, particularly in the lower limbs, occurs during the first 6 months after the injury and then plateaus over the next 12 to 16 months (Demirel et al., 1998). The drug alendronate (Fosamax) has recently been found in a 2-year clinical trial to stop bone density loss at all bone sites at which measurements were taken (Zehnder et al., 2004). The drug, a bisphosphonate, works by inhibiting bone resorption by osteoclasts.

Heterotopic ossification can range from an incidental finding on an X-ray to massive bone formation surrounding a joint, producing total ankylosis. The most common location is the hips. Heterotopic ossification is treated with range-of-motion exercises, the drug etidronate, nonsteroidal anti-inflammatory drugs (NSAIDs), and irradiation. The use of NSAIDs, especially within the first 2 months of an injury, has been found to reduce the incidence of heterotopic ossification by a factor of 2 to 3 (Banovac et al., 2004). Severe cases are treated surgically, and the chance of recurrence may be reduced by the use of the nonsurgical therapies listed above.

Depression

Depression after a spinal cord injury is common and disabling. A key longitudinal study was conducted to track more than 100 individuals with spinal cord injuries for 2 years after discharge from the hospital (Kennedy and Rogers, 2000). It found that nearly 30 percent of the individuals were depressed at the time of discharge; the rate of depression then dropped, before climbing over the next 6 months. Rates peaked at 60 percent by year's end and then declined to 16 percent by the end of the second year. The treatment of depression in any group of individuals with a chronic physical illness, particularly those with spinal cord injuries, is expected to reduce unnecessary suffering and disability and to motivate adherence to complex programs of self-care, rehabilitation, and treatment.

Effective treatments are available for depression (APA, 1994). In 1998, the Consortium for Spinal Cord Medicine published a clinical practice guideline detailing specific steps for assessment, diagnosis, and treatment of depression (PVA, 1998).

RETRAINING AND RELEARNING MOTOR TASKS

The plasticity of the nervous system, or the nervous system's ability to adapt and reorganize itself, sometimes allows the body to partially recover some of the motor function lost as a result of a spinal cord injury. As described throughout this report, a great deal of the research and clinical effort has been focused on restoring lost motor function through pharmacological or surgical methods. However, physical training and rehabilitation techniques and neuroprostheses also provide individuals with additional tools that they can use to recover from a spinal cord injury.

Body Weight Support Training

It is important that patients do not overcompensate with motor function that has been spared, thus limiting the capacity of the nervous system to adapt (Barbeau, 2003). Therefore, body weight support techniques have been developed that assist in locomotion, while minimizing compensation. One therapy that is used to improve walking in individuals in both the acute and the chronic stages of their injuries is body weight-supported treadmill training. During this therapy, individuals are placed in a harness to unload between 0 and 50 percent of their weight and are then put on a treadmill to simulate walking (Wernig et al., 1995, 1998; Protas et al., 2001; Dobkin et al., 2003a). Therapists then systematically reduce the amount of weight support, while training patients to walk on the treadmill at faster speeds.

Although this technique is promising, it is still unclear how effective body weight support treadmill training is at improving function in individuals with incomplete chronic spinal cord injuries. It is believed that body weight-supported training enhances the relearning of motor skills in the presence of spared pathways and facilitates the remaining pathways to relearn to interpret the complex sensory information associated with walking (Wernig et al., 1995; Harkema et al., 1997; Hulsebosch, 2002; Dietz and Harkema, 2004; Edgerton et al., 2004). These therapies produce a wide range of biochemical and physiological changes in the nervous system and musculature. Long term improvement in electromyogram (EMG) activity in paralytic legs has been observed (Wirz et al., 2001), which has been correlated to functional reorganization of neuronal centers in both the brain (Dobkin, 2000) and residual pathways in the spinal cord (Dietz and Harkema, 2004). Levels of neurotransmitters also change their levels in response to body weight support training (Edgerton et al., 2001). However, it is not clear if the observed physiological changes correlate with improvements in muscle control and function. To confirm these preliminary findings, an ongoing prospective large scale randomized clinical trial (The Spinal Cord Injury Locomotor Trial) has been designed to evaluate body weight-supported treadmill training and to compare that therapy with conventional physical therapy (Dobkin et al., 2003a,b). This study consists of two groups of patients, an experimental group that received body weight support and gait training, and a control group that received conventional standing and mobility training. Results from this study have not yet been published in a peer review journal; however, preliminary findings suggest that the treatment group was not associated with any improvement in the outcome measures compared to the "standard of care" gait training provided to the control group (Dobkin et al., 2003b, 2004). Three additional clinical trials are under way (NIH, 2004). Preliminary results from one of these phase II studies suggest that aggressive treadmill training may facilitate functional improvements, but this trial has not been completed and these results have yet to be published in a peer-reviewed journal (Hulsebosch, 2002).

A major difficulty with body weight support treadmill training is the effort required by therapists to guide the movements of individuals' legs (Hesse, 1999). Therefore, a number of approaches have been developed to assist, including robotic-assistive stepping devices such as the Lokomat (Hocoma AG, Volketswil Germany), in which the movements of an individual's legs are controlled by a preprogrammed physiological gait pattern. Other rhythmic leg exercises can be achieved with modified exercise bicycles.

A related approach is to incorporate functional electrical stimulation (see below) in combination with body weight-supported walking in individuals with incomplete injuries (ASIA C) (Postans et al., 2004). One study has demonstrated improvements in interlimb coordination with the use of afferent electrical stimulation during treadmill training (Field-Fote, 2001). Individuals with spinal cord injuries will likely receive the greatest benefit by combining body weight-supported treadmill training with other approaches, such as robotic devices (Dobkin and Havton, 2004), drugs, and surgery.

Functional Electrical Stimulation

Functional electrical stimulation (FES) is the approach most commonly used to artificially improve muscle function. FES devices have two key components: a control unit and stimulating electrodes. The control unit translates commands from voluntary movements or sensors into signals that are sent to the stimulating electrodes, which are taped onto the skin or surgically positioned near the specific nerves that innervate muscle groups (Bhadra et al., 2001). The stimulating electrodes provide mild shocks to muscle groups, causing them to contract (Barbeau et al., 2002). These contractions help maintain muscle mass and can initiate muscle movements, such as controlling movements of the hands or legs (Peckham et al., 2002). Modulating the magnitude of the stimulus parameters affects the strength of the muscle contraction and coordinated functional movements can be generated by controlling the relative stimulation strengths of collections of muscles (Dobkin and Havton, 2004).

FES is used in multiple ways to improve function, including cardiovascular conditioning, improving gait control and speed, restoring hand control and breathing, and controlling bowel and bladder function. FDA has approved neuroprostheses for the restoration of hand function, bowel and bladder control, and breathing, and clinicians at many spinal cord injury centers are trained in their use. In addition, an FDA-approved walking system uses a nonimplanted FES and an FES cycle ergometric device that allow periodic exercise of paralyzed leg muscles.

As noted earlier in the chapter, electrical stimulation for bladder function control involves a neuroprosthesis sold in the United States as Vocare. It is an FDA-approved medical device that provides the user with the ability to void upon demand as a result of the stimulation provided by the implanted device. Electrodes are placed on the sacral roots either intradurally (which is the most popular location in Europe) or extradurally (which is the location used more frequently in the United States). Voiding of the bladder is controlled by an implanted radio receiver controlled by an external device that delivers energy and control to the implant. This system allows individuals with spinal cord injuries to manage difficult bladder problems and drain many urine management devices (catheters and condoms). It also reduces the incidence of bladder infections. The device has been implanted in more than 1,500 patients around the world, and 90 percent of those with the implant reportedly used it 4 to 6 days per week. Thus, the cost of the device compared with that of conventional care is recovered in about 7 years (Creasey and Dahlberg, 2001).

FDA has approved a neuroprosthesis for hand control, called Free-hand, which provides two grasping patterns to individuals with C5 or C6 tetraplegia. It consists of a stimulator-receiver implanted in the chest and eight electrodes implanted at the motor points of hand and forearm muscles. Shoulder movement is used to proportionally control the degree of hand opening and closing. Fifty-one individuals with C5 or C6 tetraplegia were enrolled in a multicenter clinical study of the safety, effectiveness, and clinical impact of the Freehand system (Peckham et al., 2001). The results showed that the neuroprosthesis increased the pinch force of every subject, and it enabled 98 percent of the participants to grasp and move more objects in a standardized grasp-release test. An advanced system is under clinical investigation. This advanced system provides greater upper limb function and incorporates implanted control methods, thereby eliminating the need for the external shoulder sensor.

Tendon transfer surgery is often used either alone or in conjunction with neural prostheses (Kirshblum, 2004) for upper-extremity locomotion. This surgical procedure involves transferring one or more tendons of muscles with retained voluntary function to restore lost movements. The procedure is reversible and generally restores function equivalent to that provided by one or two spinal roots. Enhanced function is provided through additional stimulation channels, which are used to activate the muscles of the hand for fine control, elbow extension, and hand rotation. This system has been implanted in seven subjects (Peckham et al., 2002). An advanced neuroprosthesis that uses an implantable controller for restoration of hand and upper-arm control has been demonstrated to improve finger control in a group of individuals and has improved their performance of activities of daily living (Hobby et al., 2001). Recently, one participant received im-plants in both arms to further improve function.

For respiratory control, electrical stimulation can be used to stimulate the phrenic nerve, which controls the contractions of the diaphragm muscles. This technique, known as phrenic nerve pacing, was introduced in the 1960s (Escher et al., 1966). Phrenic pacing systems have allowed users to decrease or even discontinue the use of mechanical respirators and en-able more normal breathing. The technique has been applied to more than 1,000 patients worldwide and has become a clinically accepted intervention in selected individuals (DiMarco, 1999). An alternative to direct stimula-tion of the phrenic nerve has also been developed. It is less invasive, as electrodes are implanted laparoscopically into the diaphragm (DiMarco et al., 2002; Onders et al., 2004). To date, 10 individuals have received the implant, and 9 of these individuals have been able to comfortably tolerate extended periods (hours) of respirator-free pacing. If the utility of the device is confirmed in additional individuals, diaphragm pacing with intramuscular electrodes placed by laparoscopic surgery may provide a less invasive and less costly alternative to conventional phrenic nerve pacing.

The objective of some lower-extremity FES systems is to enable individuals with paraplegia to stand and transfer themselves. The functional goals associated with standing include reaching for high objects, having face-to-face interactions with other people, and transferring between surfaces independently or with minimal assistance. At present there are no commercial or FDA-approved systems for FES-aided standing; however, one implantable system has reached the multicenter clinical trial stage of development (Davis et al., 2001).

The only FDA-approved FES system for ambulation available is a surface stimulation system (Parastep). Individuals with paraplegia wear a microprocessor-stimulator unit at the waist and use a walker with controls built into the handles. This system allows these individuals to stand and walk with a reciprocal gait for limited distances. Use of the system has additional medical benefits, such as providing increased blood flow to the lower extremities, a lower heart rate at subpeak work intensities, increased muscle mass, and reduced spasticity and also has psychological benefits (Klose et al., 1997; Graupe and Kohn, 1998).

FES devices can also be used to maintain an individual's muscle fitness and potentially encourage the recovery of function. Decreased muscle mass is a secondary condition that, if left untreated, can diminish the potential for complete recovery. A common cause of muscle atrophy is the loss of motor neurons in the spinal cord that drive muscle contraction. Other, usually less severe but more widespread atrophy occurs over time because of the disuse of paralyzed but still innervated muscles. FES can help reverse disuse atrophy by stimulating muscle activity, but it relies on intact nerve-muscle connections and cannot easily be used to stimulate denervated muscles.

FES devices have received a mixed reception from both clinicians and individuals with spinal cord injuries. Originally, the controllers and stimulating electrodes were large and cumbersome and did not provide very fine control; however, technological advances are leading to reductions in the sizes of these devices and reductions in the numbers of surgical procedures required for implementation. In addition, the implanted electrodes have improved reliabilities and longevities. Some individuals with spinal cord injuries and their clinicians are dissuaded from using FES devices because of the surgical procedures required to implant the systems and, in the case of Vocare, the additional damage to the nervous system that results from the requirement to transect some of the sensory nerves that enter the spinal cord (Creasey et al., 2001). However, the potential benefit to an individual's quality of life and the decreased health care costs over the lifetime of the individual likely offset the large initial expense of FES devices (Creasey et al., 2000).

Considerable research and development have been invested in the development of computer-controlled FES devices (Taylor et al., 2002), and future advances are likely to be linked to advances in technologies and their appropriate application to individuals with spinal cord injuries. For example, numerous electrode interfaces that provide more selective activation of nerves will provide finer movements. Others use physiological principles to block neural firing and will be used to block pain and suppress spasticity. Additionally, smaller stimulators are being developed. These will provide individuals with devices that can be fully implanted.

There is also a considerable effort to develop brain-computer interfaces that can be used to convert thoughts into electrical signals that can control and stimulate muscles (Friehs et al., 2004). These interfaces are most likely to initially have impact on the most severely disabled individuals who have lost other communication channels, but retain the ability to control their cortical firing. Cortical control may be used for control of the environment and for communication by such individuals, and may also be used as an interface for robotic manipulators and FES systems. Current approaches include, from least invasive to most, extracting control information from the electroencephalogram (Keirn and Aunon, 1990; Wolpaw and McFarland, 2004), placing electrodes subcranially over the brain, or placing electrodes into the brain. Research on all approaches is ongoing both in animal models and in patients, and two-dimensional control of cursors on a monitor screen has been demonstrated. Additional technologies are being developed to assist individuals with spinal cord injuries that severely restrict their movements, including an eyeglass-type infrared-controlled computer interface (Chen et al., 1999) and a wireless environmental control system using Morse code (Yang et al., 2003).

The overall acceptance of implantable neuroprostheses in upper extremity functional restoration has been very good, with over 80 percent of patients achieving regular use of the devices (Peckham et al., 2001). In addition, more than 95 percent of those who received implants reported satisfaction with the neuroprosthesis (Polacek et al., 1999). Neuroprothesis devices, such as the Freehand system, also have the potential to reduce the overall cost of care for spinal cord injured people (Creasey et al., 2000). Although it has been a difficult challenge, some insurance companies and the U.S. Department of Veterans Affairs reimburse individuals for associated costs. Ensuring that such benefits become available to individuals with spinal cord injuries in the future will require an effective delivery model, which requires collaboration between various clinical specialties (physical medicine and rehabilitation physicians, hand surgeons, and therapists) to identify individuals who would benefit from neuroprotheses, as well as greater knowledge within the spinal cord injury community of the availability and benefits of neuroprotheses. However, the development of FES products, like pharmaceuticals, presents a financial challenge to companies, and this challenge may constrain the future development of such systems (Cavuoto, 2002; Dobkin and Havton, 2004).

REFERENCES

AANS/CNS (American Association of Neurological Surgeons/Congress of Neurological Surgeons). 2002a. Cervical spine immobilization before admission to the hospital. *Neurosurgery* 50(3 Suppl): S7-17.

AANS/CNS. 2002b. Deep venous thrombosis and thromboembolism in patients with cervical spinal cord injuries. *Neurosurgery* 50(3 Suppl): S73-80.

AANS/CNS. 2002c. Guidelines for management of acute cervical spinal injuries. Introduction. *Neurosurgery* 50(3 Suppl): S1.

Aebi M, Mohler J, Zach GA, Morscher E. 1986. Indication, surgical technique, and results of 100 surgically-treated fractures and fracture-dislocations of the cervical spine. *Clinical Orthopaedics and Related Research* (203): 244-257.

AHRQ (Agency for Healthcare Research and Quality). 1998. *National Guideline Clearinghouse*. [Online]. Available: http://www.guideline.gov/ [accessed January 10, 2005].

Anderson PCB, Gommersall L, Hayne D, Arya M, Patel HRH. 2004. New phosphodiesterase inhibitors in the treatment of erectile dysfunction. *Expert Opinion on Pharmacotherapy* 5(11): 2241-2249.

APA (American Psychiatric Association). 1994. *Diagnostic and Statistical Manual of Mental Disorders: DSM-IV*. Washington, DC: American Psychiatric Association.

Apuzzo MLJ, ed. 2002. Guidelines for the management of acute cervical spine and spinal cord injuries. *Neurosurgery* 50(3 Suppl).

Attal N, Gaude V, Brasseur L, Dupuy M, Guirimand F, Parker F, Bouhassira D. 2000. Intravenous lidocaine in central pain: A double-blind, placebo-controlled, psychophysical study. *Neurology* 54(3): 564-574.

Attal N, Guirimand F, Brasseur L, Gaude V, Chauvin M, Bouhassira D. 2002. Effects of IV morphine in central pain: A randomized placebo-controlled study. *Neurology* 58(4): 554-563.

Banovac K, Sherman AL, Estores IM, Banovac F. 2004. Prevention and treatment of heterotopic ossification after spinal cord injury. *Journal of Spinal Cord Medicine* 27(4): 376-382.

Barbeau H. 2003. Locomotor training in neurorehabilitation: Emerging rehabilitation concepts. *Neurorehabilitation & Neural Repair* 17(1): 3-11.

Barbeau H, Ladouceur M, Mirbagheri MM, Kearney RE. 2002. The effect of locomotor training combined with functional electrical stimulation in chronic spinal cord injured subjects: Walking and reflex studies. *Brain Research–Brain Research Reviews* 40(1-3): 274-291.

Behrmann DL, Bresnahan JC, Beattie MS. 1994. Modeling of acute spinal cord injury in the rat: Neuroprotection and enhanced recovery with methylprednisolone, U-74006f and YM-14673. *Experimental Neurology* 126(1): 61-75.

Benevento BT, Sipski ML. 2002. Neurogenic bladder, neurogenic bowel, and sexual dysfunction in people with spinal cord injury. *Physical Therapy* 82(6): 601-612.

Bethea JR, Castro M, Keane RW, Lee TT, Dietrich WD, Yezierski RP. 1998. Traumatic spinal cord injury induces nuclear factor-kappaB activation. *Journal of Neuroscience* 18(9): 3251-3260.

Bhadra N, Kilgore KL, Peckham PH. 2001. Implanted stimulators for restoration of function in spinal cord injury. *Medical Engineering & Physics* 23(1): 19-28.

Bowsher D. 1996. Central pain: Clinical and physiological characteristics. *Journal of Neurology, Neurosurgery & Psychiatry* 61(1): 62-69.

Bracken MB, Holford TR. 2002. Neurological and functional status 1 year after acute spinal cord injury: Estimates of functional recovery in National Acute Spinal Cord Injury Study II from results modeled in National Acute Spinal Cord Injury Study III. *Journal of Neurosurgery* 96(3 Suppl): 259-266.

Bracken MB, Collins WF, Freeman DF, Shepard MJ, Wagner FW, Silten RM, Hellenbrand KG, Ransohoff J, Hunt WE, Perot PL. 1984. Efficacy of methylprednisolone in acute spinal cord injury. *Journal of the American Medical Association* 251(1): 45-52.

Bracken MB, Shepard MJ, Collins WF, Holford TR, Young W, Baskin DS, Eisenberg HM, Flamm E, Leo-Summers L, Maroon J, et al. 1990. A randomized, controlled trial of methylprednisolone or naloxone in the treatment of acute spinal-cord injury. Results of the second National Acute Spinal Cord Injury Study. *New England Journal of Medicine* 322(20): 1405-1411.

Bracken MB, Shepard MJ, Holford TR, Leo-Summers L, Aldrich EF, Fazl M, Fehlings M, Herr DL, Hitchon PW, Marshall LF, Nockels RP, Pascale V, Perot PL Jr, Piepmeier J, Sonntag VKH, Wagner F, Wilberger JE, Winn HR, Young W. 1997. Administration of methylprednisolone for 24 or 48 hours or tirilazad mesylate for 48 hours in the treatment of acute spinal cord injury: Results of the third National Acute Spinal Cord Injury randomized controlled trial. *Journal of the American Medical Association* 277(20): 1597-1604.

Burchiel KJ, Hsu FP. 2001. Pain and spasticity after spinal cord injury: Mechanisms and treatment. *Spine* 26(24 Suppl): S146-160.

Burns AS, Rivas DA, Ditunno JF. 2001. The management of neurogenic bladder and sexual dysfunction after spinal cord injury. *Spine* 26(24 Suppl): S129-136.

Canavero S, Bonicalzi V, Pagni CA, Castellano G, Merante R, Gentile S, Bradac GB, Bergui M, Benna P, Vighetti S, Coletti Moia M. 1995. Propofol analgesia in central pain: Preliminary clinical observations. *Journal of Neurology* 242(9): 561-567.

Cardenas DD, Mayo ME. 1987. Bacteriuria with fever after spinal cord injury. *Archives of Physical Medicine and Rehabilitation* 68(5 Pt 1): 291-293.

Cardenas DD, Warms CA, Turner JA, Marshall H, Brooke MM, Loeser JD. 2002. Efficacy of amitriptyline for relief of pain in spinal cord injury: Results of a randomized controlled trial. *Pain* 96(3): 365-373.

Cavuoto J. 2002. *NeuroControl Exit Leaves Hole in Spinal Injury Market.* [Online]. Available: http://www.neurotechreports.com/pages/SCImarket.html [accessed February 8, 2005].

Charlifue SW, Gerhart KA, Menter RR, Whiteneck GG, Manley MS. 1992. Sexual issues of women with spinal cord injuries. *Paraplegia* 30(3): 192-199.

Chen D, Apple DF Jr, Hudson LM, Bode R. 1999. Medical complications during acute rehabilitation following spinal cord injury—Current experience of the model systems. *Archives of Physical Medicine and Rehabilitation* 80(11): 1397-1401.

Chen YL, Tang FT, Chang WH, Wong MK, Shih YY, Kuo TS. 1999. The new design of an infrared-controlled human-computer interface for the disabled. *IEEE Transactions on Rehabilitation Engineering* 7(4): 474-481.

Chiou-Tan FY, Eisele SG, Song JX, Markowski J, Javors M, Robertson CS. 1999. Increased norepinephrine levels during catheterization in patients with spinal cord injury. *American Journal of Physical Medicine and Rehabilitation* 78(4): 350-353.

Creasey GH, Dahlberg JE. 2001. Economic consequences of an implanted neuroprosthesis for bladder and bowel management. *American Journal of Physical Medicine and Rehabilitation* 82(11): 1520-1525.

Creasey GH, Kilgore KL, Brown-Triolo DL, Dahlberg JE, Peckham PH, Keith MW. 2000. Reduction of costs of disability using neuroprostheses. *Assistive Technology* 12(1): 67-75.

Creasey GH, Grill JH, Korsten M, U HS, Betz R, Anderson R, Walter J, Implanted Neuroprosthesis Research Group. 2001. An implantable neuroprosthesis for restoring bladder and bowel control to patients with spinal cord injuries: A multicenter trial. *Archives of Physical Medicine and Rehabilitation* 82(11): 1512-1519.

Davidoff G, Guarracini M, Roth E, Sliwa J, Yarkony G. 1987. Trazodone hydrochloride in the treatment of dysesthetic pain in traumatic myelopathy: A randomized, double-blind, placebo-controlled study. *Pain* 29(2): 151-161.

Davis JA Jr, Triolo RJ, Uhlir JP, Bhadra N, Lissy DA, Nandurkar S, Marsolais EB. 2001. Surgical technique for installing an eight-channel neuroprosthesis for standing. *Clinical Orthopaedics and Related Research* 385: 237-252.

Demirel G, Yllmaz H, Gencosmanoglu B, Kesiktas N. 1998. Pain following spinal cord injury. *Spinal Cord* 36(1): 25-28.

Derry F, Hultling C, Seftel AD, Sipski ML. 2002. Efficacy and safety of sildenafil citrate (Viagra) in men with erectile dysfunction and spinal cord injury: A review. *Urology* 60(2 Suppl 2): 49-57.

Dietz V, Harkema SJ. 2004. Locomotor activity in spinal cord-injured persons. *Journal of Applied Physiology* 96(5): 1954-1960.

Dimar JR II, Glassman SD, Raque GH, Zhang YP, Shields CB. 1999. The influence of spinal canal narrowing and timing of decompression on neurologic recovery after spinal cord contusion in a rat model. *Spine* 24(16): 1623-1633.

DiMarco AF. 1999. Diaphragm pacing in patients with spinal cord injury. *Topics in Spinal Cord Injury Rehabilitation* 5(1): 6-20.

DiMarco AF, Onders RP, Kowalski KE, Miller ME, Ferek S, Mortimer JT. 2002. Phrenic nerve pacing in a tetraplegic patient via intramuscular diaphragm electrodes. *American Journal of Respiratory and Critical Care Medicine* 166(12 Pt 1): 1604-1606.

Dobkin BH. 2000. Spinal and supraspinal plasticity after incomplete spinal cord injury: Correlations between functional magnetic resonance imaging and engaged locomotor networks. *Progress in Brain Research* 128: 99-111.

Dobkin BH, Havton LA. 2004. Basic advances and new avenues in therapy of spinal cord injury. *Annual Review of Medicine* 55: 255-282.

Dobkin BH, Apple D, Barbeau H, Basso M, Behrman A, Deforge D, Ditunno J, Dudley G, Elashoff R, Fugate L, Harkema S, Saulino M, Scott M. 2003a. Methods for a randomized trial of weight-supported treadmill training versus conventional training for walking during inpatient rehabilitation after incomplete traumatic spinal cord injury. *Neurorehabilitation & Neural Repair* 17(3): 153-167.

Dobkin BH, Apple D, Barbeau H, Basso M, Behrman A, Deforge D, Ditunno J, Dudley G, Elashoff R, Fugate L, Harkema S, Saulino M, Scott M. 2003b. Randomized trial of weight-supported treadmill training versus conventional training for walking during patient rehabilitation after incomplete traumatic spinal cord injury. *Journal of Rehabilitation Research & Development* 40(6 Suppl 3): 32.

Dobkin BH, Apple D, Barbeau H, Basso M, Behrman A, Deforge D, Ditunno J, Dudley G, Elashoff R, Fugate L, Harkema S, Saulino M, Scott M. 2004. Walking-related gains over the first 12 weeks of rehabilitation for incomplete traumatic spinal cord injury: The SCILT randomized clinical trial. *Neurologie & Rehabilitation* 10(4): 179-187.

Drewes AM, Andreasen A, Poulsen LH. 1994. Valproate for treatment of chronic central pain after spinal cord injury: A double-blind cross-over study. *Paraplegia* 32(8): 565-569.

Edgerton VR, Leon RD, Harkema SJ, Hodgson JA, London N, Reinkensmeyer DJ, Roy RR, Talmadge RJ, Tillakaratne NJ, Timoszyk W, Tobin A. 2001. Retraining the injured spinal cord. *Journal of Physiology* 533(1): 15-22.

Edgerton VR, Tillakaratne NJT, Bigbee AJ, de Leon RD, Roy RR. 2004. Plasticity of the spinal circuitry after injury. *Annual Review of Neuroscience* 27: 145-167.

Eide PK, Stubhaug A, Stenehjem AE, Hodge CJ, Burchiel KJ. 1995. Central dysesthesia pain after traumatic spinal cord injury is dependent on N-methyl-D-aspartate receptor activation. *Neurosurgery* 37(6): 1080-1087.

Elliot S. 2002. Sexual dysfunction and infertility in men with spinal cord disorders. In: Lin V, Cardenas DD, Cutter NC, Frost FS, Hammond MC, Lindblom LB, Perkash I, Waters R, eds. *Spinal Cord Medicine: Principles and Practice*. New York: Demos Medical Publishing. Pp. 349-368.

Escher DJ, Furman S, Solomon N, Schwedel JB. 1966. Transvenous pacing of the phrenic nerves. *American Heart Journal* 72(2): 283-284.

Faden AI, Jacobs TP, Holaday JW. 1981. Thyrotropin-releasing hormone improves neurologic recovery after spinal trauma in cats. *New England Journal of Medicine* 305(18): 1063-1067.

Fehlings MG, Spine Focus Panel. 2001. Summary statement: The use of methylprednisolone in acute spinal cord injury. *Spine* 26(24 Suppl): S55.

Fehlings MG, Sekhon LH, Tator C. 2001. The role and timing of decompression in acute spinal cord injury: What do we know? What should we do? *Spine* 26(24 Suppl): S101-110.

Field-Fote EC. 2001. Combined use of body weight support, functional electric stimulation, and treadmill training to improve walking ability in individuals with chronic incomplete spinal cord injury. *Archives of Physical Medicine and Rehabilitation* 82(6): 818-824.

Finnerup NB, Jensen TS. 2004. Spinal cord injury pain—Mechanisms and treatment. *European Journal of Neurology* 11(2): 73-82.

Finnerup NB, Sindrup SH, Bach FW, Johannesen IL, Jensen TS. 2002. Lamotrigine in spinal cord injury pain: A randomized controlled trial. *Pain* 96(3): 375-383.

Friehs GM, Zerris VA, Ojakangas CL, Fellows MR, Donoghue JP. 2004. Brain-machine and brain-computer interfaces. *Stroke* 35(11 Suppl 1): 2702-2705.

Garfin SR, Shackford SR, Marshall LF, Drummond JC. 1989. Care of the multiply injured patient with cervical spine injury. *Clinical Orthopaedics and Related Research* 239: 19-29.

Garraway SM, Petruska JC, Mendell LM. 2003. BDNF sensitizes the response of lamina II neurons to high threshold primary afferent inputs. *European Journal of Neuroscience* 18(9): 2467-2476.

Geisler FH, Coleman WP, Grieco G, Poonian D, Sygen Study Group. 2001. Recruitment and early treatment in a multicenter study of acute spinal cord injury. *Spine* 26(24 Suppl): S58-67.

Glickman S, Kamm MA. 1996. Bowel dysfunction in spinal-cord-injury patients. *Lancet* 347(9016): 1651-1653.

Graupe D, Kohn KH. 1998. Functional neuromuscular stimulator for short-distance ambulation by certain thoracic-level spinal-cord-injured paraplegics. *Surgical Neurology* 50(3): 202-207.

Hachen HJ. 1974. Emergency transportation in the event of acute spinal cord lesion. *Paraplegia* 12(1): 33-37.

Hains BC, Klein JP, Saab CY, Craner MJ, Black JA, Waxman SG. 2003. Upregulation of sodium channel $Na_v1.3$ and functional involvement in neuronal hyperexcitability associated with central neuropathic pain after spinal cord injury. *Journal of Neuroscience* 23(26): 8881-8892.

Harkema SJ, Hurley SL, Patel UK, Requejo PS, Dobkin BH, Edgerton VR. 1997. Human lumbosacral spinal cord interprets loading during stepping. *Journal of Neurophysiology* 77(2): 797-811.

Herman RM, D'Luzansky SC, Ippolito R. 1992. Intrathecal baclofen suppresses central pain in patients with spinal lesions. A pilot study. *Clinical Journal of Pain* 8(4): 338-345.

Hesse S. 1999. Treadmill training with partial body weight support in hemiparetic patients: Further research needed. *Neurorehabilitation & Neural Repair* 13(3): 179-181.

Hobby J, Taylor PN, Esnouf J. 2001. Restoration of tetraplegic hand function by use of the neurocontrol Freehand system. *Journal of Hand Surgery—British* 26(5): 459-464.

Hulsebosch CE. 2002. Recent advances in pathophysiology and treatment of spinal cord injury. *Advances in Physiology Education* 26(1-4): 238-255.

Hulsebosch CE. 2003. Central sensitization and pain after spinal cord injury. *Seminars in Pain Medicine* 1(3): 159-170.

Hurlbert RJ. 2000. Methylprednisolone for acute spinal cord injury: An inappropriate standard of care. *Journal of Neurosurgery: Spine* 93(1 Suppl): 1-7.

Jackson AB, Wadley V. 1999. A multicenter study of women's self-reported reproductive health after spinal cord injury. *Archives of Physical Medicine and Rehabilitation* 80(11): 1420-1428.

Kaplan SA, Chancellor MB, Blaivas JG. 1991. Bladder and sphincter behavior in patients with spinal cord lesions. *Journal of Urology* 146(1): 113-117.

Kawasaki Y, Kohno T, Zhuang Z-Y, Brenner GJ, Wang H, Van Der Meer C, Befort K, Woolf CJ, Ji R-R. 2004. Ionotropic and metabotropic receptors, protein kinase A, protein kinase C, and Src contribute to C-fiber-induced ERK activation and cAMP response element-binding protein phosphorylation in dorsal horn neurons, leading to central sensitization. *Journal of Neuroscience* 24(38): 8310-8321.

Keirn ZA, Aunon JI. 1990. A new mode of communication between man and his surroundings. *IEEE Transactions on Biomedical Engineering* 37(12): 1209-1214.

Kennedy P, Rogers BA. 2000. Anxiety and depression after spinal cord injury: A longitudinal analysis. *Archives of Physical Medicine and Rehabilitation* 81(7): 932-937.

Kerr BJ, Bradbury EJ, Bennett DL, Trivedi PM, Dassan P, French J, Shelton DB, McMahon SB, Thompson SW. 1999. Brain-derived neurotrophic factor modulates nociceptive sensory inputs and NMDA-evoked responses in the rat spinal cord. *Journal of Neuroscience* 19(12): 5138-5148.

Kirk PM, King RB, Temple R, Bourjaily J, Thomas P. 1997. Long-term follow-up of bowel management after spinal cord injury. *SCI Nursing* 14(2): 56-63.

Kirshblum S. 1999. Treatment alternatives for spinal cord injury related spasticity. *Journal of Spinal Cord Medicine* 22(3): 199-217.

Kirshblum S. 2004. New rehabilitation interventions in spinal cord injury. *Journal of Spinal Cord Medicine* 27(4): 342-350.

Klose KJ, Jacobs PL, Broton JG, Guest RS, Needham-Shropshire BM, Lebwohl N, Nash MS, Green BA. 1997. Evaluation of a training program for persons with SCI paraplegia using the Parastep 1 ambulation system. Part 1. Ambulation performance and anthropometric measures. *Archives of Physical Medicine and Rehabilitation* 78(8): 789-793.

Loubser PG, Donovan WH. 1991. Diagnostic spinal anaesthesia in chronic spinal cord injury pain. *Paraplegia* 29(1): 25-36.

Mao J, Price DD, Mayer DJ. 1995. Mechanisms of hyperalgesia and morphine tolerance: A current view of their possible interactions. *Pain* 62(3): 259-274.

McDonald JW, Becker D. 2003. Spinal cord injury: Promising interventions and realistic goals. *American Journal of Physical Medicine and Rehabilitation* 82(10 Suppl): S38-49.

Mirza SK, Chapman JR. 2001. Principles of management of spine injury. In: Rockwood CA, Green DP, Heckman JD, Bucholz RW, eds. *Rockwood and Green's Fractures in Adults*. 5th ed. Philadelphia: Lippincott Williams & Wilkins. Pp. 1295-1324.

NIH (National Institutes of Health). 2004. *Clinical Trials*. [Online]. Available: http://www. clinicaltrials.gov/ [accessed August 18, 2004].

Onders RP, Aiyar H, Mortimer JT. 2004. Characterization of the human diaphragm muscle with respect to the phrenic nerve motor points for diaphragmatic pacing. *American Surgeon* 70(3): 241-247.

Peckham PH, Keith MW, Kilgore KL, Grill JH, Wuolle KS, Thrope GB, Gorman P, Hobby J, Mulcahey MJ, Carroll S, Hentz VR, Wiegner A, Implantable Neuroprosthesis Research Group. 2001. Efficacy of an implanted neuroprosthesis for restoring hand grasp in tetraplegia: A multicenter study. *Archives of Physical Medicine and Rehabilitation* 82(10): 1380-1388.

Peckham PH, Kilgore KL, Keith MW, Bryden AM, Bhadra N, Montague FW. 2002. An advanced neuroprosthesis for restoration of hand and upper arm control using an implantable controller. *Journal of Hand Surgery* 27(2): 265-276.

Pitts LH, Ross A, Chase GA, Faden AI. 1995. Treatment with thyrotropin-releasing hormone (TRH) in patients with traumatic spinal cord injuries. *Journal of Neurotrauma* 12(3): 235-243.

Polacek L, Wuolle KS, Van Doren CL, Bryden AM, Peckham HP, Keith MW, Kilgore KL, Grill JH. 1999. Satisfaction with and usage of a hand neuroprosthesis. *Archives of Physical Medicine and Rehabilitation* 80(2): 206-213.

Postans NJ, Hasler JP, Granat MH, Maxwell DJ. 2004. Functional electric stimulation to augment partial weight-bearing supported treadmill training for patients with acute incomplete spinal cord injury: A pilot study. *Archives of Physical Medicine and Rehabilitation* 85(4): 604-610.

Protas EJ, Holmes SA, Qureshy H, Johnson A, Lee D, Sherwood AM. 2001. Supported treadmill ambulation training after spinal cord injury: A pilot study. *Archives of Physical Medicine and Rehabilitation* 82(6): 825-831.

PVA (Paralyzed Veterans of America). 1998. *Consortium for Spinal Cord Medicine—Depression Following Spinal Cord Injury: A Clinical Practice Guideline for Primary Care Physicians*. Washington, DC: Paralyzed Veterans of America.

PVA. 2000. *Consortium for Spinal Cord Medicine—Pressure Ulcer Prevention and Treatment Following Spinal Cord Injury: A Clinical Practice Guideline for Healthcare Professionals*. Washington, DC: Paralyzed Veterans of America.

PVA. 2001. *Consortium for Spinal Cord Medicine—Acute Management of Autonomic Dysreflexia: Individuals with Spinal Cord Injury Presenting to Health-Care Facilities*. Washington, DC: Paralyzed Veterans of America.

PVA. 2002. *Consortium for Spinal Cord Medicine*. [Online]. Available: http://www.pva.org/ res/cpg/devgde.htm [accessed January 11, 2004].

Siddall PJ, Molloy AR, Walker S, Mather LE, Rutkowski SB, Cousins MJ. 2000. The efficacy of intrathecal morphine and clonidine in the treatment of pain after spinal cord injury. *Anesthesia & Analgesia* 91(6): 1493-1498.

Sidi AA, Becher EF, Reddy PK, Dykstra DD. 1990. Augmentation enterocystoplasty for the management of voiding dysfunction in spinal cord injury patients. *Journal of Urology* 143(1): 83-85.

Silber JS, Vaccaro AR. 2001. Summary statement: The role and timing of decompression in acute spinal cord injury: Evidence-based guidelines. *Spine* 26(24 Suppl): S110.

Sipski ML, Rosen RC, Alexander CJ, Hamer RM. 2000. Sildenafil effects on sexual and cardiovascular responses in women with spinal cord injury. *Urology* 55(6): 812-815.

Sonksen J, Sommer P, Biering-Sorensen F, Ziebe S, Lindhard A, Loft A, Andersen AN, Kristensen JK. 1997. Pregnancy after assisted ejaculation procedures in men with spinal cord injury. *Archives of Physical Medicine and Rehabilitation* 78(10): 1059-1061.

Spinal Cord Medicine Consortium. 1998. Clinical practice guidelines: Neurogenic bowel management in adults with spinal cord injury. *Journal of Spinal Cord Medicine* 21(3): 248-293.

Tai Q, Kirshblum S, Chen B, Millis S, Johnston M, DeLisa JA. 2002. Gabapentin in the treatment of neuropathic pain after spinal cord injury: A prospective, randomized, double-blind, crossover trial. *Journal of Spinal Cord Medicine* 25(2): 100-105.

Tator CH, Fehlings MG. 1991. Review of the secondary injury theory of acute spinal cord trauma with emphasis on vascular mechanisms. *Journal of Neurosurgery* 75(1): 15-26.

Tator CH, Duncan EG, Edmonds VE, Lapczak LI, Andrews DF. 1993. Changes in epidemiology of acute spinal cord injury from 1947 to 1981. *Surgical Neurology* 40(3): 207-215.

Taylor DM, Tillery SIH, Schwartz AB. 2002. Direct cortical control of 3D neuroprosthetic devices. *Science* 296(5574): 1829-1832.

Vierck CJ Jr, Siddall P, Yezierski RP. 2000. Pain following spinal cord injury: Animal models and mechanistic studies. *Pain* 89(1): 1-5.

von Heijne M, Hao JX, Sollevi A, Xu XJ, Wiesenfeld-Hallin Z. 2000. Marked enhancement of anti-allodynic effect by combined intrathecal administration of the adenosine A1-receptor agonist R-phenylisopropyladenosine and morphine in a rat model of central pain. *Acta Anaesthesiologica Scandinavica* 44(6): 665-671.

Wernig A, Muller S, Nanassy A, Cagol E. 1995. Laufband therapy based on "rules of spinal locomotion" is effective in spinal cord injured persons. *European Journal of Neuroscience* 7(4): 823-829.

Wernig A, Nanassy A, Muller S. 1998. Maintenance of locomotor abilities following Laufband (treadmill) therapy in para- and tetraplegic persons: Follow-up studies. *Spinal Cord* 36(11): 744-749.

Wiesenfeld-Hallin Z, Aldskogius H, Grant G, Hao JX, Hokfelt T, Xu XJ. 1997. Central inhibitory dysfunctions: Mechanisms and clinical implications. *Behavioral and Brain Sciences* 20(3): 420-425.

Wirz M, Colombo G, Dietz V. 2001. Long term effects of locomotor training in spinal humans. *Journal of Neurology, Neurosurgery & Psychiatry* 71(1): 93-96.

Wolpaw JR, McFarland DJ. 2004. Control of a two-dimensional movement signal by a noninvasive brain-computer interface in humans. *Proceedings of the National Academy of Sciences (U.S.A.)* 101(51): 17849-17854.

Yang CH, Chuang LY, Yang CH, Luo CH. 2003. Morse code application for wireless environmental control systems for severely disabled individuals. *IEEE Transactions on Neural Systems & Rehabilitation Engineering* 11(4): 463-469.

Yarkony GM, Heinemann AW. 1995. Pressure ulcers. In: Stover SL, DeLisa JA, Whiteneck GG, eds. *Spinal Cord Injury: Clinical Outcomes from the Model Systems*. Gaithersburg, MD: Aspen Publications.

Yezierski RP. 2000. Pain following spinal cord injury: Pathophysiology and central mechanisms. *Progress in Brain Research* 129: 429-449.

Zehnder Y, Risi S, Michel D, Knecht H, Perrelet R, Kraenzlin M, Zach GA, Lippuner KJ. 2004. Prevention of bone loss in paraplegics over 2 years with alendronate. *Journal of Bone and Mineral Research* 19(7): 1067-1074.

5

PROGRESS TOWARD NEURONAL REPAIR AND REGENERATION

As is apparent from the information presented in the previous chapter, in the past several decades there has been significant progress in improving patient survival and emergency care and in expanding the range of rehabilitative options. During this same time period, the breadth and depth of neuroscience discoveries relevant to spinal cord injury have widely expanded the horizons of potential therapies. What once was dogma—that the central nervous system cannot regenerate—has been dismissed. This newly discovered potential for central nervous system (CNS) regeneration and repair has opened up numerous therapeutic targets and opportunities.

The new challenge facing researchers is to harness the expanding knowledge to develop effective treatments to protect and repair the spinal cord and improve or restore altered and lost function. To address this challenge, researchers must focus on a set of strategies to prevent further tissue loss, maintain the health of living cells and replace cells that have died through apoptosis or necrosis, grow axons and ensure functional connections, and reestablish synapses that restore the neural circuits required for functional recovery.

This chapter highlights the inroads that are being made in experimental settings to develop therapies that will reduce the effects of acute, secondary, and chronic injury and eventually provide cures. As research proceeds to refine and improve current therapies, it also generates creative approaches for curing spinal cord injuries. The research strategies and therapeutic approaches described here will both benefit from and inform basic and clinical research efforts from many related fields of neuroscience, bioengineering, and rehabilitative research.

ACUTE INJURY

Reduction of Edema and Free-Radical Attack

A complex series of biochemical reactions that cause ischemia and edema, followed by necrosis and inflammation, occur as a result of a spinal cord injury. Each reaction could provide a target for early intervention and treatment. The key is to pick out, from among the myriad of reactions, the dominant and most specific players and then target them for treatment.

Many different therapeutic approaches have been tested in vitro or with animal models of spinal cord injury (Table 5-1). Some are aimed at

TABLE 5-1 Examples of Strategies to Reduce the Effects of Acute Spinal Cord Injuries Tested with Animal Models

Strategy	Examples of Therapeutic Classes or Agents
Reduce ischemia	• Antivasospasm agents • Protein kinase inhibitors • Steroids • Prevent disruption to the blood-spinal cord barrier • Mild to moderate regional hypothermia
Reduce calcium influx	• Blockers of ion channels or exchangers
Reduce edema and formation of free radicals	• Antioxidant enzymes, including free-radical scavengers (e.g., superoxide dismutase, glutathione peroxidase, catalase, and melatonin) • Inhibitors of nitric oxide synthase
Control inflammation or enhance protective immunity	• Steroids and other anti-inflammatories (e.g., COX-2 inhibitors and anti-inflammatory cytokines) • Activated macrophages and monocytes • Inhibitors of immune cell infiltration of the CNS • Antibodies against integrin on the vascular surface to prevent egress of neutrophils
Reduce tissue loss	• Cell transplantation (e.g., Schwann cells and olfactory ensheathing cells) • Increase intercellular cyclic AMP levels

TABLE 5-2 Strategies to Block Cell Death

- Block formation of free radicals
- Block key proteases (e.g., caspases and calpain)
- Block cytochrome *c* release
- Block glutamate receptors
- Promote adequate circulation
- Combination (multipotential) therapies

SOURCE: Dobkin and Havton, 2004.

reducing ischemia (from the onset of injury), some are aimed at later events, and some are aimed at more than one event.

An emerging strategy, based on more than a decade of study with animal models, takes aim at the formation of free radicals, a crucial step in the onset of necrosis and apoptosis (see the next section) (Table 5-2) (Sugawara and Chan, 2003). Parallel lines of research on stroke and other neurological conditions are being conducted, with opportunities for collaborative efforts.

Control of Inflammation or Enhancement of Protective Immunity

The immune system's response to injury has both protective and damaging effects, depending on the cell type, location, and concentration; the timing of the injury; and a host of other factors. One strategy that has been examined is to boost the protective effects of the immune system by injecting animals with T cells that inhibit a protein found in myelin (Hauben et al., 2000). This strategy was found to result in the death of fewer nerve cells. In another attempt to strengthen the immune response, macrophages were implanted into rats at the site of the lesion and distally into the parenchyma (Rapalino et al., 1998). The macrophages were derived from fractions of blood enriched with peripheral blood monocytes incubated with segments of sciatic nerve. Rats injected with the activated macrophages showed improved axon regrowth and motor function. A clinical trial based on the results of the work by Rapalino and colleagues was then initiated (Bomstein et al., 2003; Proneuron Biotechnologies, 2004), and a multisite phase II clinical trial is now being conducted; the results have not yet been published.

One contrasting strategy—to blunt the damaging effects of the immune system—is potentially possible with immunosuppressant drugs, such as cyclosporin A and FK506 (tacrolimus). Transplant surgeons have used immunosuppressants to prevent organ rejection for many years, and in recent years these agents have successfully been used as neuroprotective agents in animal models of stroke and traumatic brain injury (Kaminska et al., 2004). The drugs are now being tested in animals with spinal cord injuries (Madsen et al., 1998; Bavetta et al., 1999; Diaz-Ruiz et al., 1999, 2000; Nottingham et al., 2002; Akgun et al., 2004). Although their mechanisms of action are not fully known, they may reduce glial cell responses and inflammation (Kaminska et al., 2004).

One promising therapy is based on a set of experiments designed to decrease the infiltration of neutrophils and to delay the entry of monocytes into the spinal cord after an injury (Gris et al., 2004). After a spinal cord injury, monocytes and neutrophils bind to a specific protein, VCAM-1, or the CD11d subunit of the CD11d/CD18 integrin on the interior of blood vessels and then egress into the spinal cord. These actions contribute to the inflammatory response and cause considerable secondary damage. Antibodies to VCAM-1 have been developed (Mabon et al., 2000) and have been found to significantly reduce the numbers of macrophages and neutrophils at the site of injury when they are administered to rodents after a spinal cord injury. Rats that received this antibody also showed improved proprioception and locomotion, significant decreases in autonomic dysreflexia, and less pain (Mabon et al., 2000; Bao et al., 2004). If the results of these experiments are validated, this therapy could be successfully translated into a clinical trial.

Researchers and clinicians have also explored the possibility of cooling the spinal cord. The purpose of this treatment is to minimize the damage caused by apoptosis and the secondary effects of inflammation (Dimar et al., 1999). This approach, which uses extreme levels of total body hypothermia, was extensively studied in the 1960s and 1970s but lost favor in the 1980s because of potential adverse effects, including kidney failure (Inamasu et al., 2003). However, new methods of introducing mild hypothermia have been developed, and hypothermia treatment is once again being considered as a potential treatment for traumatic brain injuries and spinal cord injuries (Dietrich et al., 1994; Yu et al., 2000). Of particular interest are techniques that are under development to precisely control hypothermia to the area of injury beyond several hours (Robertson et al., 1986; Kida et al., 1994; Marsala et al., 1997; Dimar et al., 2000).

In patients with cardiovascular and traumatic brain injuries, mild to moderate hypothermia has been reported to improve outcomes (Marion et al., 1997; Jiang et al., 2000; Hypothermia After Cardiac Arrest Study Group, 2002; Bernard et al., 2002). Two studies have examined the efficacy of spinal cord cooling in 18 patients with complete spinal cord injuries (Bricolo et al., 1976; Hansebout et al., 1984). Each of those studies demonstrated that the patients had rates of recovery of sensory and motor functions that were better than expected (Koons et al., 1972; Tator and Deecke, 1973; Negrin, 1975); however, in the 20 years that have followed there has been a limited number of clinical trials that have examined this treatment, but they do appear to support the benefit of hypothermia. A 2003 review of all published laboratory experiments of induced hypothermia for the treatment of traumatic spinal cord injuries showed that it offers no benefit for severe injuries but does result in improvements in functional outcomes in individuals with mild to moderate traumatic spinal cord injuries (Inamasu et al., 2003). Induced hypothermia has also been demonstrated to provide functional improvement in rats with ischemic spinal cord injuries (Dimar et al., 2000).

SECONDARY INJURY

Rescue of Neural Tissue at Risk of Apoptotic Cell Death

Neurons near the site of injury may be spared during the acute phase of injury, but they are at risk of dying during the secondary phase. Thus, another target of therapies for spinal cord injuries is to suppress the wave of apoptotic cell death that expands the scope of injury well beyond its original site. Apoptosis involves a complex sequence of biochemical reactions launched inside the cell by a variety of signals, including excessive calcium influx (see Chapter 2). A range of strategies is being tested to prevent apoptosis, primarily in animal models. The strategies fall under the umbrella term *neuroprotection*, because their goal is to shore up the nervous system's defenses against the cascade of biochemical threads. Some strategies (e.g., inhibition of free radicals) may block not only apoptosis but also necrosis (Kondo et al., 1997). To add to the complexity, the death of the cell can also lead to the death of an adjacent cell; for example, apoptosis of oligodendrocytes may also induce death of the neurons that they ensheath or adjacent astrocytes (Hulsebosch, 2002). Apoptosis depends heavily on caspases, a group of intracellular proteins that cleave and thereby disable other proteins. Of this group of proteins, caspase-3 and caspase-9 are thought to be dominant players in spinal cord injury-induced apoptosis (Eldadah and Faden, 2000). Inhibition of caspases may therefore be key to preventing apoptosis. Several clinical trials of caspase inhibitors for the treatment of other illnesses are under way (NIH, 2004).

Another protease, calpain, also plays a role earlier in the biochemical cascade that leads to spinal cord injury-induced apoptosis and thus represents another target for the treatment of spinal cord injuries. Calpain inhibition has successfully prevented neuron death in animal models of spinal cord injury (Ray et al., 2003). Finally, a drug already on the market, the antibiotic minocycline, may alleviate the impact of a spinal cord injury by inhibiting the release of cytochrome *c* (Teng et al., 2004), a molecule also associated with apoptosis (Di Giovanni et al., 2003).

Glutamate, a neurotransmitter that is released in excess amounts during a spinal cord injury, can cause potassium to enter the cell, resulting in the death of nearby neurons by necrosis or apoptosis. Glutamate, however, must first bind to receptor proteins that also act as potassium and calcium gates before these ions can enter neurons. Researchers have studied drugs that block glutamate receptors in the hope of preventing excess potassium and calcium from entering and killing the neuron (Lea and Faden, 2003). The results of human clinical trials of glutamate receptor blockade outside the field of spinal cord injury, however, have been disappointing, with little evidence of efficacy (Muir and Lees, 2003). Some blocking strategies have induced rather than prevented cell death (Lea and Faden, 2003). The key to neuroprotection may be more selective targeting of glutamate receptor subtypes, some of which are responsible for activation (e.g., metabotropic glutamate receptors) and others of which are responsible for inhibition (e.g., ionotropic glutamate receptors) (Lea and Faden, 2003; Movsesyan et al., 2004).

The effects of erythropoietin in mediating tissue protection after a spinal cord injury have also been explored in laboratory experiments. Erythropoietin is a protein that is primarily responsible for stimulating red blood cell production; however, in animals given erythropoietin immediately after a spinal cord injury, the rate of survival of the neurons responsible for controlling movements increased and the treatment resulted in benefits to neurological function (Celik et al., 2002; Brines et al., 2004). Ongoing studies are attempting to replicate and further explore this approach.

Restoration of Trophic Support

Neurons need more than oxygen to survive and flourish. Their sustenance depends on trophic factors, which are small proteins secreted by neighboring cells that come into contact with neuronal cell bodies, dendrites, and areas along the length of the axons. Several trophic factors have successfully been introduced by injection or by minipumps in animal models of spinal cord injury: brain-derived neurotrophic factor (BDNF), neurotrophic factor-3 (NT-3), glial-derived neurotrophic factor (GDNF), nerve growth factor (NGF), and fibroblast growth factor (FGF), among others (Xu et al., 1995a; Bamber et al., 2001; Jones et al., 2001; Schwab, 2002). The key is to ensure the delivery of the most appropriate factors, as different classes of neurons depend on different trophic factors and some trophic factors may have deleterious effects, such as inducing sensory neurons to become hypersensitive to pain (Krenz and Weaver, 2000). Also key is placement of the appropriate factor at the best anatomical site to deliver levels high enough and continuously enough to keep neurons alive and promote their regrowth. Methods of delivering trophic factors include transplantation to the site of injury of cells that have been genetically engineered to release high concentrations of growth factors (Conner et al., 2001; Grill et al., 1997; Menei et al., 1998). Investigators have also found that combination therapy may be the most effective. For example, in a multipronged effort to rescue neurons and promote their regrowth, marrow stromal cells delivered in combination with growth factors and cyclic AMP have been found to be more effective than each individual treatment alone (Lu et al., 2004).

CHRONIC INJURY

Removal of Barriers to Axon Regrowth

After spinal cord injury there are many barriers that prevent the regrowth of axons. Several experimental therapeutic strategies take aim at these events, including treatment with antibodies directed to growth-inhibiting molecules (Schnell and Schwab, 1990), the use of mechanisms to interfere with the signaling pathways activated by inhibitory molecules (Cai et al., 1999), prevention or removal of the glial scar (Stichel et al., 1999), enzyme treatment to remove inhibitory proteoglycan molecules (Bradbury et al., 2002), transplantation of growth-promoting cells (Xu et al., 1995b, 1997; McDonald et al., 1999), and administration of growth-promoting molecules (Ramer et al., 2000).

A glial scar is a pathological hallmark of the chronic phase of injury. The scar may physically block axonal penetration or may release inhibitory molecules that block axon regrowth (Fawcett and Asher, 1999; Silver and Miller, 2004). Wholesale efforts to disrupt the scar by removing glial cells altogether or stopping them from proliferating produce widespread excitotoxicity and complications that arise due to the loss of certain neurotrophic factors (Fawcett and Asher, 1999). Furthermore, elimination of glial cells removes their positive role in nervous system recovery.

Several approaches to reducing the impact of the scar have been tested with animal models. The most promising of these approaches may be blockade or degradation of the inhibitory molecules rather than destruction of the glial cells that produce and secrete them. One experiment targeted the large class of inhibitors known as chondroitin sulfate proteoglycans (CSPGs) (Bradbury et al., 2002). Molecules of this class are up-regulated by the injury and are released by astrocytes within the glial scar. CSPGs are soluble molecules that, once released, contribute to a meshwork around neurons known as the extracellular matrix. CSPGs have been found to block axon regrowth both in vitro and in animal models (Fawcett and Asher, 1999; Silver and Miller, 2004) by increasing the activity of the enzyme protein kinase C (PKC) (Sivasankaran et al., 2004). It has been shown that the administration of PKC inhibitors to rats with spinal cord injuries improves axon regeneration and myelination (Sivasankaran et al., 2004). In another rodent model, researchers degraded CSPGs by administering an enzyme, chondroitinase ABC. Administration of this enzyme promoted the regrowth of axons from spinal cord neurons into grafts of peripheral nerve into the spinal cord (Yick et al., 2004) and growth of CNS axons from grafts of Schwann cells into the spinal cord (Chau et al., 2004). The enzyme treatment also improved locomotion and proprioception (Bradbury et al., 2002; Yick et al., 2004).

Schwab (2004) and colleagues pioneered another line of research with animal models that targets the inhibitory molecule Nogo-A, which is expressed on the surface of myelin-forming oligodendrocytes. In 1990, it had been shown that antibodies to Nogo-A led to the regrowth of injured axons over long distances (Schnell and Schwab, 1990). A decade later, after the gene for Nogo-A had been cloned, the researchers developed a safer and more focused strategy: production of large quantities of a partially humanized version of a fragment of the antibody in vitro and then injection of this new antibody as a pure reagent (Brosamle et al., 2000). The results of experiments with mice that lack the Nogo gene (a strategy known as gene knockout) examining axon regrowth and improved gait after injury have varied (Kim et al., 2003). However, experiments performed with rats have shown that injection of the Nogo antibody promotes long-distance axonal regeneration and functional regeneration (Brosamle et al., 2000). A clinical trial of the Nogo antibody is being planned.

Because Nogo-A and other inhibitory agents exert their effects through the Nogo receptor, a protein that sits on the external membrane of axons, blockade of the Nogo receptor is another potential way to boost regrowth. GrandPre and colleagues (2002) applied the small peptide NEP1-40 to the injured spinal cord. NEP1-40 binds to, but fails to activate, the Nogo receptor. Those investigators found that receptor blockade leads to substantial regrowth of the disrupted axons. Because Nogo-A and other inhibitory substances (e.g., myelin-associated glycoprotein) act through the same receptor, receptor blockade has the advantage of simultaneously inhibiting more than one inhibitory substance. A follow-up experiment successfully adapted NEP1-40 for injection up to 2 weeks after a spinal cord injury, with some recovery of locomotion (Li and Strittmatter, 2003).

A related strategy being explored would target Nogo inhibition at the growing tip of the axon. Once the Nogo receptor is activated, it works through several intermediate reactions within the cell, known as signaling pathways, to block axon regrowth. When researchers targeted one of those intermediate reactions, and thus interrupted the signaling pathway, they found axon regrowth and the recovery of function (Fournier et al., 2003). This treatment was with an agent that inhibited Rho-associated kinase

(ROCK), an enzyme that appears to dismantle the cell's internal scaffolding necessary for the growing tip of the axon (Amano et al., 2000). By inhibiting its destructive action, researchers believe that they can prevent the collapse of the growing tip and thus promote axonal extension. A phase I/II clinical trial is currently under way to evaluate the safety, pharmacokinetics, and efficacy of an antagonist to ROCK, Cethrin, in promoting neurogeneration and neuroprotection.

Promotion of Axon Regrowth and Guidance

For most of the last century, the dogma was that regrowth of nerve axons occurred only in the peripheral nervous system and not in the CNS. Landmark experiments in the early 1980s revolutionized thinking about nerve cells' capacity for long-distance regeneration. The experiments showed that CNS axon regrowth and connectivity could occur if the CNS environment was changed to match that normally present in peripheral nerves (David and Aguayo, 1981; Keirstead et al., 1989). The previous section highlighted techniques used to overcome the inhibitory environment. This section highlights the axon itself and what treatments might directly boost its regrowth. In reality, the distinction between eliminating the inhibitory effects of glial cells and promoting axon regrowth is blurred, and the techniques are closely intertwined.

The promotion of axon regrowth depends, first, on saving the entire neuron from apoptotic cell death (see above). Survival of the whole cell and then promotion of axon regrowth depend on the presence of growth factors in the immediate environment. The majority of these projections remain very short and local to the immediate site of injury. For unknown reasons, however, some fibers are capable of growing long distances around the lesion site. Nevertheless, axon regrowth does not result in improved function unless the axons can stimulate and inhibit the correct cellular target, whether it is in the brain, the spinal cord, or the periphery. If incorrect synapses are formed, pain and spasticity rather than restoration of normal walking and other functions can ensue.

Axon regrowth can also be stimulated by a variety of growth factors and other agents that enhance growth. Agents found to be successful in animal models are the purine nucleotide inosine (Benowitz et al., 1999) and cyclic AMP (Neumann et al., 2002; Qiu et al., 2002). Elevation of cyclic AMP levels by prevention of its normal breakdown can also induce regrowth (Pearse et al., 2004). Whether these agents work directly on the growing tip or more indirectly through the cell's nucleus is not fully known.

Axon regrowth may be necessary, but not sufficient, to regenerate a functional neuronal circuit capable of controlling movements or responding to stimuli. It is also critical that the regrowing axons find their correct target cells. During the normal development of an embryo, axons need to be guided to their appropriate targets through the combination of actions of attractive and repulsive axon guidance molecules, such as netrins, semaphorins, slits, and ephrins. Many of these guidance molecules arise from glia (astrocytes and oligodendrocytes), which act as guideposts, and intermediate target cells that steer a growing axon to its appropriate target (Chotard and Salecker, 2004). Each of these molecules also has at least one complementary receptor on the axon. When the guidance molecule and receptor interact, the receptor transmits a signal to the growing axon to either keep growing or avoid the area. These groups of molecules act in complex ways to guide developing axons. Axon guidance relies on the interplay of many different guidance molecules and receptors. Furthermore, the concentration gradients of the molecules also significantly influence the effects of the molecules on steering the axon in a specific direction.

The complexity of this mechanism is also underscored by the example of diffusible netrin molecules that, depending on the receptor on the axon with which they interact, can act as either an attractant molecule (Keino-Masu et al., 1996) or a repulsive molecule (Leonardo et al., 1997). Much information has been garnered about how these molecules affect axonal targeting in the developing nervous system; however, studies are under way to determine whether injured axons in the adult CNS are able to reexpress their receptors for these guidance molecules and whether the axonal targets can once again express their guidance cues (Koeberle and Bahr, 2004). Studies to date demonstrate that the expression patterns of many guidance molecules and receptors are the same during nervous system development and after an injury; but some are very different, and these differences could have important consequences on the correct targeting of a growing axon. For instance, the level of expression of a specific class of ephrins (ephrin-Bs) appears to be decreased in the brain, which could limit reinnervation by regenerating axons (Hindges et al., 2002). To overcome this, methods are being developed to examine the effectiveness of using gene therapy strategies and scaffolds (discussed below) to express different combinations of guidance molecules. These guidance molecules could be used as physical conduits that promote regrowth (Dobkin and Havton, 2004).

Gene Therapy

Gene therapy is another treatment strategy that has great potential to provide the injured spinal cord with the specific gene products—proteins—that it needs to promote functional recovery. Gene therapy is not a current treatment for spinal cord injuries but is being studied with animal models of spinal cord injury. The concept is to transfer into the spinal cord a gene encoding a therapeutic protein, such as a growth factor or an axon guidance molecule, or to transplant cells modified to incorporate the gene. When the gene is expressed, the cell makes the desired protein. An advantage of gene therapy over cell replacement therapy is that a specific gene or set of genes can be introduced and the amount (or dose) of the protein can be controlled, which is extremely important in maintaining the fine balance of natural proteins surrounding injured nerve cells and helping guide their growth or regrowth toward target cells in the brain or spinal cord. One of the greatest problems with most therapies is that the dose cannot be readily fine-tuned at the site of injury or along the path of the regrowing axons. Gene therapy can potentially overcome that obstacle.

Gene therapy can be used to modulate the amount of protein in a number of ways. One method is to introduce a second gene called a promoter gene along with the therapeutic gene. The promoter gene's purpose is to turn the therapeutic gene on and off. The promoter gene's action can also be regulated, for example, with a well-tolerated drug. In one novel example, researchers inserted a promoter gene responsive to the drug tetracycline next to the therapeutic gene, which in this case was the gene for NGF. To activate the production of NGF, the researchers then added a drug similar to tetracycline to the mice's drinking water. Once it was consumed, the drug turned on the promoter gene, which, in turn, drove the expression of NGF (Blesch et al., 2001). When the researchers wished to minimize or stop the production of NGF, they reduced the dose or removed the drug from the drinking water, thus regulating the amount of NGF needed to stimulate axonal growth.

Research to date has focused on the introduction of genes for growth factors (FGF and GDNF) and neurotrophins (BDNF, NGF, NT-3, and NT-4/5). These therapeutic genes are first inserted into fibroblasts (skin cells) in a culture dish. The genetically modified fibroblasts are then implanted directly into the injured area of the spinal cord (a technique known as ex vivo gene therapy). Although most of the research has focused on fibroblasts, other types of cells can be genetically modified, such as stem cells, oligodendrocytes, and Schwann cells. A similar strategy for introducing genes that is being explored is gene therapy. A few important issues for both these strategies are the types of genes to be introduced, how expression of the gene can be limited to specific cell types (which is normally done by using specific gene promoters such as GFAP for astrocytes), and how the gene can be introduced into the cell. One common method of introducing genes is through the use of viruses, but this method can be problematic, because some viruses (such as retroviruses) can only be inserted into dividing cells and most neurons do not divide. Other viruses are used because they specifically target the nervous system, or they can be used to introduce genes into nondividing neurons, but they may also attract a more general immune response that has its own detrimental effects.

Using gene therapy, spinal cord injury researchers have succeeded in introducing growth factors that have led to some recovery of function in rodent models (Blesch and Tuszynski, 2004; Hendriks et al., 2004). The experiments have thus far established the potential value of gene therapy, which can be used alone or in combination with other therapies.

Bridging Gaps with Transplantation

Spinal cord injury not only leaves a glial cell scar but also leaves a physical gap. As early as 1906, a peripheral nerve was transplanted into the brain to see if CNS axons would regrow in an environment that was known to be supportive of axonal growth in the peripheral nervous system. Seven decades later, Richardson and colleagues (1980) found that months after they inserted a segment of a peripheral nerve into a gap in the spinal cord, the cut axons had regrown into the implanted nerve from both stumps of the severed spinal cord. This technique has been validated in studies with optic nerve neurons, which travel long distances between the eye and the brain. When peripheral nerve grafts were attached to the optic nerve stump, retinal axons were induced to regenerate long distances within the grafts and were capable of making functional connections when the grafts ended near their correct targets in the brain (Carter et al., 1989). Similar techniques have been used in the spinal cord. For example, researchers have induced some neuronal regeneration by transplanting peripheral nerve and Schwann cells inside a polymer tube to fill a complete or partial gap in the spinal cords (Bunge, 2001). Today, scientists are continuing to develop a number of different types of bridges that consist not only of peripheral nerves or Schwann cells, but also olfactory ensheathing cells (OECs), stem cells, marrow stromal cells, trophic factors, biomaterials, or some combination thereof.

A new generation of scaffolds is being developed for the broad field of tissue engineering (Holmes, 2002). The ideal scaffold for use in the repair of a spinal cord injury would be attractive to regenerating axons, a physical conduit for entry and exit, nontoxic and nonimmunogenic, versatile enough to house a wide range of drugs or cell types, and degradable over a time window sufficient for regrowth (Geller and Fawcett, 2002). The types of materials that may potentially be used as scaffolds include naturally occurring materials (e.g., collagen), organic polymers, and inorganic materials. Even more innovative scaffolds are materials that are injected as liquids and that then self-assemble into fibers with diameters of less than 1 micrometer (Silva et al., 2004).

Restoration of Impulse Conduction in Demyelinated Axons

Healthy nerve cells transmit information by conducting impulses along the lengths of their membranes. Impulses are carried by the movement of charged particles (ions) through cellular channels in the axonal membrane, the most prominent being positively charged sodium (Na^+) and potassium (K^+) ions. This process is facilitated by the myelin sheath, which acts as an insulator to expedite impulse transmission. Myelin is often destroyed by the injury, although nerve axons may remain intact, and so several therapeutic strategies take aim at the surviving axons by endowing them with the capacity to transmit impulses in the absence of myelin (Chudler, 2004).

One approach is to transplant cells capable of myelination into demyelinated lesions (Kocsis et al., 2002, 2004). Several studies with animal models of spinal cord injury have provided evidence that implanted Schwann cells (cultured and purified) can remyelinate demyelinated axons, restore conduction, and improve function (Bunge and Wood, 2004).

Restoration of functional conduction across the membrane is still possible, without myelin, by altering channel activity. The drug 4-aminopyridine (fampridine) has been found to be effective in improving conduction in demyelinated axons in animal models (Shi and Blight, 1997). However, the results obtained with a sustained-release form of the drug in human clinical trials have been only modest. One trial showed negative results (van der Bruggen et al., 2001), but other small trials showed some improvements in individuals' motor function and sensory function (pinprick and light touch) and reductions in spasticity (muscle tone) and pain (Qiao et al., 1997; Potter et al., 1998). The results for the two primary end points—spasticity and global impression of functioning—of the largest and most recent clinical trial (a phase III trial) did not reach statistical significance, according to the sponsor's website (the results are not yet published). The study did show, however, a positive trend toward less spasticity (Acorda Therapeutics, 2004; Hayes et al., 2004).

Another therapeutic approach is to target sodium channels in a subtype-specific manner. When axons within the spinal cord are demyelinated, as in individuals with multiple sclerosis, the body inserts new sodium channels into the membrane of axons that have lost their myelin (Craner et al., 2004a,b). This is one example of plasticity, the body's natural way of trying to adapt to changed conditions and compensating for lost function. Plasticity is not always beneficial, however. Neurons have 10 distinct sodium channels, each of which has different physiological properties. This represents a subtlety of neuronal design that permits different types of neurons to produce different patterns of impulses within the nervous system (Waxman, 2000). Some types of channels produce background levels of activity that can be interpreted by the brain as pain, whereas others allow large fluxes of sodium that can trigger axonal degeneration. The development of medications that selectively enhance or inhibit the actions of specific subtypes of sodium channels may make it possible to adjust the balance of the channels to preserve normal axon function without silencing them.

Restoration of Sensory Function

The loss of sensory modalities can be as debilitating as the loss of motor function. Although sensory function was not previously a substantial focus of spinal cord injury research, scientists are now making progress in understanding what contributes to the loss of sensation and developing treatments to restore sensory modalities, including touch, temperature, pain, proprioception, and feedback control of movements.

Proprioception is an often overlooked sensation that is critical in coordinating walking and other movements (Box 5-1). Muscles and joints have special sensory neurons designed to signal the CNS about muscle length, the velocity of movements, and the load (or force) being applied. This sensory input is continually used to convey positional sense (awareness of position of the body in space), to trigger spinal reflexes, and to prepare for effective control over movement. Sensory neurons carrying proprioceptive information course from the muscles and joints directly into the spinal cord. There they project to motor neurons in the spinal cord or they course to the brain (through several synapses). The fibers forming the first part of the pathway, from the muscles to the spinal cord, appear to possess recep-

---

BOX 5-1
A Personal Perspective on the Loss of Proprioception

One of the defects of spinal cord injury not often discussed or appreciated is loss of proprioception. As a C5-6 quadriplegic, I have no sense of where my lower limbs are placed and a minimal sense of the positioning of my upper extremities. I can move my arms and legs and can actually walk with braces and someone making sure I don't fall over because of proprioception/balance. I move my legs particularly only if I can see where they are and where they are going. I literally cannot move my legs without visual sensing of position. I expect that lack of proprioception is an important aspect of motor function and its return after spinal cord injury is an important aspect of regaining function.

—Robert Schimke, Professor Emeritus
of Biology, Stanford University

tors for a specific neurotrophic factor known as NT-3 (McMahon et al., 1994).

In one of the first experiments of its kind, researchers applied NT-3 directly onto the spinal cords of rats (intrathecally) whose sensory fibers had been cut near the entry point into the spinal cord. The cut end of the nerve regrew into the spinal cord and reconnected with target cells at the appropriate level. Not only were the new synapses anatomically correct, but proprioceptive functioning was restored behaviorally and physiologically (Ramer et al., 2002). In a separate set of experiments, patients with a disease that causes demyelination in the peripheral nervous system were given NT-3. This treatment led to improved sensation, a return of the reflexes, and peripheral axon regeneration (Sahenk, 2003). Thus, there is a need to explore the use of neurotrophic factors for promotion of the regrowth of the sensory fibers.

STEM CELLS AND OTHER CELL-BASED THERAPIES

Cell-based therapies hold great potential as a means of replacing cells and restoring function that has been lost because of a disease or an injury. The application of cell-based therapies to spinal cord injuries is a natural outgrowth of research in other fields, such as cancer, diabetes, and heart disease. Hematopoietic stem cell-based therapies are now being used routinely to treat certain cancers and are being tested for use in regenerative medicine, for example, to replace insulin-secreting cells destroyed by juvenile diabetes or muscle cells destroyed by heart attacks. Therapies are being developed to restore function in individuals with spinal cord injuries by transplanting many different types of cells, including Schwann cells and OECs to restore nerve conduction, genetically engineered cells to restore trophic support and support regrowth, and stem cells that have the capacity to improve function through a number of mechanisms (Hulsebosch, 2002).

The Promise of Schwann Cells and Olfactory Ensheathing Cells

For more than a decade, researchers have known that Schwann cells, the ensheathing cells ordinarily found only in the peripheral nervous system, migrate into the spinal cord after it is injured. Thus, Schwann cells may be used in potential therapies for spinal cord injuries whether they are endogenous or transplanted (Bunge and Wood, 2004). There they may help stimulate axonal growth and myelinate the newly grown axons. The use of Schwann cells is attractive because they are readily accessible and proliferate rapidly in cell culture—up to 100,000 times—and do not trigger an immune response, as long as the individual's own Schwann cells are used. One problem, however, is that regrowing axons do not exit and grow substantially beyond the site of the Schwann cell implant without the use of other interventions. This problem has led to research focusing on combination strategies, discussed later in this chapter, and has spurred the use of another type of ensheathing cell, OECs. These are specialized types of glial cells that wrap bundles of sensory nerve fibers as they extend from the olfactory mucosa of the nose to the brain's olfactory center (the olfactory bulb) into the outer layer of the olfactory bulb (for a review, see Raisman, 2001). One role of OECs is to form channels to guide the axonal growth of olfactory neurons from the nose to the brain (Williams et al., 2004). Olfactory neurons are unusual because they are continually being replenished by stem cells in the nasal mucosa throughout adulthood. Axons of the new neurons need to be steered toward their destination by the OECs. Although OECs do not normally myelinate individual axons in vivo, they can become myelinating cells when they are grown in tissue culture under certain conditions (Devon and Doucette, 1992). As a result, OECs are viewed as prime candidates to guide axon regrowth and to replace the myelin in the axons of individuals with spinal cord injuries.

Several experiments have found that when cultured OECs are implanted into an injured spinal cord, they support the regrowth of axons over long distances and restore function (Li et al., 1997, 1998; Ramon-Cueto et al., 1998, 2000; Radtke et al., 2004). Compared to Schwann cells, OECs were not as effective, after implantation into a contused spinal cord, in inducing long-distance axon regrowth and myelination and improving locomotion (Takami et al., 2002), although they may not have survived well in the lesion milieu. An advantage of OECs is that they intermingle more readily with astrocytes and may be more migratory in the spinal cord than Schwann cells. The disadvantages of OECs are that they do not readily expand in large numbers when they are cultured and are not as readily accessible as Schwann cells. Internationally researchers are attempting to implant fetal olfactory cells into individuals with spinal cord injuries. However, well-designed clinical trials to evaluate this approach have yet to be performed, and there are concerns about safety and efficacy (see Chapter 6) (Lev, 2004; Judson, 2005). Nevertheless, although both Schwann cells and OECs appear to improve function, the mechanisms are not fully understood.

The Promise of Stem Cells

Stem cell therapy holds a seemingly boundless potential for the repair of spinal cord injuries, but research is still in the early stages. The interest arises from stem cells' defining characteristics: their ability to replace themselves by cell division and their versatility, that is, their ability to mature into one or other more specialized cell types (NRC, 2002).

Stem cell biology is a quickly evolving field, and much remains to be learned about the use of stem cells in regenerative therapies for spinal cord injuries. Important advances in the understanding of the biology of stem cells are being made in many areas of research. It is becoming clear that many types of adult stem cells have a multilineage potential to give rise to cells that during development are normally derived from a different lineage. For instance, stem cells found in adult bone marrow (Orlic et al., 2001) and liver (Malouf et al., 2001) are capable of generating muscle cells in the heart, and adult hepatic stem cells have the capacity to transdifferentiate into pancreatic endocrine hormone-producing cells (Yang et al., 2002). Recently, numerous reports have described the regenerative capability of a number of stem cell sources, including pancreatic islet tissue from the spleen (Kodama et al., 2005). Evidence also suggests that neuronal cells can be derived not only from neuronal stem cells but also from mesenchymal stem cells (Smith, 2004), bone marrow stem cells (Brazelton et al., 2000; Mezey et al., 2000), stem cells surrounding the heart (Drapeau et al., 2004), and other types of stem cells. Therefore, it is critical that researchers developing stem cell-based therapies to restore function after a spinal cord injury integrate knowledge garnered from other fields of stem cell biology.

Since the early 1990s it has been known that stem cells with the capacity to form neurons and glial cells also reside in the nervous system (Gage, 2000). Stem cells might be used in the repair of spinal cord injury by replacing spinal cord cells lost to injury or to rescue the host's spinal cord cells from dying during the second wave of degeneration. Most of the unresolved questions surrounding stem cell research deal with the safety of the transplant procedure itself, the health and survival of the cells, the ability to induce stem cells to differentiate into a stable cell type, the side effects of the process, and the level of functioning that results. Further research in this area is needed to answer these questions.

Over the past 5 years, a number of studies, mostly with animal models, have successfully transplanted pure or highly enriched cultures of stem cells for the treatment of spinal cord injuries. Most of those studies found that the stem cells survived after transplantation and led to some degree of myelination, axon regrowth, and functional improvement, directly or indirectly (Table 5-3). Because the methods used varied widely, it is difficult to compare the results of the different studies. For the most part, however, when the recovery of function was measured, it was only modest at best.

The most commonly studied adult stem cells for the treatment of spinal cord injuries and other neurological conditions are neural stem cells. They are prime candidates for repair of the spinal cord after an injury because they can be isolated and can mature into neurons or glia (oligodendrocytes and astrocytes) in vitro and in vivo (Yandava et al., 1999; Uchida et al., 2000). However, as indicated above, other types of stem cells—including mesenchymal cells, bone marrow cells, and stem cells derived from the

Teng et al. (2002)	Rats	Neural stem cells from neonatal mouse cell line	To replace neurons and glia and to channel their growth with scaffolding	The combination therapy (scaffold and stem cells) led to functional recovery of animals with spinal cord injuries. Stem cells did not differentiate, but they supported host axon regrowth and functional recovery.
Lu et al. (2003)	Rats	Neural stem cells from neonatal mouse cell line	To secrete trophic factors for host's axon regrowth	Neural stem cells secreted trophic factors in vivo and induced host sensory and motor axons to regrow. The cells were implanted into the spinal cords of animals with spinal cord injuries.
Mikami et al. (2004)	Mice	Dendritic cells	To act as antigen-presenting cells in the immune system	Implanted cells induced neural stem cells and progenitor cells to proliferate, differentiate, and survive and improved locomotor function.
Fujiwara et al. (2004)	Rats	Neural stem cells from fetal rat hippocampus	To develop a less invasive delivery method	Stem cells were injected intravenously. They migrated to the spinal cord lesion site and differentiated there into neurons and glia.

tissue surrounding the heart—may give rise to neuronal cells; and numerous research avenues need to be explored. Additionally, there is much to learn about the mechanisms that direct stem cells to differentiate and mature (e.g., plasticity, fusion, and transdifferentiation), and it is likely that the observations of the mechanism of action from the study of stem cell-based therapies for a wide range of health outcomes will be able to be directly translated to the development of therapeutic interventions to promote spinal cord repair and regeneration.

DEVELOPING NEW INTERVENTIONS AND COMBINATION THERAPEUTIC STRATEGIES

This chapter and others have identified many possible targets for therapeutic interventions and many possible therapeutic approaches. As researchers gain additional insights into the mechanisms of neuronal repair and regeneration, efforts to move these discoveries into clinically meaningful therapies will continue.

One of the major themes arising from this chapter is that, owing to its complexity, a spinal cord injury is unlikely to be cured by a single therapy. The biological processes involved in regaining sensory or motor functions, preventing or eliminating pain, and retraining and relearning motor tasks are so diverse that treatment strategies that use a combination of therapies will almost certainly be required. A balance between destructive and regenerative events in the aftermath of a spinal cord injury dictates the clinical course and outcome; therapeutic approaches will likewise need to address the multiple and complex therapeutic targets and health problems. This is analogous to childhood leukemia, once a uniformly fatal disease. Investigators tested one drug after another, with only marginal effects on life expectancy. Ultimately, a carefully crafted combination of drugs resulted in a total cure rate of more than 50 percent (NAS, 1997).

In light of the complicated dynamics, some of the most promising and intriguing studies that were recently published and are described in this chapter have drawn on the combined potencies of more than one therapy. One study, for example, showed that a combination therapy that targets both the neuronal cell body and its axons was more effective than either therapy alone (Lu et al., 2004). Another study implanted scaffolds seeded with stem cells (Teng et al., 2002). The concept behind that study was that the scaffold would set the stage by providing a conduit for growth and the stem cells would release soluble factors to stimulate growth. With the combination, axons regrew and restored some of the lost function. A third study boosted the cell-signaling molecules needed for axon regrowth and replacement of myelin. It showed that functional recovery could be achieved with rolipram, which boosts cyclic AMP levels, combined with an injection of cyclic AMP and grafts of Schwann cells (Pearse et al., 2004). Rolipram plus embryonic tissue transplants also promote axonal regeneration and functional recovery (Nikulina et al., 2004).

This chapter has dealt with more than a dozen approaches that can be used to treat or reverse the impact of a spinal cord injury. Each approach, if successful, would likely only restore partial function, but theoretically they can be pursued together with others to provide maximal recovery of function. For example, cell-based therapies that replace myelin could be combined with treatment with agents that promote axon regrowth, such as neurotrophic factors.

One of the major challenges with the development of combination therapies is determination of the specific therapies that can be combined safely and that in concert will provide the greatest efficacy for the treatment of spinal cord injuries. This is a major impediment, because for most complications associated with a spinal cord injury there are multiple experimental approaches to alleviate the complication. Although it is possible for different combinations of drugs to be combined by trial and error, greater progress can be made if specific research efforts are devoted to developing and implementing a mechanism that can be used to select the most likely components that will be required for combination therapies. This requires a strategic approach for screening and assessing the potentials of compounds and therapies to be components of a combination therapy. A second major challenge is determining the appropriate order to apply each of the individual therapies in combinations to maximize the therapeutic value of each treatment.

The National Institute of Neurological Disorders and Stroke (NINDS) should play a lead role in developing a strategic approach to the development of combination therapeutic strategies. Furthermore, NINDS, in conjunction with other federal agencies, nonprofit organizations, research centers, and pharmaceutical companies, should examine the challenges that will arise in designing and conducting clinical trials of combination therapies. Some of the issues that need to be addressed include study design and regulatory implications. Other fields of research (e.g., cancer and HIV-AIDS) have dealt with some of the issues involved in testing combination therapies, and lessons should be learned from those efforts.

PRIORITIES FOR SPINAL CORD INJURY RESEARCH

More knowledge is needed on the optimal targets and pathways on which intervention efforts should be focused. There is still much to be learned about the basic biology of spinal cord injuries (Chapter 2), and as discussed throughout this chapter, numerous potential therapeutic targets are involved in the complex processes of maintaining cell and tissue viability and promoting axonal growth and synaptic integrity to achieve improved and appropriate function (Table 5-4). The addition of information to the body of knowledge on neurological circuitry and mechanisms will be of benefit not only to improving function after a spinal cord injury but also to developing therapies for other neurological diseases and conditions. In the past several decades the breadth and depth of neuroscience discoveries relevant to spinal cord injury have widely expanded the horizons of potential therapies. These new opportunities require increased research support by federal and state agencies, academic organizations, pharmaceutical and device companies, and nonprofit organizations. Further details on the nature and extent of the funding and infrastructure for spinal cord injury research are provided in Chapter 7.

A note of caution is needed, as one of the concerns regarding experimental therapies for spinal cord injuries has been the willingness by some patients to try unvalidated experimental therapies before the interventions have been thoroughly tested for safety and efficacy in methodologically rigorous studies. The committee urges the careful consideration and thorough study of new therapies with the utmost attention to patient safety.

TABLE 5-4 Priorities for Spinal Cord Injury Research

Develop neuroprotection therapies: identify interventions that promote neuroprotective mechanisms that preserve the spinal cord.

Promote axonal sprouting and growth: enhance understanding of the molecular mechanisms that promote and inhibit axonal regeneration—including the roles of glia (astrocytes and oligodendrocytes), scar formation, and inflammation and inhibitory molecules—and develop therapeutic approaches to promote growth.

Steer axonal growth: determine the molecular mechanisms that direct axons to their appropriate targets and regulate the formation and maintenance of appropriate synaptic connections.

Reestablish essential neuronal and glial circuitry: advance the understanding of the molecular mechanisms that regulate the formation and maintenance of the intricate neuronal and glial circuitry, which controls the complex multimodal function of the spinal cord, including autonomic, sensory, and motor functions. Increase knowledge of the mechanisms that control locomotion, including the differences in the central pattern generator between bipeds and quadrupeds.

Prevent acute and chronic complications: develop interventions that prevent and reverse the evolution of events that lead to the wide range of outcomes that result from chronic injury and disability after a spinal cord injury.

Maintain maximal potential for recovery: expand the understanding of the requirements for proper postinjury care and rehabilitation that are needed to maintain the maximal potential for full recovery.

The committee emphasizes the need to use a multifaceted approach to furthering the goal of curing spinal cord injuries. Strategies need to be developed to provide an organized approach to testing therapies in combination. The committee also recognizes that advances in science rely on novel breakthroughs, including those from other fields of research, and that there is a critical need to increase the awareness of spinal cord injury researchers of developments in other fields relevant to spinal cord injuries and to expand innovative approaches to spinal cord injury research. The discussion throughout this chapter emphasizes both the potential for progress and the numerous unknowns in the development of therapies. As more is learned about the pathways of the molecular and cellular events that result from a spinal cord injury, further therapeutic targets can be identified and approaches to promoting repair and restoring function can be refined.

RECOMMENDATIONS

Recommendation 5.1: *Increase Efforts to Develop Therapeutic Interventions*
The National Institutes of Health, other federal and state agencies, nonprofit organizations, and the pharmaceutical and medical device industries should increase research funding and efforts to develop therapeutic interventions that will prevent or reverse the physiological events that lead to chronic disability and interventions that are applicable to chronic spinal cord injuries. Specifically, research is needed to

• improve understanding of the basic mechanisms and identify suitable targets to promote neuroprotection, foster axonal growth, enhance axonal guidance, regulate the maintenance of appropriate synaptic connections, and reestablish functional neuronal and glial circuitry; and
• enhance understanding of proper postinjury care and rehabilitation, such as retraining, relearning, and the use of neuroprostheses, to create the groundwork required to maintain and enhance the maximal potential for full recovery.

Recommendation 5.2: *Develop a Strategic Plan for Combination Therapeutic Approaches*
The National Institute of Neurological Disorders and Stroke should develop a strategic plan to screen and assess the potential for compounds and therapies to be used in combination to treat acute and chronic spinal cord injuries.

REFERENCES

Acorda Therapeutics. 2004. *Pipeline Clinical Stage—Fampridine-SR.* [Online]. Available: http://www.acorda.com/pipeline_fampridine_sci1.asp [accessed August 18, 2004].

Akgun S, Tekeli A, Kurtkaya O, Civelek A, Isbir SC, Ak K, Arsan S, Sav A. 2004. Neuroprotective effects of Fk-506, L-carnitine and Azathioprine on spinal cord ischemia-reperfusion injury. *European Journal of Cardio-Thoracic Surgery* 25(1): 105-110.

Akiyama Y, Radtke C, Kocsis JD. 2002. Remyelination of the rat spinal cord by transplantation of identified bone marrow stromal cells. *Journal of Neuroscience* 22(15): 6623-6630.

Amano M, Fukata Y, Kaibuchi K. 2000. Regulation and functions of Rho-associated kinase. *Experimental Cell Research* 261(1): 44-51.

Bamber NI, Li H, Lu X, Oudega M, Aebischer P, Xu XM. 2001. Neurotrophins BDNF and NT-3 promote axonal re-entry into the distal host spinal cord through Schwann cell-seeded mini-channels. *European Journal of Neuroscience* 13(2): 257-268.

Bao F, Chen Y, Dekaban GA, Weaver LC. 2004. An anti-Cd11d integrin antibody reduces cyclooxygenase-2 expression and protein and DNA oxidation after spinal cord injury in rats. *Journal of Neurochemistry* 90(5): 1194-1204.

Bavetta S, Hamlyn PJ, Burnstock G, Lieberman AR, Anderson PN. 1999. The effects of FK506 on dorsal column axons following spinal cord injury in adult rats: Neuroprotection and local regeneration. *Experimental Neurology* 158(2): 382-393.

Benowitz LI, Goldberg DE, Madsen JR, Soni D, Irwin N. 1999. Inosine stimulates extensive axon collateral growth in the rat corticospinal tract after injury. *Proceedings of the National Academy of Sciences (U.S.A.)* 96(23): 13486-13490.

Bernard SA, Gray TW, Buist MD, Jones BM, Silvester W, Gutteridge G, Smith K. 2002. Treatment of comatose survivors of out-of-hospital cardiac arrest with induced hypothermia. *New England Journal of Medicine* 346(8): 557-563.

Blesch A, Tuszynski MH. 2004. Gene therapy and cell transplantation for Alzheimer's disease and spinal cord injury. *Yonsei Medical Journal* 45(Suppl): 28-31.

Blesch A, Conner JM, Tuszynski MH. 2001. Modulation of neuronal survival and axonal growth in vivo by tetracycline-regulated neurotrophin expression. *Gene Therapy* 8(12): 954-960.

Bomstein Y, Marder JB, Vitner K, Smirnov I, Lisaey G, Butovsky O, Fulga V, Yoles E. 2003. Features of skin-coincubated macrophages that promote recovery from spinal cord injury. *Journal of Neuroimmunology* 142(1-2): 10-16.

Bradbury EJ, Moon LD, Popat RJ, King VR, Bennett GS, Patel PN, Fawcett JW, McMahon SB. 2002. Chondroitinase ABC promotes functional recovery after spinal cord injury. *Nature* 416(6881): 636-640.

Brazelton TR, Rossi FM, Keshet GI, Blau HM. 2000. From marrow to brain: Expression of neuronal phenotypes in adult mice. *Science* 290(5497): 1775-1779.

Bricolo A, Ore GD, Da Pian R, Faccioli F. 1976. Local cooling in spinal cord injury. *Surgical Neurology* 6(2): 101-106.

Brines M, Grasso G, Fiordaliso F, Sfacteria A, Ghezzi P, Fratelli M, Latini R, Xie QW, Smart J, Su-Rick CJ, Pobre E, Diaz D, Gomez D, Hand C, Coleman T, Cerami A. 2004. Erythropoietin mediates tissue protection through an erythropoietin and common beta-subunit heteroreceptor. *Proceedings of the National Academy of Sciences (U.S.A.)* 101(41): 14907-14912.

Brosamle C, Huber AB, Fiedler M, Skerra A, Schwab ME. 2000. Regeneration of lesioned corticospinal tract fibers in the adult rat induced by a recombinant, humanized IN-1 antibody fragment. *Journal of Neuroscience* 20(21): 8061-8068.

Bunge MB. 2001. Bridging areas of injury in the spinal cord. *Neuroscientist* 7(4): 325-339.

Bunge MB, Wood PM. 2004. Transplantation of Schwann cells and olfactory ensheathing cells to promote regeneration in the CNS. In: Selzer ME, Clarke S, Cohen LG, Dincan PW, Gage FH, eds. *Textbook of Neural Repair and Rehabilitation.* Cambridge, United Kingdom: Cambridge University Press.

Cai D, Shen Y, De Bellard M, Tang S, Filbin MT. 1999. Prior exposure to neurotrophins blocks inhibition of axonal regeneration by MAG and myelin via a cAMP-dependent mechanism. *Neuron* 22(1): 89-101.

Carter DA, Bray GM, Aguayo AJ. 1989. Regenerated retinal ganglion cell axons can form well-differentiated synapses in the superior colliculus of adult hamsters. *Journal of Neuroscience* 9(11): 4042-4050.

Celik M, Gokmen N, Erbayraktar S, Akhisaroglu M, Konakc S, Ulukus C, Genc S, Genc K, Sagiroglu E, Cerami A, Brines M. 2002. Erythropoietin prevents motor neuron apoptosis and neurologic disability in experimental spinal cord ischemic injury. *Proceedings of the National Academy of Sciences (U.S.A.)* 99(4): 2258-2263.

Chau CH, Shum DK, Li H, Pei J, Lui YY, Wirthlin L, Chan YS, Xu XM. 2004. Chondroitinase ABC enhances axonal regrowth through Schwann cell-seeded guidance channels after spinal cord injury. *FASEB Journal* 18(1): 194-196.

Chotard C, Salecker I. 2004. Neurons and glia: Team players in axon guidance. *Trends in Neurosciences* 27(11): 655-661.

Chudler. 2004. *Lights, Camera, Action Potential.* [Online]. Available: http://faculty.washington.edu/chudler/ap.html [accessed August 12, 2004].

Conner JM, Darracq MA, Roberts J, Tuszynski MH. 2001. Non-tropic actions of neurotrophins: Subcortical NGF gene delivery reverses age-related degeneration of primate cortical cholinergic innervation. *Proceedings of the National Academy of Sciences (U.S.A.)* 98(4): 1941-1946.

Craner MJ, Hains BC, Lo AC, Black JA, Waxman SG. 2004a. Co-localization of sodium channel $Na_v1.6$ and the sodium-calcium exchanger at sites of axonal injury in the spinal cord in EAE. *Brain* 127(2): 294-303.

Craner MJ, Newcombe J, Black JA, Hartle C, Cuzner ML, Waxman SG. 2004b. Molecular changes in neurons in multiple sclerosis: Altered axonal expression of $Na_v1.2$ and $Na_v1.6$ sodium channels and $Na^+/Ca2^+$ exchanger. *Proceedings of the National Academy of Sciences (U.S.A.)* 101(21): 8168-8173.

David S, Aguayo AJ. 1981. Axonal elongation into peripheral nervous system "bridges" after central nervous system injury in adult rats. *Science* 214(4523): 931-933.

Devon R, Doucette R. 1992. Olfactory ensheathing cells myelinate dorsal root ganglion neurites. *Brain Research* 589(1): 175-179.

Di Giovanni S, Knoblach SM, Brandoli C, Aden SA, Hoffman EP, Faden AI. 2003. Gene profiling in spinal cord injury shows role of cell cycle in neuronal death. *Annals of Neurology* 53(4): 454-468.

Diaz-Ruiz A, Rios C, Duarte I, Correa D, Guizar-Sahagun G, Grijalva I, Ibarra A. 1999. Cyclosporin-A inhibits lipid peroxidation after spinal cord injury in rats. *Neuroscience Letters* 266(1): 61-64.

Diaz-Ruiz A, Rios C, Duarte I, Correa D, Guizar-Sahagun G, Grijalva I, Madrazo I, Ibarra A. 2000. Lipid peroxidation inhibition in spinal cord injury: Cyclosporin-A vs methylprednisolone. *Neuroreport* 11(8): 1765-1767.

Dietrich WD, Alonso O, Busto R, Globus MY, Ginsberg MD. 1994. Post-traumatic brain hypothermia reduces histopathological damage following concussive brain injury in the rat. *Acta Neuropathologica (Berlin)* 87(3): 250-258.

Dimar JR, Glassman SD, Raque GH, Zhang YP, Shields CB. 1999. The influence of spinal canal narrowing and timing of decompression on neurologic recovery after spinal cord contusion in a rat model. *Spine* 24(16): 1623-1633.

Dimar JR, Shields CB, Zhang YP, Burke DA, Raque GH, Glassman SD. 2000. The role of directly applied hypothermia in spinal cord injury. *Spine* 25(18): 2294-2302.

Dobkin BH, Havton LA. 2004. Basic advances and new avenues in therapy of spinal cord injury. *Annual Review of Medicine* 55: 255-282.

Drapeau J, El-Helou V, Clement R, Bel-Hadj S, Gosselin H, Trudeau LE, Villeneuve L, Calderone A. 2004. Nestin-expressing neural stem cells identified in the scar following myocardial infarction. *Journal of Cell Physiology*. [Online]. Available: http://www3.interscience.wiley.com/cgi-bin/abstract/109858358/ABSTRACT [accessed February 27, 2005]

Eldadah BA, Faden AI. 2000. Caspase pathways, neuronal apoptosis, and CNS injury. *Journal of Neurotrauma* 17(10): 811-829.

Fawcett JW, Asher RA. 1999. The glial scar and central nervous system repair. *Brain Research Bulletin* 49(6): 377-391.

Fournier AE, Takizawa BT, Strittmatter SM. 2003. Rho kinase inhibition enhances axonal regeneration in the injured CNS. *Journal of Neuroscience* 23(4): 1416-1423.

Fujiwara Y, Tanaka N, Ishida O, Fujimoto Y, Murakami T, Kajihara H, Yasunaga Y, Ochi M. 2004. Intravenously injected neural progenitor cells of transgenic rats can migrate to the injured spinal cord and differentiate into neurons, astrocytes and oligodendrocytes. *Neuroscience Letters* 366(3): 287-291.

Gage FH. 2000. Mammalian neural stem cells. *Science* 287(5457): 1433-1438.

Geller HM, Fawcett JW. 2002. Building a bridge: Engineering spinal cord repair. *Experimental Neurology* 174(2): 125-136.

GrandPre T, Li S, Strittmatter SM. 2002. Nogo-66 receptor antagonist peptide promotes axonal regeneration. *Nature* 417(6888): 547-551.

Grill R, Murai K, Blesch A, Gage FH, Tuszynski MH. 1997. Cellular delivery of neurotrophin-3 promotes corticospinal axonal growth and partial functional recovery after spinal cord injury. *Journal of Neuroscience* 17(14): 5560-5572.

Gris D, Marsh DR, Oatway MA, Chen Y, Hamilton EF, Dekaban GA, Weaver LC. 2004. Transient blockade of the Cd11d/Cd18 integrin reduces secondary damage after spinal cord injury, improving sensory, autonomic, and motor function. *Journal of Neuroscience* 24(16): 4043-4051.

Hansebout RR, Tanner JA, Romero-Sierra C. 1984. Current status of spinal cord cooling in the treatment of acute spinal cord injury. *Spine* 9(5): 508-511.

Hauben E, Butovsky O, Nevo U, Yoles E, Moalem G, Agranov E, Mor F, Leibowitz-Amit R, Pevsner E, Akselrod S, Neeman M, Cohen IR, Schwartz M. 2000. Passive or active immunization with myelin basic protein promotes recovery from spinal cord contusion. *Journal of Neuroscience* 20(17): 6421-6430.

Hayes KC, Potter PJ, Hsieh JT, Katz MA, Blight AR, Cohen R. 2004. Pharmacokinetics and safety of multiple oral doses of sustained-release 4-aminopyridine (fampridine-SR) in subjects with chronic, incomplete spinal cord injury. *Archives of Physical Medicine and Rehabilitation* 85(1): 29-34.

Hendriks WTJ, Ruitenberg MJ, Blits B, Boer GJ, Verhaagen J. 2004. Viral vector-mediated gene transfer of neurotrophins to promote regeneration of the injured spinal cord. *Progress in Brain Research* 146: 451-476.

Hindges R, McLaughlin T, Genoud N, Henkemeyer M, O'Leary DD. 2002. EphB forward signaling controls directional branch extension and arborization required for dorsal-ventral retinotopic mapping. *Neuron* 35(3): 475-487.

Holmes TC. 2002. Novel peptide-based biomaterial scaffolds for tissue engineering. *Trends in Biotechnology* 20(1): 16-21.

Hulsebosch CE. 2002. Recent advances in pathophysiology and treatment of spinal cord injury. *Advances in Physiology Education* 26(1-4): 238-255.

Hypothermia After Cardiac Arrest Study Group. 2002. Mild therapeutic hypothermia to improve the neurologic outcome after cardiac arrest. *New England Journal of Medicine* 346(8): 549-556.

Inamasu J, Nakamura Y, Ichikizaki K. 2003. Induced hypothermia in experimental traumatic spinal cord injury: An update. *Journal of the Neurological Sciences* 209(1-2): 55-60.

Jiang J, Yu M, Zhu C. 2000. Effect of long-term mild hypothermia therapy in patients with severe traumatic brain injury: 1-year follow-up review of 87 cases. *Journal of Neurosurgery* 93(4): 546-549.

Jones LL, Oudega M, Bunge MB, Tuszynski MH. 2001. Neurotrophic factors, cellular bridges and gene therapy for spinal cord injury. *Journal of Physiology (London)* 533(1): 83-89.

Judson HF. 2005. The Problematic Dr. Huang Hongyun. *Technology Review* 5(1): 1-5.

Kaminska B, Gaweda-Walerych K, Zawadzka M. 2004. Molecular mechanisms of neuroprotective action of immunosuppressants—Facts and hypotheses. *Journal of Cellular & Molecular Medicine* 8(1): 45-58.

Keino-Masu K, Masu M, Hinck L, Leonardo ED, Chan SS, Culotti JG, Tessier-Lavigne M. 1996. Deleted in colorectal cancer (DCC) encodes a netrin receptor. *Cell* 87(2): 175-185.

Keirstead SA, Rasminsky M, Fukuda Y, Carter DA, Aguayo AJ, Vidal-Sanz M. 1989. Electrophysiologic responses in hamster superior colliculus evoked by regenerating retinal axons. *Science* 246(4927): 255-257.

Kida Y, Takano H, Kitagawa H, Tsuji H. 1994. Effects of systemic or spinal cord cooling on conductive spinal evoked potentials. *Spine* 19(3): 341-345.

Kim JE, Li S, GrandPre T, Qiu D, Strittmatter SM. 2003. Axon regeneration in young adult mice lacking Nogo-A/B. *Neuron* 38(2): 187-199.

Kocsis JD, Akiyama Y, Lankford KL, Radtke C. 2002. Cell transplantation of peripheral-myelin-forming cells to repair the injured spinal cord. *Journal of Rehabilitation Research & Development* 39(2): 287-298.

Kocsis JD, Akiyama Y, Radtke C. 2004. Neural precursors as a cell source to repair the demyelinated spinal cord. *Journal of Neurotrauma* 21(4): 441-449.

Kodama S, Davis M, Faustman DL. 2005. Diabetes and stem cell researchers turn to the lowly spleen. *Science of Aging Knowledge Environment*. [Online]. Available: http://sageke.sciencemag.org/cgi/content/full/2005/3/pe2 [accessed February 27, 2005].

Koeberle PD, Bahr M. 2004. Growth and guidance cues for regenerating axons: Where have they gone? *Journal of Neurobiology* 59(1): 162-180.

Kondo T, Reaume AG, Huang TT, Carlson E, Murakami K, Chen SF, Hoffman EK, Scott RW, Epstein CJ, Chan PH. 1997. Reduction of CuZn-superoxide dismutase activity exacerbates neuronal cell injury and edema formation after transient focal cerebral ischemia. *Journal of Neuroscience* 17(11): 4180-4189.

Koons DD, Gildenberg PL, Dohn DF, Henoch M. 1972. Local hypothermia in the treatment of spinal cord injuries. Report of seven cases. *Cleveland Clinic Quarterly* 39(3): 109-117.

Krenz NR, Weaver LC. 2000. Nerve growth factor in glia and inflammatory cells of the injured rat spinal cord. *Journal of Neurochemistry* 74(2): 730-739.

Lea PM, Faden AI. 2003. Modulation of metabotropic glutamate receptors as potential treatment for acute and chronic neurodegenerative disorders. *Drug News & Perspectives* 16(8): 513-522.

Leonardo ED, Hinck L, Masu M, Keino-Masu K, Ackerman SL, Tessier-Lavigne M. 1997. Vertebrate homologues of *C. elegans* UNC-5 are candidate netrin receptors. *Nature* 386(6627): 833-838.

Lev M. 2004, August 27. Fetal-cell surgery raises hopes, fears. A procedure that involves aborted fetuses is drawing spinal-injury patients from the U.S., but a lack of clinical trials concerns researchers. *Chicago Tribune*. p. C4.

Li S, Strittmatter SM. 2003. Delayed systemic Nogo-66 receptor antagonist promotes recovery from spinal cord injury. *Journal of Neuroscience* 23(10): 4219-4227.

Li Y, Field PM, Raisman G. 1997. Repair of adult rat corticospinal tract by transplants of olfactory ensheathing cells. *Science* 277(5334): 2000-2002.

Li Y, Field PM, Raisman G. 1998. Regeneration of adult rat corticospinal axons induced by transplanted olfactory ensheathing cells. *Journal of Neuroscience* 18(24): 10514-10524.

Liu S, Qu Y, Stewart TJ, Howard MJ, Chakrabortty S, Holekamp TF, McDonald JW. 2000. Embryonic stem cells differentiate into oligodendrocytes and myelinate in culture and after spinal cord transplantation. *Proceedings of the National Academy of Sciences (U.S.A.)* 97(11): 6126-6131.

Lu P, Jones LL, Snyder EY, Tuszynski MH. 2003. Neural stem cells constitutively secrete neurotrophic factors and promote extensive host axonal growth after spinal cord injury. *Experimental Neurology* 181(2): 115-129.

Lu P, Yang H, Jones LL, Filbin MT, Tuszynski MH. 2004. Combinatorial therapy with neurotrophins and cAMP promotes axonal regeneration beyond sites of spinal cord injury. *Journal of Neuroscience* 24(28): 6402-6409.

Mabon PJ, Weaver LC, Dekaban GA. 2000. Inhibition of monocyte/macrophage migration to a spinal cord injury site by an antibody to the integrin alphaD: A potential new anti-inflammatory treatment. *Experimental Neurology* 166(1): 52-64.

Madsen JR, MacDonald P, Irwin N, Goldberg DE, Yao GL, Meiri KF, Rimm IJ, Stieg PE, Benowitz LI. 1998. Tacrolimus (FK506) increases neuronal expression of GAP-43 and improves functional recovery after spinal cord injury in rats. *Experimental Neurology* 154(2): 673-683.

Malouf NN, Coleman WB, Grisham JW, Lininger RA, Madden VJ, Sproul M, Anderson PA. 2001. Adult-derived stem cells from the liver become myocytes in the heart in vivo. *American Journal of Pathology* 158(6): 1929-1935.

Marion DW, Penrod LE, Kelsey SF, Obrist WD, Kochanek PM, Palmer AM, Wisniewski SR, DeKosky ST. 1997. Treatment of traumatic brain injury with moderate hypothermia. *New England Journal of Medicine* 336(8): 540-546.

Marsala M, Galik J, Ishikawa T, Yaksh TL. 1997. Technique of selective spinal cord cooling in rat: Methodology and application. *Journal of Neuroscience Methods* 74(1): 97-106.

McDonald JW, Liu XZ, Qu Y, Liu S, Mickey SK, Turetsky D, Gottlieb DI, Choi DW. 1999. Transplanted embryonic stem cells survive, differentiate and promote recovery in injured rat spinal cord. *Nature Medicine* 5(12): 1410-1412.

McMahon SB, Armanini MP, Ling LH, Phillips HS. 1994. Expression and coexpression of Trk receptors in subpopulations of adult primary sensory neurons projecting to identified peripheral targets. *Neuron* 12(5): 1161-1171.

Menei P, Montero-Menei C, Whittemore SR, Bunge RP, Bunge MB. 1998. Schwann cells genetically modified to secrete human BDNF promote enhanced axonal regrowth across transected adult rat spinal cord. *European Journal of Neuroscience* 10(2): 607-621.

Mezey E, Chandross KJ, Harta G, Maki RA, McKercher SR. 2000. Turning blood into brain: Cells bearing neuronal antigens generated in vivo from bone marrow. *Science* 290(5497): 1779-1782.

Mikami Y, Okano H, Sakaguchi M, Nakamura M, Shimazaki T, Okano HJ, Kawakami Y, Toyama Y, Toda M. 2004. Implantation of dendritic cells in injured adult spinal cord results in activation of endogenous neural stem/progenitor cells leading to de novo neurogenesis and functional recovery. *Journal of Neuroscience Research* 76(4): 453-465.

Movsesyan VA, Stoica BA, Faden AI. 2004. mGLuR5 activation reduces beta-amyloid-induced cell death in primary neuronal cultures and attenuates translocation of cytochrome C and apoptosis-inducing factor. *Journal of Neurochemistry* 89(6): 1528-1536.

Muir KW, Lees KR. 2003. Excitatory amino acid antagonists for acute stroke. *Cochrane Database of Systematic Reviews* (3): CD001244.

NAS (National Academy of Sciences). 1997. *Curing Childhood Leukemia.* [Online]. Available: http://www.beyonddiscovery.org/includes/DBFile.asp?ID=80 [accessed November 11, 2004].

Negrin J Jr. 1975. Spinal cord hypothermia: Neurosurgical management of immediate and delayed post-traumatic neurologic sequelae. *New York State Journal of Medicine* 75(13): 2387-2392.

Neumann S, Bradke F, Tessier-Lavigne M, Basbaum AI. 2002. Regeneration of sensory axons within the injured spinal cord induced by intraganglionic cAMP elevation. *Neuron* 34(6): 885-893.

NIH (National Institutes of Health). 2004. *Clinical Trials.* [Online]. Available: http://www.clinicaltrials.gov [accessed August 18, 2004].

Nikulina E, Tidwell JL, Dai HN, Bregman BS, Filbin MT. 2004. The phosphodiesterase inhibitor rolipram delivered after a spinal cord lesion promotes axonal regeneration and functional recovery. *Proceedings of the National Academy of Sciences (U.S.A.)* 101(23): 8786-8790.

Nottingham S, Knapp P, Springer J. 2002. FK506 treatment inhibits caspase-3 activation and promotes oligodendroglial survival following traumatic spinal cord injury. *Experimental Neurology* 177(1): 242-251.

NRC (National Research Council). 2002. *Stem Cells and the Future of Regenerative Medicine.* Washington, DC: National Academy Press.

Orlic D, Kajstura J, Chimenti S, Jakoniuk I, Anderson SM, Li B, Pickel J, McKay R, Nadal-Ginard B, Bodine DM, Leri A, Anversa P. 2001. Bone marrow cells regenerate infarcted myocardium. *Nature* 410(6829): 701-705.

Pearse DD, Pereira FC, Marcillo AE, Bates ML, Berrocal YA, Filbin MT, Bunge MB. 2004. cAMP and Schwann cells promote axonal growth and functional recovery after spinal cord injury. *Nature Medicine* 10(6): 610-616.

Potter PJ, Hayes KC, Segal JL, Hsieh JT, Brunnemann SR, Delaney GA, Tierney DS, Mason D. 1998. Randomized double-blind crossover trial of fampridine-SR (sustained release 4-aminopyridine) in patients with incomplete spinal cord injury. *Journal of Neurotrauma* 15(10): 837-849.

Proneuron Biotechnologies. 2004. *ProCord—An Experimental Procedure for Spinal Cord Injuries.* [Online]. Available: http://www.proneuron.com/clinicalstudies%5Cindex.html [accessed November 11, 2004].

Qiao J, Hayes KC, Hsieh JT, Potter PJ, Delaney GA. 1997. Effects of 4-aminopyridine on motor evoked potentials in patients with spinal cord injury. *Journal of Neurotrauma* 14(3): 135-149.

Qiu J, Cai D, Dai H, McAtee M, Hoffman PN, Bregman BS, Filbin MT. 2002. Spinal axon regeneration induced by elevation of cyclic AMP. *Neuron* 34(6): 895-903.

Radtke C, Akiyama Y, Brokaw J, Lankford KL, Wewetzer K, Fodor WL, Kocsis JD. 2004. Remyelination of the nonhuman primate spinal cord by transplantation of H-transferase transgenic adult pig olfactory ensheathing cells. *FASEB Journal* 18(2): 335-337.

Raisman G. 2001. Olfactory ensheathing cells—Another miracle cure for spinal cord injury? *Nature Reviews Neuroscience* 2(5): 369-375.

Ramer MS, Priestley JV, McMahon SB. 2000. Functional regeneration of sensory axons into the adult spinal cord. *Nature* 403(6767): 312-316.

Ramer MS, Bishop T, Dockery P, Mobarak MS, O'Leary D, Fraher JP, Priestley JV, McMahon SB. 2002. Neurotrophin-3-mediated regeneration and recovery of proprioception following dorsal rhizotomy. *Molecular & Cellular Neurosciences* 19(2): 239-249.

Ramon-Cueto A, Plant GW, Avila J, Bunge MB. 1998. Long-distance axonal regeneration in the transected adult rat spinal cord is promoted by olfactory ensheathing glia transplants. *Journal of Neuroscience* 18(10): 3803-3815.

Ramon-Cueto A, Cordero MI, Santos-Benito FF, Avila J. 2000. Functional recovery of paraplegic rats and motor axon regeneration in their spinal cords by olfactory ensheathing glia. *Neuron* 25(2): 425-435.

Rapalino O, Lazarov-Spiegler O, Agranov E, Velan GJ, Yoles E, Fraidakis M, Solomon A, Gepstein R, Katz A, Belkin M, Hadani M, Schwartz M. 1998. Implantation of stimulated homologous macrophages results in partial recovery of paraplegic rats. *Nature Medicine* 4(7): 814-821.

Ray SK, Matzelle DD, Sribnick EA, Guyton MK, Wingrave JM, Banik NL. 2003. Calpain inhibitor prevented apoptosis and maintained transcription of proteolipid protein and myelin basic protein genes in rat spinal cord injury. *Journal of Chemical Neuroanatomy* 26(2): 119-124.

Richardson PM, McGuinness UM, Aguayo AJ. 1980. Axons from CNS neurons regenerate into PNS grafts. *Nature* 284(5753): 264-265.

Robertson CS, Foltz R, Grossman RG, Goodman JC. 1986. Protection against experimental ischemic spinal cord injury. *Journal of Neurosurgery* 64(4): 633-642.

Sahenk Z. 2003 (October 21). *Neurotrophin-3 Treatment Promotes Nerve Regeneration and Improvements in Sensory Function in Patients with CMT1A.* Paper presented at the 128th Annual Meeting of the American Neurological Association, San Francisco, CA.

Schnell L, Schwab ME. 1990. Axonal regeneration in the rat spinal cord produced by an antibody against myelin-associated neurite growth inhibitors. *Nature* 343(6255): 269-272.

Schwab ME. 2002. Increasing plasticity and functional recovery of the lesioned spinal cord. *Progress in Brain Research* 137: 351-359.

Schwab ME. 2004. Nogo and axon regeneration. *Current Opinion in Neurobiology* 14(1): 118-124.

Shi R, Blight AR. 1997. Differential effects of low and high concentrations of 4-aminopyridine on axonal conduction in normal and injured spinal cord. *Neuroscience* 77(2): 553-562.

Silva GA, Czeisler C, Niece KL, Beniash E, Harrington DA, Kessler JA, Stupp SI. 2004. Selective differentiation of neural progenitor cells by high-epitope density nanofibers. *Science* 303(5662): 1352-1355.

Silver J, Miller JH. 2004. Regeneration beyond the glial scar. *Nature Reviews Neuroscience* 5(2): 146-156.

Sivasankaran R, Pei J, Wang KC, Zhang YP, Shields CB, Xu XM, He Z. 2004. PKC mediates inhibitory effects of myelin and chondroitin sulfate proteoglycans on axonal regeneration. *Nature Neuroscience* 7(3): 261-268.

Smith LE. 2004. Bone marrow-derived stem cells preserve cone vision in retinitis pigmentosa. *Journal of Clinical Investigation* 114(6): 755-757.

Stichel CC, Hermanns S, Luhmann HJ, Lausberg F, Niermann H, D'Urso D, Servos G, Hartwig HG, Muller HW. 1999. Inhibition of collagen IV deposition promotes regeneration of injured CNS axons. *European Journal of Neuroscience* 11(2): 632-646.

Sugawara T, Chan PH. 2003. Reactive oxygen radicals and pathogenesis of neuronal death after cerebral ischemia. *Antioxidants & Redox Signaling* 5(5): 597-607.

Takami T, Oudega M, Bates ML, Wood PM, Kleitman N, Bunge MB. 2002. Schwann cell but not olfactory ensheathing glia transplants improve hindlimb locomotor performance in the moderately contused adult rat thoracic spinal cord. *Journal of Neuroscience* 22(15): 6670-6681.

Tator CH, Deecke L. 1973. Value of normothermic perfusion, hypothermic perfusion, and durotomy in the treatment of experimental acute spinal cord trauma. *Journal of Neurosurgery* 39(1): 52-64.

Teng YD, Lavik EB, Qu X, Park KI, Ourednik J, Zurakowski D, Langer R, Snyder EY. 2002. Functional recovery following traumatic spinal cord injury mediated by a unique polymer scaffold seeded with neural stem cells. *Proceedings of the National Academy of Sciences (U.S.A.)* 99(5): 3024-3029.

Teng YD, Choi H, Onario RC, Zhu S, Desilets FC, Lan S, Woodard EJ, Snyder EY, Eichler ME, Friedlander RM. 2004. Minocycline inhibits contusion-triggered mitochondrial cytochrome C release and mitigates functional deficits after spinal cord injury. *Proceedings of the National Academy of Sciences (U.S.A.)* 101(9): 3071-3076.

Uchida N, Buck DW, He D, Reitsma MJ, Masek M, Phan TV, Tsukamoto AS, Gage FH, Weissman IL. 2000. Direct isolation of human central nervous system stem cells. *Proceedings of the National Academy of Sciences (U.S.A.)* 97(26): 14720-14725.

van der Bruggen MA, Huisman HB, Beckerman H, Bertelsmann FW, Polman CH, Lankhorst GJ. 2001. Randomized trial of 4-aminopyridine in patients with chronic incomplete spinal cord injury. *Journal of Neurology* 248(8): 665-671.

Waxman SG. 2000. The neuron as a dynamic electrogenic machine: Modulation of sodium-channel expression as a basis for functional plasticity in neurons. *Philosophical Transactions of the Royal Society of London, Series B: Biological Sciences* 355(1394): 199-213.

Williams SK, Franklin RJ, Barnett SC. 2004. Response of olfactory ensheathing cells to the degeneration and regeneration of the peripheral olfactory system and the involvement of the neuregulins. *Journal of Comparative Neurology* 470(1): 50-62.

Xu XM, Guenard V, Kleitman N, Aebischer P, Bunge MB. 1995a. A combination of BDNF and NT-3 promotes supraspinal axonal regeneration into Schwann cell grafts in adult rat thoracic spinal cord. *Experimental Neurology* 134(2): 261-272.

Xu XM, Guenard V, Kleitman N, Bunge MB. 1995b. Axonal regeneration into Schwann cell-seeded guidance channels grafted into transected adult rat spinal cord. *Journal of Comparative Neurology* 351(1): 145-160.

Xu XM, Chen A, Guenard V, Kleitman N, Bunge MB. 1997. Bridging Schwann cell transplants promote axonal regeneration from both the rostral and caudal stumps of transected adult rat spinal cord. *Journal of Neurocytology* 26(1): 1-16.

Yandava BD, Billinghurst LL, Snyder EY. 1999. "Global" cell replacement is feasible via neural stem cell transplantation: Evidence from the dysmyelinated shiverer mouse brain. *Proceedings of the National Academy of Sciences (U.S.A.)* 96(12): 7029-7034.

Yang L, Li S, Hatch H, Ahrens K, Cornelius JG, Petersen BE, Peck AB. 2002. In vitro transdifferentiation of adult hepatic stem cells into pancreatic endocrine hormone-producing cells. *Proceedings of the National Academy of Sciences (U.S.A.)* 99(12): 8078-8083.

Yick LW, So KF, Cheung PT, Wu WT. 2004. Lithium chloride reinforces the regeneration-promoting effect of chondroitinase ABC on rubrospinal neurons after spinal cord injury. *Journal of Neurotrauma* 21(7): 932-943.

Yu CG, Jimenez O, Marcillo AE, Weider B, Bangerter K, Dietrich WD, Castro S, Yezierski RP. 2000. Beneficial effects of modest systemic hypothermia on locomotor function and histopathological damage following contusion-induced spinal cord injury in rats. *Journal of Neurosurgery: Spine* 93(1 Suppl): 85-93.

6

DEVELOPING NEW
THERAPEUTIC INTERVENTIONS:
FROM THE LABORATORY TO THE CLINIC

Moving from an experimental therapy in the laboratory to an approved treatment for patient use involves a prescribed series of steps that validate and ensure the safety and efficacy of the therapeutic intervention (Table 6-1). Although these steps in the drug and device development and approval process are time-consuming and expensive, they are designed and regulated to ensure patient safety.

This chapter discusses the challenges and opportunities involved in developing therapeutic interventions to treat spinal cord injuries. The chapter describes major steps along the research pipeline and discusses the issues involved in translating experimental therapies into clinical practice. Finally, the unique challenges of designing and implementing clinical trials of treatments and therapies for both acute and chronic spinal cord injuries and the tools needed to improve the efficiencies of clinical trials are discussed.

The development of new medications or devices that target a specific complication, such as preventing or reducing neuropathic pain, can take an average of 15 years (Quest for new cures, 2003; PhRMA, 2004a). It often takes at least 3 years, and often upwards of 7 years, for a potential therapeutic compound to be identified and for the preclinical research to be conducted. During this stage, potential therapies are tested, refined, and verified by using multiple in vitro and in vivo assessment assays. Once a likely intervention is identified, it moves through a set of clinical trials that examine the drug's safety and efficacy in humans (Table 6-1). Using statistical methods, researchers can analyze the results of each phase to identify differences between the outcomes displayed by the test population, which received an experimental therapy, and the outcomes of a control popula-

TABLE 6-1 The Research Pipeline

	Stage	Purpose	Average Time in Stage (years)	Test Population	Success Rate
Laboratory	Discovery and preclinical testing	File patent (20 yr); assess safety, biological activity, and formulations; and verify effectiveness	3 to 7	Laboratory and animal studies	5 of 5,000 (0.1%) compounds that are screened enter clinical trials
	File investigational new drug application (IND) with FDA				
Clinic	Phase I clinical trial	Determine safety and dosage	2 to 3	20 to 100 healthy volunteers	75% enter Phase II
	Phase II clinical trial	Evaluate effectiveness, look for side effects	2 to 4	100 to 500 volunteer patients	61.2% enter Phase III
	Phase III clinical trial	Confirm effectiveness, monitor adverse reactions from long-term use	1 to 4	1,000 to 5,000 volunteer patients	86.8% file NDA
	File new drug application (NDA) with FDA				
	FDA	Review process and approval	1 to 2		1 approved out of original 5,100 compounds (0.02 % overall success rate)
	Phase IV clinical trial	Additional postmarketing testing required by FDA			

SOURCE: Adapted from PhRMA (2004b); Quest for new cures (2003).

tion, which most often received a sham or a placebo treatment. If a clinical trial is designed and performed correctly, clinicians can use the results obtained with a limited number of participants to guide a treatment for an entire patient population (Matthew, 2001).

Phase I clinical trials are used to determine safety and an appropriate treatment dosage and regimen and, in some cases, are used to perform preliminary analysis of the biological activity of the intervention. Phase II and phase III clinical trials evaluate the efficacy of the new intervention and examine adverse effects in studies with larger populations. In the end, a novel drug that has entered a phase I clinical trial has only an approximately 30 to 40 percent chance of successfully completing a phase III clinical trial and being approved by the Food and Drug Administration (FDA) (Harding, 2004). Phase IV clinical trials are required by the FDA for additional analysis of long-term risks and benefits.

As described in Chapters 4 and 5, a range of approaches relating to the treatment of spinal cord injuries are being explored, including efforts to prevent or reduce the adverse consequences during the acute phase of the injury and combination strategies designed to remyelinate nerve fibers, promote nerve fiber growth, and prevent cell death. During the development and verification of new therapies, researchers and regulators make decisions regarding when the data are sufficient to indicate that the intervention is efficacious and safe and can move on to the next stage of the process. The challenge is to develop therapies in a timely fashion without undermining future scientific endeavors and, most importantly, without endangering patient safety.

CRITERIA FOR VALIDATING A NOVEL THERAPY

The spinal cord injury research community is making substantial progress in developing novel therapies that may soon be ready for clinical trials. However, many of the alternative therapies that individuals with spinal cord injuries are using are not recommended options or standards of care because they have not been proven to be safe and efficacious (see Appendix F). An overriding concern that arises when a researcher contemplates translating a successful laboratory therapy to the clinical setting is the extent of preclinical data needed to justify proceeding with testing in studies with humans (Ramer et al., 2000; Kleitman, 2004). A coordinated and methodical approach is needed to verify the safety and effectiveness of therapies and treatments that are proceeding through the research pipeline. A 2003 article published in the *Journal of Rehabilitation Research & Development* describes a set of criteria that should be considered before a treatment can enter into a clinical trial (Table 6-2) (Dietrich, 2003). To meet these criteria, the author recommends that a coordinated effort among the spinal cord injury research community be mobilized to quickly respond to new scientific findings. As discussed in detail in Chapter 7, an enhanced research infrastructure and network is needed to facilitate collaborative research efforts.

Verification of a Therapy's Preclinical Effectiveness in Replicated Studies with Animals

Preclinical testing provides data on whether a therapeutic intervention holds promise for the treatment of spinal cord injuries in humans. However, because the nature and severity of spinal cord injuries vary between individuals, a wide spectrum of behavioral and functional deficits exist, with no one outcome occurring among those with spinal cord injuries.

An emphasis on the replication of preclinical studies (replication studies) between laboratories is needed. Difficulties in getting replication studies

TABLE 6-2 Criteria for Drug Therapies Entering a Clinical Trial

- The therapeutic window is not unrealistically restrictive.
- The therapy improves both structural and functional outcomes.
- The study is clinically relevant and has been replicated in an independent laboratory.
- Improvements are seen in multiple animal models, with clinically relevant end points.
- Major findings are published in reputable peer-reviewed journals.
- The safety of the treatment has been confirmed.

SOURCE: Adapted from Dietrich, 2003.

published and concerns over constraints in meeting the needs of the sponsoring funding agencies may be among the reasons for the lack of replication studies. The spinal cord injury research community needs to embrace and encourage these studies, which can be incorporated into broader studies that not only replicate a previous study but also include novel elements in the experiment. The National Institute of Neurological Disorders and Stroke (NINDS) identified the need for these types of studies by establishing the Facilities of Research Excellence in Spinal Cord Injury (FOR-SCI) funding mechanism in 2002 (NINDS, 2002). The Miami Project to Cure Paralysis is one of the two recipients of a FOR-SCI contract and is conducting studies to review and replicate studies in the areas of neuroprotection and axonal regeneration after a spinal cord injury. The second FOR-SCI contract is with the Reeve-Irvine Research Center and stipulates a focus on interventions to promote regeneration in the chronic setting. Similar contracts should be established for replication studies in other areas of relevant research.

Furthermore, it is critical that research findings, including those from replication studies and studies with negative or inconclusive results, be published in peer-reviewed journals with details about the study design, quantitative end points, and statistical analyses (Dietrich, 2003). Not only should positive study conclusions be presented, but a forum also should be generated to enable peer review of negative conclusions, especially those pertaining to replication studies. These efforts would enable the scientific community to scrutinize the data and would provide information to the spinal cord injury patient population on the results of preclinical and clinical testing of all novel therapies.

Safety Concerns in Moving to Tests with Humans

The safety of human subjects is of paramount concern when decisions are made about when and how to test therapeutic interventions in studies with humans. International codes of ethics, including the Declaration of Helsinki (World Medical Association, 2004), indicate that before an experimental therapy is tried in humans, a high standard of consensus about the appropriateness of a therapy should be established in the scientific community through laboratory and animal experiments (Sugarman, 1999). In 2001, the American Society for Neural Transplantation and Repair developed a set of guidelines that recommend that safety studies be conducted in the best available model—or in the case of spinal cord injuries, multiple models—before the therapy is tested in humans (Redmond et al., 2001). Failure to do so can put the study subjects at undue risk. Specifically, animal models should be used to examine potential toxicities and harmful complications (Dietrich, 2003).

Furthermore, the safety and efficacy of a novel therapy in relation to those of the alternatives available in a particular situation must also be considered (Sugarman, 1999). If no treatments are available and the patient population has a life-threatening condition, bioethicists have argued that "it seems reasonable to pursue experimental alternatives that may be somehow unsafe" (Sugarman, 1999).

Additional bioethical criteria that need to be considered to ensure that it is appropriate to move an experimental therapy from the laboratory bench to clinical trials include the following (Dekkers and Boer, 2001; Sugarman and McKenna, 2003):

- the study should address an important research question that cannot be answered by use of an alternative study design;
- the scientific community has reached a consensus about the safety of the proposed experiment on the basis of the findings from preclinical studies;
- evidence that the intervention might ultimately be beneficial is sufficient;
- the clinical trial design is based on sound science and has minimal risks and maximal benefits, the outcomes are measurable and meaningful, and the selection of subjects is fair; and
- valid informed consent is obtained from each participant.

Concerns have been raised about the experimental therapies that are being requested and tried by individuals with spinal cord injuries, even though the interventions have not been assessed for safety and efficacy in

---

BOX 6-1
Experimental Olfactory Ensheathing Cell Implants

In recent years, more than 500 individuals with spinal cord injuries (including approximately 100 American patients) have been treated in Beijing, China, with an experimental therapy that involves surgically implanting olfactory ensheathing cells (see Chapter 5) above and below the site of injury (Lev, 2004). These individuals have been willing to spend more than $25,000 each for this procedure (Lev, 2004). Anecdotal reports relate that some individuals appear to regain partial function within days after the surgery, whereas other reports indicate that patients have severe infections shortly after the procedure (Huang et al., 2003; Lev, 2004).

The scientific community has not received reports on whether standard preclinical testing has been performed and whether outcomes assessment measures have been collected from every patient, and little is known about whether long-term follow-up is being conducted (Huang et al., 2003). It is therefore unclear to what extent individuals with spinal cord injuries regain function after the procedure. There is general agreement, including from the lead physician performing this procedure, that the improvement occurs too soon after surgery for it to be a direct result of the olfactory ensheathing cells, neuronal regeneration, or remyelination of the remaining neurons. The benefit may be attributable to decompression of the spinal cord, a placebo effect of the surgery, or an as yet unidentified mechanism. The mechanism of recovery needs to be further elucidated.

This procedure has raised many issues for individuals with spinal cord injuries and the research community. Individuals with spinal cord injuries argue that they should be able to make decisions regarding their own health. Many scientists and health care professionals are worried, however, that this is an invasive, costly, and potentially dangerous procedure that has not yet been validated (Lev, 2004).

A phase I clinical trial of this intervention is under way in Australia and, when it is completed, will provide a better understanding of the safety and efficacy of olfactory ensheathing cell transplants. Until the results of the clinical trials are obtained, however, the spinal cord injury community should be cautioned against receiving such therapies. As Rosenfeld and Gillett have noted, "[s]tem-cell-based technology offers amazing possibilities for the future . . . but [t]he experimental basis of stem-cell or OEC [olfactory ensheathing cell] transplantation should be sound before these techniques are applied to humans with spinal cord injury" (Rosenfeld and Gillett, 2004).

---

clinical trials (Box 6-1). Because of the devastating outcomes of a spinal cord injury, many individuals with such injuries are willing to try therapies that they think may have promise, even if there is the potential for adverse health effects. The challenge for the research community is to better inform individuals about clinical trials and to accelerate the development of interventions while carefully considering patient safety.

LESSONS LEARNED FROM PREVIOUS CLINICAL TRIALS OF SPINAL CORD INJURY INTERVENTIONS

Over the past 5 years, nearly 300 publications in peer-reviewed journals have elucidated the results of clinical trials of interventions for spinal cord injuries (see Appendix G). The majority of these trials are associated with therapies for chronic complications, particularly bowel and bladder problems, exercise and locomotion; spasticity and muscle control; and sexual function; and only a handful have assessed therapies for use during the acute phase of the injury (Figure 6-1). In addition, only a few large-scale phase II and III clinical trials have been conducted, in part because of the absence of therapies that are ready for that stage of the research process (Ellaway et al., 2004).

A 2004 review concluded that many of the most-cited clinical trials of interventions for spinal cord injuries had methodological limitations that hinder interpretation of their results and the ability to generalize their

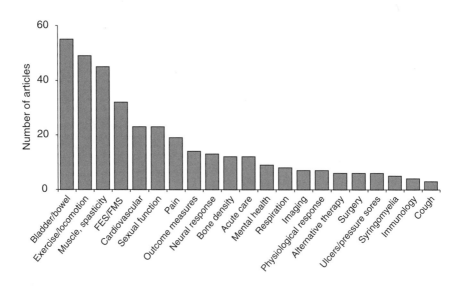

FIGURE 6-1 Publications on clinical trials for interventions for spinal cord injuries (1998 to 2003).
Multiple articles may result from the same clinical trial. A particular article may address multiple secondary conditions. As such, they are counted separately under each category. Abbreviations: FES = functional electrical stimulation; FMS = functional magnetic stimulation.

findings (Dobkin and Havton, 2004). In addition, as noted above, one of the issues raised in discussing clinical trials in this field is the use of alternative therapies that are highly experimental and that are not based on completed clinical trials or that are based on trials whose results are only putative (see Appendix F).

The International Spinal Research Trust (ISRT) recently asserted that continued advances in research laboratories will result in more experimental therapies being ready for clinical trials in the next few years. Furthermore, ISRT concluded that to meet this demand, new well-designed clinical trials that use novel tools to assess the effects of a treatment on the outcomes will need to be developed (Ellaway et al., 2004).

Useful lessons for future trials can be learned from the series of clinical trials that assessed the ability of methylprednisolone to improve the recovery of individuals after a spinal cord injury, including the original three National Acute Spinal Cord Injury Study (NASCIS) trials (Bracken et al., 1984, 1990, 1997) (see Appendix E). Although the authors of the NASCIS trials concluded that methylprednisolone should be a standard treatment for acute spinal cord injuries, many clinicians question its efficacy because of issues regarding the statistical analysis used to assess the improvements to the central nervous system and concern over adverse complications. The limitations of the studies in addressing some of the potential confounding variables may limit the extent to which the results of the studies can be generalized to all individuals with acute spinal cord injuries (Hanigan and Anderson, 1992; Bracken, 2000; Hurlbert, 2000; Dumont et al., 2001). For example, the NASCIS II trial did not include details about other interventions used (e.g., radiology, surgical manipulations, or the extent of rehabilitative therapies) that may have contributed to improvements or recovery (Hanigan and Anderson, 1992). Concerns have also been raised about the robustness of the statistical analysis and the heterogeneity of the injured population used in the studies, which made the baselines of the different populations difficult to compare (Bracken and Holford, 2002). Furthermore, although it was concluded that the NASCIS II and III trials were "well designed and well executed," post hoc analysis of these trials "failed to demonstrate improvement in primary outcome measures" (motor scores, pinprick scores, and light-touch scores) (Hurlbert, 2000). Consequently, it has been stated that the data describing improved recovery with methylprednisolone treatment are weak and that the improvements observed may represent random events (Hurlbert, 2000). Some have also suggested that it should not be a recommended treatment (Hurlbert, 2000). However, concerns about the potential legal ramifications of not using methylprednisolone may cause some physicians to continue to treat their patients with the medication. To strengthen future trials, it is important to learn from the experiences of the NASCIS studies and other similar studies.

CHALLENGES IN CONDUCTING CLINICAL TRIALS OF SPINAL CORD INJURY INTERVENTIONS

The emergency nature of the incidents that cause spinal cord injuries, the heterogeneity of the resulting injuries and functional limitations, the longitudinal time course, the absence of standardized outcome measures, and the diverse community and the small number of individuals who receive such injuries all contribute to unique challenges in designing and conducting clinical trials of interventions for the treatment of spinal cord injuries.

Obtaining Informed Consent for Acute-Care Clinical Trials

Immediately after a spinal cord injury the body triggers a cascade of responses that can further injure the spinal cord and cause additional complications (see Chapter 2). Many of these changes occur within the first few hours after the injury. For a treatment to be effective at preventing the majority of the complications that arise during the acute stage of the injury, it must be provided to a patient soon after the injury; this period of time is generally thought to be 8 hours (Clifton et al., 2002).

To ensure that a patient is fully aware of the potential benefits and hazards of participating in a clinical trial, federal regulations require that patients provide informed consent before the experimental treatment is initiated. For patients who do not have the capacity to give informed consent, legal proxy can be obtained from a family member or a guardian. Therefore, obtaining informed consent for most clinical trials that examine interventions in the chronic stage of spinal cord injury has not been a major hurdle. However, experimental interventions are being developed that will require clinical trials involving patients in an emergency setting who may be unable to provide informed consent.

However, obtaining informed consent in emergency-care situations has been fraught with challenges. In many cases, interventions need to be administered as soon as possible after the injury and there is no time to wait for a patient to recover sufficiently or for a legal proxy to be obtained (Smithline and Gerstle, 1998). In 1996, revisions to the federal informed-consent regulations were made to allow a limited waiver for informed consent in the case of clinical trials of emergency-care interventions or other similar situations (DHHS, 1996; Smithline and Gerstle, 1998; Clifton et al., 2002). The previous regulations allowed for a waiver of informed consent only if the patient would receive no more than a minimal additional risk by entering into the trial. In the new language, the definition of the risk of the research was changed to "reasonable in relation to what is known about the medical condition of the potential class of subjects" (DHHS, 1996).

This change in language has made a significant difference in the ability of clinical trials of emergency medical treatments to proceed.

An illustration of the need for careful consideration of the design of clinical trials for acute-care interventions is found in the National Acute Brain Injury Study: Hypothermia trial. That study, which was initiated in 1994, before the new waiver consent rules were implemented, examined whether cooling the brain to 33°C within 8 hours of the injury could prevent further secondary damage. No positive effect was found; however, the details of the study design demonstrated the need for timely waiver consent (Clifton et al., 2002). During the first 9 months of the study, on average, it took close to 12 hours to obtain informed consent, initiate the treatment, and achieve the target temperature. However, after the new regulations were passed and the study design was changed to include waiver of consent if a responsible family member could not be located within 1.5 hours after admission of the injured patient to the hospital, the average time dropped to 7.9 hours (Clifton et al., 2002). The authors argue that it would be "impractical and unjust to perform studies of acute brain injury without use of waiver consent when the treatment window is less than six hours" (Clifton et al., 2002). Many similar issues apply to clinical trials for the emergency treatment of spinal cord injuries, and informed-consent waiver guidelines should be developed and standardized for use in clinical trials of interventions for acute care for spinal cord injuries.

Challenges in Patient Recruitment

Clinical trials require an adequate number of participants to ensure that the study groups are representative of the larger patient population and to overcome the variations in results unrelated to the intervention (Pocock, 1983). Furthermore, it is important that the control groups be as homogeneous as possible so that valid comparisons can be made. The combination of these two requirements results in narrow eligibility criteria and, thus, can result in longer patient accrual times (NRC, 1993).

For example, when Acorda was recruiting individuals with spinal cord injuries for a phase III trial of 4-aminopyridine (fampridine), it was estimated that about 1,200 patients would have to be screened to locate 400 patients who met the broad eligibility requirements (inclusion criteria) for the study (Blight, 2004). This process can be much more difficult for trials that have stricter inclusion criteria. The number of potential patients is made even smaller because few individuals enroll in clinical trials. For example, according to the National Cancer Institute, only 2 to 3 percent of cancer patients are ever enrolled in clinical trials (IOM, 1999). It is not totally clear why these numbers are so low, even though the general population is increasingly aware of clinical trials. However, the eligibility requirements are often strict and many patients have concerns about sharing personal information with researchers.

As described throughout this report, individuals with spinal cord injuries are presented with countless challenges in their everyday lives that make it difficult for them to travel. Depending on the severity of the injury and the resources available in their communities, an individual's ability to travel independently may be further limited. Furthermore, for some individuals the travel necessary for participation in a clinical trial would be a significant expense. These challenges may limit the number of individuals available for a clinical trial, although there are opportunities to use existing regional patient care centers to facilitate access to clinical trials.

To increase the number of individuals with spinal cord injuries as potential clinical trial participants, health care professionals must be aware of ongoing clinical trials so that they can educate their patients about the available options and the benefits of participating in clinical trials. Efforts to increase the dissemination of information to both health care professionals and individuals with spinal cord injuries are needed.

Spontaneous Recovery Can Complicate Interpretation of Results

As discussed in Chapter 1, a small number of patients with incomplete injuries and paraplegia recover some function, particularly bowel and bladder function, usually within the first year after the injury (Maynard et al., 1979; Ditunno et al., 2000). Thus, the potential for the recovery of function that is not due to the intervention complicates the interpretation of clinical trial results and necessitates careful attention to the matching of a control group and the population receiving the intervention.

NEXT STEPS IN DESIGNING AND CONDUCTING CLINICAL TRIALS

Although investigators performing clinical trials of interventions for spinal cord injuries are presented with unique challenges, many tools and techniques can be used to maximize participation and improve data analysis.

Utilize Statistical Methodologies for Addressing Small Numbers of Patients and Heterogeneity of Outcomes

The limited number of individuals who qualify for clinical trials of interventions for spinal cord injuries and the heterogeneity of the nature and the severity of their injuries make it difficult to conduct multiple large-scale, randomized, controlled clinical trials. Furthermore, for studies that examine cell- or gene-based interventions, standard research designs—which often require large numbers of research participants to achieve adequate statistical power—may not always be possible or appropriate. Therefore, clinical trials may need to be performed with a small sample of patients (small "*n*" trials). Depending on the clinical end points and the magnitude of the effects desired, a small "*n*" trial may involve only a few patients or as many as 100 patients. Statistical methodologies (e.g., sequential analysis, hierarchical models, Bayesian analysis, and decision analysis) can be used to provide substantial evidence of efficacy in studies with small sample sizes (Table 6-3) (IOM, 2001). If it is necessary to perform a clinical trial with a small population of participants, a recent Institute of Medicine (IOM) report (2001) recommended that the following steps be followed:

- clearly define the research question;
- tailor the study design by giving careful consideration to alternative methods and involve statisticians early in the design process;
- clarify sample characteristics and methods for reporting the results of clinical trials with small sample sizes;
- perform corroborative analyses to evaluate the consistency and robustness of the results; and
- exercise caution in the interpretation of the results before attempting to extrapolate or generalize the findings.

The use of small "*n*" methodologies can be especially useful for phase I clinical trials that investigate the safety and dosage of new medications or

TABLE 6-3 Appropriate Contexts in Which to Consider a Clinical Trial with a Small Population

Context	Example
A new drug or procedure will be used for the first time in human subjects.	A traditional phase I study may be used to determine the maximum tolerated dose of a new drug.
The number of subjects available for study is extremely limited.	The investigator wishes to study changes in bone mineral density in astronauts during extended stays in space.
The study population is small, isolated, or unique.	The investigator is studying health outcomes unique to a small isolated tribe or in patients with a rare disease.

SOURCE: IOM, 2001.

devices in studies with a small number of patients. Phase II and phase III clinical trials can be performed with small samples of patients, but they usually involve larger sample sizes. As stated in the recent IOM report, "[a] small clinical trial often guides the design of a subsequent trial. Therefore, a key question will be what information from the current trial will be of greatest value in designing the next one?" (IOM, 2001). Many of these methodologies have not been field tested in situations typical of spinal cord injury clinical trials; therefore, it may be appropriate to develop a research initiative to gather experienced clinical trialists to provide recommendations on how small "n" clinical trials could be effectively applied to spinal cord injury clinical trials.

Clinical trials of neuroprostheses provide examples of trials that use a relatively small number of subjects to provide a statistically significant result. These trials are characterized by outcomes that are often clear and immediate. Furthermore, as demonstrated by the examples in Box 6-2, the subject can serve as his or her own control. This allows the outcomes obtained postoperatively with the neuroprosthesis off and on to be compared with the individual's performance before implementation of the neuroprosthesis. Study designs for clinical trials of neuroprostheses can therefore be successful with only a small number of subjects, and FDA has considered this type of study design to be acceptable in the steps leading to the premarketing approval of neuroprostheses.

Increasing Clinicians' Expertise in Conducting Clinical Trials

Designing, implementing, and conducting a large-scale clinical trial that has adequate controls and that can provide statistically significant outcomes data require health care professionals who are well trained in clinical trial methodology. This ensures that the therapies are administered in an appropriately controlled fashion, that surveys are properly conducted, and that the findings of the surveys and outcome measures are properly assessed. NINDS has recently recognized the need to provide intensive training in this area and is in the process of developing a course for clinical fellows and junior faculty in neurology or a neurosurgical subspecialty on the principles of clinical trial methodologies for neurology research.

Use of Multicenter Trials and Centralized Institutional Review Boards

In an effort to maximize the number of participants who can qualify for a trial, many large-scale clinical trials are designed by creating collaborative efforts between multiple research centers and trauma hospitals (Box 6-3). However, multicenter trials are costly and can be difficult to implement (NRC, 1993). Furthermore, a careful study design, careful study implemen-

---

BOX 6-2
Clinical Trials of Neuroprostheses That Use
Small Numbers of Patients

Clinical trials of neuroprostheses can be designed so that a small number of patients can provide the information needed to provide proof of the efficacy of the prosthesis. The individual's performance before use of the neuroprosthesis can be compared with the individual's postoperative performance with the neuroprosthesis off and on. Studies are performed to assess the changes in performance over time to ensure the stable performance of the neuroprosthesis (a minimum of 12 months).

A trial to examine a system for restoring hand grasp and release in people with C5-C6 tetraplegia assessed outcomes in each of three domains: impairment, disability, and handicap (Peckham et al., 2001). The hypothesis was that the person would have improvements in strength and range of motion of the hand (impairment measures); ability to grasp more objects in a standard pick-and-place test (disability measure); and ability to perform more activities of daily living (handicap measure). The protocol called for preoperative measurement of performance and postoperative measurement of performance with the neuroprosthesis off and on. Power analysis predicted that statistical significance would be achieved with less than 20 subjects, because the impact of the intervention was a significant restoration of capabilities when the device was on compared with the individual's capabilities (nearly no function) in either the preoperative state or in the postoperative state with the device off. FDA allowed the application for premarketing approval to be submitted with less than 30 subjects.

In a second clinical trial of a bladder neuroprosthesis, the individual's performance was determined in the same three states described above: preoperatively and postoperatively with the prosthesis off and on (Creasey et al., 2001). A similar power analysis predicted that the study would achieve statistical significance with less than 20 subjects, and this was achieved for the primary outcome measure of the amount of residual urine in the bladder. Additional secondary measures were also evaluated.

---

tation, and proper training of the participating physicians and nurses are required to ensure that the same standards of care and assessment are provided to each participant, regardless of where they receive the treatment being evaluated in the trial.

One large hurdle for multicenter trials has been the necessity of receiving the approval of the institutional review board (IRB) of each of the many research centers participating in the trial. The responsibility of the IRB is to ensure that human subjects are protected from all unnecessary harms associated with the study; however, for those responsible for conducting a multicenter trial, the task of obtaining IRB approval from multiple institutions is often time-consuming and cumbersome. As a solution to this problem, central IRBs began receiving accreditation in 2003. The

---

BOX 6-3
Corticosteroids for the Treatment of Head Injury:
The Role of Large-Scale, Randomized Clinical Trials

For more than 30 years, corticosteroids, including methylprednisolone, have been used to treat head injuries. Corticosteroids were given to patients to help control posttraumatic inflammatory changes, which are believed to contribute to neuronal degeneration. The use of this treatment was based on randomized clinical trials that included no more than a few hundred patients in each trial and a total of approximately 2,000 patients (Roberts et al., 2004). Meta-analysis of these trials suggested that the absolute risk of death in the corticosteroid-treated groups was about 1 to 2 percent lower than that for the controls (Alderson and Roberts, 1997).

To confirm this benefit, researchers initiated the corticosteroid randomization after significant head injury (CRASH) trial. The CRASH trial included close to 20,000 patients who were recruited from more than 239 hospitals in 49 countries. The levels of coordination and integration of the data required in this trial are a model for future large multicenter trials. The CRASH trial analyzed the effects of early administration of a 48-hour infusion of methylprednisolone on the risk of death and disability after a head injury (Roberts et al., 2004). The CRASH trial found that the risk of death from all causes within 2 weeks of treatment was 3 percent higher in patients taking the corticosteroids than in those receiving a placebo.

This study has two major limitations. First, the data were based on 2 weeks of follow-up data. The 6-month follow-up data have not yet been published. Second, the main cause of death was not noted; therefore, it is not known how many of the deaths were specifically due to the corticosteroid treatment.

This study demonstrates the potential hazards of establishing treatments when a large randomized clinical trial has not been performed. As commented in an editorial published with the article, "[t]he key message of CRASH, however, is that applying treatments with unproven effectiveness is like flying blindly. In the future, we should avoid trusting in underpowered clinical trials with surrogate rather than clinical endpoints, and transferring evidence from one disease to another" (Sauerland and Maegele, 2004).

---

private-industry sponsors of clinical trials prefer to use central IRBs for multicenter clinical trials, because a single process of review and approval can be used and the average time required to obtain approval is reduced (Loh and Meyer, 2004). However, the results of a survey of 125 major medical schools in the United States found that concerns about institutional liability and the loss of local representation in the review process are detracting from the use of central IRBs (Loh and Meyer, 2004). To increase academic and industry collaborations and reduce the administrative burden on local IRBs, the National Cancer Institute (NCI) developed a pilot program, the NCI Central Institutional Review Board (CIRB), which conducts a complete review of the trial but also allows local IRBs to focus on the implementation and specific issues related to the local conduct of

> **BOX 6-4**
> **Synopsis of the National Cancer Institute**
> **Central Institutional Review Board Process**
>
> 1. The CIRB receives a completed application, protocol, informed-consent form, and related materials from the cooperative group conducting the clinical trial through NCI.
> 2. The full board conducts an initial review and approves the protocol.
> 3. After the protocol is activated by the cooperative group, all review documents are posted on a website for access by the participating institutions.
> 4. A local investigator at a participating institution decides to enroll subjects in a CIRB-approved protocol. Either the investigator or the local IRB downloads the application packet to facilitate review.
> 5. The local IRB chair or subcommittee conducts a facilitated review, concentrating on issues specific to the local context.
> 6. The local IRB notifies the CIRB administrative office through the website of its acceptance of the protocol.
> 7. The CIRB becomes the IRB of record for the protocol and is responsible for continuing review as well as review of subsequent amendments and any serious adverse events reported by the individual centers performing the trial.
> 8. The local IRB is responsible for reviewing serious adverse events that occur locally and oversight of the local conduct of the study.
>
> SOURCE: Adapted from NCI, 2004.

the study (Box 6-4). This model system could be expanded for use in multicenter clinical trials in areas of research other than cancer, including spinal cord injury research.

Coordination of Care and Cure Efforts

It is important that ongoing efforts related to patient care and rehabilitation after a spinal cord injury be coordinated with efforts in developing therapeutic interventions for spinal cord injuries. A number of sites and systems can be used to conduct clinical trials of interventions for spinal cord injuries. The Model Spinal Cord Injury Systems of Care, funded by the National Institute on Disability and Rehabilitation Research (see Chapter 7), offers the resources of 16 hospitals and rehabilitation centers across the country with a known patient base and the staff and facilities that could be enlisted to conduct clinical trials. The resources of the Model Spinal Cord Injury Systems of Care have been used to conduct clinical trials of the drugs 4-aminopyridine (fampridine) and sildenafil (Viagra) (Northwest Regional Spinal Cord Injury System, 2000). In addition, most major hospital centers and health maintenance organizations also have rehabilitation and treatment centers and unique patient registry resources. The U.S. Department of Veterans Affairs (VA) Spinal Cord Injury Service is another extensive resource with a large patient population and health care professionals with clinical expertise in rehabilitation medicine. VA, which has a number of clinics throughout the United States, has an already established infrastructure that could be used to help clinical trial administrators educate and recruit members of the community into clinical trials. Furthermore, VA has a Cooperative Studies Program to promote clinical trials throughout the VA health care system.

Standardization of Clinical Trial Outcome Measures

Currently, clinicians have more than 30 assessment tests and surveys that they can use to examine individuals with spinal cord injuries and assess their progress toward recovery (Table 6-4; see also Appendix D). Each of the individual measures in these tests and surveys focuses on a specific area of function or quality of life. However, a standard set of outcome measures is not available. This is particularly problematic in multicenter clinical trials, in which data from multiple centers must be compared to determine the efficacy of a treatment intervention. Furthermore, a single assessment scale that could provide a standardized rating of the severity of an injury and assess an individual's progress toward recovery would be useful for researchers, clinicians, and individuals with spinal cord injuries.

One of the most frequently used scales is the American Spinal Injury Association Impairment Scale, which measures the degree of paralysis and loss of sensation (Ditunno et al., 1994). This five-point scale scores the effect of an injury on the basis of muscle strength and the severity of loss of sensory function and has been widely adopted to establish a standardized language for describing an individual's spinal cord injury (Young, 2002) (see Chapter 2). However, the scale's minimal resolution prevents sensitivity to small but significant changes in function (NINDS, 2003; Ellaway et al., 2004). Furthermore, the scale is focused on motor function and does not address bowel, bladder, and other functional limitations and does not assess quality of life and activities of daily living.

There is a need to develop a common set of integrated outcome measures specifically designed to assess a patients' recovery and response to treatments and experimental therapies. The ISRT clinical initiative recommended a set of tests to ensure appropriate evaluation of the physiology of individuals with spinal cord injuries before and after treatments; however, this set has yet to be incorporated into a standard of care for all individuals with spinal cord injuries (Table 6-5). Five European spinal cord injury centers are collaborating to develop a standardized protocol for outcomes

TABLE 6-4 Tools to Assess Spinal Cord Injury in Humans

Functional recovery

American Spinal Injury Association (ASIA) International Standards for
Neurological Classification
- Analyzes the effect that the injury has on both motor and sensory systems
- Is based on the extent of injury and muscle strength
- Uses an alphabetical score from A (the most severe) to E (the least severe)
- Insensitive to small but significant changes in motor and sensory functions
- May not be sensitive enough to detect even several spinal levels of
  regeneration in thoracic injuries
- Does not specifically address functions that affect a patient's quality of life
- Does not assess pain, bowel, bladder, or sexual function

Functional Independence Measure (FIM)
- Is an 18-item, seven-level ordinal scale
- Is designed to assess areas of dysfunction in activities that commonly occur
- The scale has few cognitive, behavioral, and communication-related functional
  items
- Is not specific for spinal cord injuries but is designed to assess neurological,
  musculoskeletal, and other disorders

Functional Assessment Measure (FAM)
- Was developed to augment the FIM
- Specifically addresses functional areas that are relatively less emphasized in
  FIM, including cognitive, behavioral, communication, and community
  functioning measures
- The scale has few cognitive, behavioral, and communication-related functional
  items
- Is not specific for spinal cord injuries but is designed to assess neurological,
  musculoskeletal, and other disorders

Spinal Cord Independence Measure (SCIM)
- Is specifically designed to assess spinal cord injuries and to be sensitive to
  changes
- Analyzes self-care, respiration, and sphincter management and mobility
- Is more sensitive than FIM for spinal cord injuries

Electrophysiology
- Assesses MEPs or SSEP
- Stimulates corresponding cortical areas of the brain and records the response
  in target nerves to see if connections are still functional
- Is correlated to impairment of locomotor activity
- Is noninvasive
- Electrical activity may not coordinate with function
- Hard to assess subtle but critical improvements to circuitry
- Does not assess pain, bowel, bladder, or sexual function

Continued

TABLE 6-4 Continued

Quality of life

Activities of Daily Living (ADL)
- Measures basic tasks of everyday living
- Is used as a predictor of admission to nursing homes and hospitals
- Lots of variation, depending on which items are measured and how a disabling condition is classified

SF-12, SF-36, and SF-54
- Measure changes in quality of life, mental health, pain, and social function
- Reflect the individual's perceptions and preferences about physical, emotional, and social well-being
- Hard to detect changes in quality of life over time
- Questions about walking can be construed as offensive to individuals with spinal cord injuries

International Classification of Impairment, Disabilities, and Handicaps (ICIDH)
- Was designed by the World Health Organization to classify the consequences of disease and their implications on the patient's life
- Defines impairment, disabilities, and handicaps
- ICIDH-2 incorporates disability as a dynamic process and holds that environmental factors can influence the impairment

Needs Assessment Checklist (NAC)
- Is used as a rehabilitation outcome measure designed specifically for spinal cord injury population
- Uses a 4-point scale
- Consists of 199 behavioral indicators that assess patient achievement in nine categories required for maintenance of health and quality of living
- Is not subject to floor or ceiling effects

NOTE: MEPs = motor evoked potential; SSEP = somatosensory evoked potential.

assessment (Curt et al., 2004). In addition, the International Collaboration on Repair Discoveries (ICORD) has recently published a set of guidelines for clinical trials (ICORD, 2004) and is in the process of developing clinical outcome measures for each type of intervention.

Given the heterogeneity between individuals in terms of the types and severities of their spinal cord injuries (see Table 1-2 and Chapter 2), not only is a common set of outcome measures required, but an integrated rating scale for the assigned set of outcome measures should also be designed. This will improve efforts to define clinical trial end points, monitor the progression of an individual's treatment, and examine the effects of the treatment intervention on the multiple complications associated with a spinal cord injury.

TABLE 6-5 ISRT's Set of Standard Tests to Assess Patient Outcomes

- Conventional clinical and neurological assessments
- Dynamometry for appropriate muscles
- Tests for motor-evoked potential responses to transcranial magnetic stimulation
- Tests for reflexes in paraspinal muscles
- Quantitative sensory testing, including electrical sensory perceptual threshold
- Tests for sympathetic skin response

The heterogeneity of spinal cord injuries not only provides a reason for developing this scale but also presents challenges. These challenges can be addressed, however, by looking at similar rating scales that have been developed for other neurological disorders that have variable severities, including the Amyotrophic Lateral Sclerosis Functional Rating Scale (ALSFRS) and the Unified Parkinson's Disease Rating Scale (UPDRS). ALSFRS is used to assess 10 behaviors, including swallowing, speaking, and movement, by using four to five defined functional status end points for each behavior. For example, in the handwriting evaluation, the choices are

- normal;
- slow or sloppy, all words are legible;
- not all words are legible;
- able to grip pen but unable to write; and
- unable to grip pen.

UPDRS was developed in 1987 in response to the need for a rating scale that could monitor the longitudinal progression of Parkinson's disease (Fahn et al., 1987). Like ALSFRS, this scale includes groups of questions devoted to motor function, activities of daily living, and behavior and mood. The scale is used to quantify an individual's total disability and can be used to monitor the progression of the disease.

Currently, both the ISRT and the Christopher Reeve Paralysis Foundation are in the process of developing new assessment techniques for use in large-scale clinical trials of interventions for spinal cord injuries. Coordination and collaboration are needed to develop a standard set of assessment measures to ensure valid comparisons of data between these and other groups. This effort could benefit from a consensus conference, similar to the World Federation of Neurology Airlie House Therapeutic Trials in ALS workshop (Munsat, 1995), that could be sponsored by the New York State

Spinal Cord Injury Trust, to develop a set of outcome measures for spinal cord injury.

Ensuring Independent Evaluations

Investigator bias, either deliberate or unintended, can also significantly affect the interpretation of the results and analysis of the outcomes of clinical trials. Although independent peer review is designed to address these concerns, not every study, especially early-phase trials, enters peer review. Furthermore, reviewers are rarely given access to patients so that the reviewers can conduct their own evaluations, and the reviewers do not usually have access to the raw data from the study. Because of potential conflicts, it is important that evaluation of the findings from the trial be performed by unbiased coinvestigators or others researchers who were not part of the study. In response to concerns regarding patient safety, the policy of the National Institutes of Health requires that multisite clinical trials of interventions that may involve a risk to the participant establish a data safety monitoring board that is independent of IRBs and that is responsible for ensuring that the clinical trial is conducted with the highest regard for patient safety and ethical standards and to ensure the credibility of the clinical trial and the validity of the study results.

Increasing Industry Involvement

The level of investment in research and development on interventions for spinal cord injuries by the pharmaceutical and medical device industries is difficult to determine. A number of clinical trials of medications have focused on improving bowel, bladder, and sexual function (see Appendix G); and the Pharmaceutical Research and Manufacturers of America's New Medications in Development database indicates that a number of medications for alleviating neuropathic pain are in phase I and phase II clinical trials (PhRMA, 2004a).

The potential financial incentives for industry to invest in the research and development of interventions to treat spinal cord injuries may be limited for a number of reasons, including the following:

- Further research is needed on the basic mechanisms of neuronal injury and repair to target therapeutic approaches.
- Only recently have the science and experimental methodology reached the stage at which the screening of large numbers of candidate drugs and compounds is possible.
- Spinal cord injury is not a single outcome; rather, the types of

injuries vary, injury occurs at different locations on the spinal cord, and the severities of the injuries vary widely.

• Because of the relatively small numbers of potential patients—an estimated 247,000 people in the United States have a spinal cord injury, and an estimated 11,000 new cases occur each year—and because of the heterogeneity of the secondary complications, the population of individuals with spinal cord injuries is small and is further fragmented, making the market for medications and other therapeutic interventions for spinal cord injuries even smaller.

Additionally, a variety of other issues confront the development of any new therapeutic product:

• Financial costs. It is estimated that it costs an average of $800 million to go through the drug development and approval process from the identification of a drug target through FDA approval of an efficacious product (Tufts Center for the Study of Drug Development, 2001). The expense of launching a new drug is even more expensive, and the cost increased 55 percent from 1995 to 2002 (FDA, 2004b).

• Time. The drug and device development process is also very time-consuming. For example, it takes on average 12 to 15 years before a drug is ready to market to the general patient population. As a result, from the time that a compound is discovered and a 20-year patent is filed, it takes on average 17 to 18 years for a pharmaceutical company to recoup its costs.

• Competition. The therapy could be displaced by a newer and more effective treatment before the company realizes a profit.

One mechanism used to provide incentives to pharmaceutical companies is the Orphan Drug Act (P.L. 97-414). Signed into law in 1983 to stimulate the research, development, and approval of drugs for the treatment of rare diseases (defined as conditions that affect 200,000 people or less in the United States), the federal legislation provides two major incentive mechanisms: sponsors are granted 7 years of marketing exclusivity after approval of the orphan drug product, and sponsors receive tax incentives for clinical research on the product.

In 2004, 21 years since the legislation was enacted, only approximately 200 drugs and biological products have qualified for orphan drug status (FDA, 2004a). It is unclear whether the incentives provided by the Orphan Drug Act are sufficient to attract pharmaceutical industry investment in therapeutic interventions for spinal cord injuries. For diseases that affect more than 200,000 people, it is possible to obtain orphan drug status for interventions needed by certain patient subgroups for specific indications.

This has been the case for spinal cord injury; for example, Acorda was granted orphan drug status in developing the drug 4-aminopyridine (fampridine) to treat spasticity, since spasticity affects less than 200,000 individuals with chronic spinal cord injuries. In addition, Proneuron received orphan drug status for its autologous incubated macrophage therapy (Procord), which is designed to improve motor and sensory neurological outcomes in individuals with acute complete spinal cord injuries.

Some of the health outcomes of a spinal cord injury—such as spasticity, chronic pain, and pressure sores—also affect individuals with other diseases and conditions. The existence of these larger markets offers a potentially greater incentive for the private sector to invest in research and development. For example, medications to alleviate spasticity would benefit not only individuals with spinal cord injuries but also individuals with multiple sclerosis. This is especially compelling for interventions for the alleviation of pressure sores, a chronic problem affecting many elderly and bed-ridden patients.

To increase the amount of industry investment in spinal cord injury research, mechanisms need to be developed to provide incentives and overcome impediments. Public-private partnerships, joint postdoctoral internships between industry and academia, and other mechanisms that would facilitate collaborative efforts and move the science closer to clinical applications should be explored. As an initial step in this process, a conference or workshop is needed to bring together the relevant stakeholders to discuss current barriers and develop collaborative approaches and incentives. One topic could be modifying the standards used to obtain "orphan" status to be based on the percentage of the United States population affected by the disease or disorder rather than the total number of affected individuals. Discussions are needed among the range of stakeholders in the development of new therapeutics for spinal cord injuries, including federal and state health agencies; professional societies in neuroscience and clinical medicine; academic institutions; basic and clinical researchers; and biotechnology, medical device, and pharmaceutical companies.

Coordination and Expansion of Spinal Cord Injury Registries and Databases

Registries are online systems for storing and relating information about individuals (Box 6-5). A population-based spinal cord injuries registry would collect standardized information on the incidence, type, and causes of spinal cord injuries for a geographically defined population, including spinal cord injury mortality among cases not seen or admitted for hospital care. This information would allow greater insights into how spinal cord injuries might be prevented but would be of limited use in the development

BOX 6-5
Model Patient Registries

The Center for International Blood and Marrow Transplant Research administers a database of clinical information on recipients of blood and bone marrow transplants that includes data on patients throughout the treatment process, beginning with the time of diagnosis and continuing through all subsequent phases: the time of administration of chemotherapy, the phase of decision making to perform a transplant, the time that the patient receives high-dose myeloablative therapy, the time that the patient is reinfused with stem cells, the immediate posttransplantation period, the complications that occur immediately posttransplantation, and eventually, the posttransplantation outcomes, such as disease remission. As is the case for spinal cord injury clinical trials, relatively few patients are eligible for clinical trials of bone marrow transplants. In addition to collecting data from an international network of transplant centers, the registry facilitates multicenter collaborations among the researchers and clinicians at those centers. They disseminate information to physicians, patients, researchers in other fields, and the general public. University researchers and pharmaceutical companies also use the data in the database as control groups, although they are charged for use of the data. In addition, the registry has a contract with the National Marrow Donor Program to oversee patient advocacy.

The Consortium of Multiple Sclerosis Centers established The North American Research Consortium on Multiple Sclerosis (NARCOMS): Multiple Sclerosis Patient Registry in 1993 to speed the development of new therapies and health care services by facilitating research on multiple sclerosis and reducing the time and cost of research studies. The registry is a database consisting of functional, accessible information that investigators use to develop research strategies and survey issues related to multiple sclerosis. As of June 2004, the number of registry participants reached more than 24,000. Online enrollment has recently become available for this registry. The availability of the website has made it easier and faster for participants to enroll. The goal of the registry is to develop a computerized database with 35,000 participants who will be monitored over time by the use of semiannual updates.

In 1973 the National Cancer Institute initiated the Surveillance, Epidemiology, and End Results (SEER) Program, which currently collects and publishes cancer incidence and survival data from 14 population-based cancer registries. Included in the SEER database is information on more than 3 million cancer cases, and approximately 170,000 new cases are added each year. Since the inception of the SEER Program quality control has been an integral part of the effort and the quality and completeness of the data is evaluated each year. A valuable innovation in the SEER registry is that it provides web-based access to registry data and analytic tools that can be used by both researchers and policy makers.

of treatments. At the other end of the spectrum, a spinal cord injury registry could record specific outcome measures for individuals with spinal cord injuries and track those outcome measures over time, including data about the outcomes of specific treatments. This type of registry could be used to understand the effectiveness of specific treatments, including practices or programs for improving functional outcomes and quality of life. Spinal cord injury registries could also provide a mechanism for identifying and contacting potential participants regarding clinical trials or notifying individuals about new therapeutic interventions.

By knowing the prevalence of certain conditions and outcomes, it is possible to determine how many individuals in each study group will be needed for accurate determination of whether a treatment is really safe or effective or whether an apparent effect was due to chance. Most importantly, a spinal cord injury registry would increase the level of understanding of the natural course of injury and repair, which in turn would allow the design of meaningful clinical trials.

At present there is no nationwide coordination of spinal cord injury registries. However, several efforts that have the potential to fill this gap are under way or are being initiated. The Model Spinal Cord Injury Care Systems database has more than 25,000 initial hospitalization records for individuals with spinal cord injuries and is the largest available resource specifically focused on spinal cord injuries (Nobunaga et al., 1999). The Trauma Care Systems Planning and Development Act of 1990 (P.L. 101-590) stipulates that states receiving federal assistance for trauma care must establish a central data reporting and analysis system for trauma care data. Thus far, 38 states have general trauma registries that allow them to assess the incidence and prevalence of various traumatic injuries (including traumatic brain injury and spinal cord injury) and to develop prevention programs. The Department of Veterans Affairs has initiated efforts to centralize its registry of veterans with spinal cord injuries (VA, 2002). To facilitate multicenter clinical trials, the Christopher Reeve Clinical Trials Network is also developing an extensive patient database in coordination with five European rehabilitation centers that receive patients from acute-care hospitals.

For spinal cord injuries, there are issues regarding the logistics of obtaining informed consent from people whose personal health information will be used in the registry. Because a willingness to participate is often influenced by the individual's condition, all conditions may not be accurately represented in the registry. For example, the authors of a prospective study of the feasibility of establishing a registry of stroke patients in Canada concluded that the registry was virtually useless because so few people agreed to participate and those few who did agree tended to be the least severely injured, which resulted in a registry with a highly biased sample of the general population of stroke victims (Ingelfinger and Drazen, 2004; Tu et al., 2004). Although the experiences of researchers and clinicians who work with individuals with spinal cord injuries suggest that they are overall quite willing, and even eager, to participate in similar registries, the issue of sampling bias is too important to leave unexamined in any patient registry.

Important considerations in designing databases include:

- scalability (it must be able to grow);
- flexibility (it must be able to accommodate different types of data and be modifiable as needs evolve or new measures are incorporated); and
- reliability (data entry practices must be consistent and verification of accuracy must be performed on an ongoing basis; often, the same patient is entered into the registry twice or the nature and the extent of data entry practices differ between sites).

Globally, data registries are at risk of significant bias because of privacy issues that have made the collection and use of health data more difficult for researchers (Ingelfinger and Drazen, 2004). Although such restrictions are generally imposed because of legitimate interests in protecting individuals from the misuse of their personal information, research efforts intended to help patients have also been restricted as an unintended consequence. The implementation of the Health Insurance Portability and Accountability Act Privacy Rule in 2003 imposed new restrictions on how patient health information can be shared among researchers. Although some of those requirements can be waived, most IRBs have been reluctant to do so. Other countries have imposed similar laws.

There are also concerns about the use of a legacy database—one that has already been created, often with a different application in mind. These databases are often out of date, the information is difficult to verify, and the structure of the database may be incompatible with new formats, potentially resulting in information exchanges that corrupt the new or the old system. This has been accomplished in other cases by establishing standard templates for health data, such as the Health Level Seven (HL7) project or Integrating the Healthcare Enterprise. Few data registries have reached their maximum potential, and spinal cord injury researchers would be well advised to seek input from successful pioneers in registry development.

Efforts should be made to develop standardized protocols for patient registry systems so that registries can be coordinated and used to assist in identifying candidates for participation in clinical trials and provide information on upcoming clinical trials to individuals with spinal cord injuries (see Chapter 7). This may require the establishment of a new set of databases that are flexible and capable of being integrated.

The coordination of all this information will provide an invaluable tool for spinal cord injury research, will facilitate increased participation in clinical trials, and will provide data sets that can be used for studies investigating the long-term treatment outcomes from therapeutic interventions and the safety of those interventions.

ACCELERATING PROGRESS

Neither the scientific community nor the community of individuals with spinal cord injuries is content with the limited therapeutic options currently available for the treatment of spinal cord injuries. There is an obvious and urgent need to identify and test new interventions and to accelerate the pace of research, particularly in moving laboratory findings to clinical practice. A spinal cord injury involves serious and traumatic adverse changes to the human body, and an extensive research effort is needed to develop treatment approaches for the range of health outcomes that individuals with spinal cord injuries face.

Challenges arise in dealing with new experimental therapies that look promising but that are not yet in clinical trials with human subjects. Some individuals are willing to take chances on interventions that may endanger their safety but that may also offer the possibility of functional improvements. Efforts are needed to assist these individuals in understanding the current status of clinical trials. This includes identifying those trials open for the recruitment of participants and providing information on the potential health risks of experimental therapies.

RECOMMENDATIONS

Recommendation 6.1: *Facilitate Clinical Trials*
Mechanisms should be implemented that will facilitate the implementation of clinical trials while observing the established standards for the protection of human subjects in clinical research, including:

- Utilize and coordinate existing facilities and resources in acute care, chronic care, and rehabilitation to support multicenter clinical trials.
- The use of central institutional review board mechanisms in conjunction with local institutional review boards should be explored to facilitate coordinated multicenter studies.
- Patient registries and databases should be coordinated and expanded to improve mechanisms to conduct clinical trials and facilitate patient recruitment by increasing awareness of ongoing clinical trials among potential participants.
- A set of standardized clinical outcome measures should be devel-

oped. This may include a rating scale that is capable of integrating functional outcomes from different spheres of disability.

• Clinical trial design should be a multidisciplinary effort and should incorporate, as appropriate, small "*n*" methodologies for early-phase clinical trials to ensure the rapid advancement of new therapies. Initial clinical trials that are promising should then be followed up with larger-scale clinical trials.

Recommendation 6.2: *Increase Industry Involvement*
The National Institutes of Health and the Food and Drug Administration (in collaboration with state and other federal agencies, professional societies, academic institutions, nonprofit organizations, and the pharmaceutical and medical device industries) should explore mechanisms that can be used to link federal, state, academic, and nonprofit efforts with those of industry with the goal of increasing the investment and involvement of the private sector in the development of therapeutic interventions for spinal cord injuries.

REFERENCES

Alderson P, Roberts I. 1997. Corticosteroids in acute traumatic brain injury: Systematic review of randomised controlled trials. *British Medical Journal* 314(7098): 1855-1859.

Berry C, Kennedy P. 2003. A psychometric analysis of the Needs Assessment Checklist (NAC). *Spinal Cord* 41(9): 490-501.

Blight A. 2004, February 24. *Challenges of Conducting Clinical Trials on Spinal Cord Injury in Industry*. Presentation at the Institute of Medicine Workshop on Translational and Clinical Research Workshop, Washington, DC. Institute of Medicine Committee on Spinal Cord Injury.

Bracken MB. 2000. Methylprednisolone and spinal cord injury. *Journal of Neurosurgery—Spine* 93(1 Suppl): 175-179.

Bracken MB, Holford TR. 2002. Neurological and functional status 1 year after acute spinal cord injury: Estimates of functional recovery in National Acute Spinal Cord Injury Study II from results modeled in National Acute Spinal Cord Injury Study III. *Journal of Neurosurgery* 96(3 Suppl): 259-266.

Bracken MB, Collins WF, Freeman DF, Shepard MJ, Wagner FW, Silten RM, Hellenbrand KG, Ransohoff J, Hunt WE, Perot PL. 1984. Efficacy of methylprednisolone in acute spinal cord injury. *Journal of the American Medical Association* 251(1): 45-52.

Bracken MB, Shepard MJ, Collins WF, Holford TR, Young W, Baskin DS, Eisenberg HM, Flamm E, Leo-Summers L, Maroon J. 1990. A randomized, controlled trial of methylprednisolone or naloxone in the treatment of acute spinal-cord injury. Results of the second National Acute Spinal Cord Injury Study. *New England Journal of Medicine* 322(20): 1405-1411.

Bracken MB, Shepard MJ, Holford TR, Leo-Summers L, Aldrich EF, Fazl M, Fehlings M, Herr DL, Hitchon PW, Marshall LF, Nockels RP, Pascale V, Perot PL Jr, Piepmeier J, Sonntag VKH, Wagner F, Wilberger JE, Winn HR, Young W. 1997. Administration of methylprednisolone for 24 or 48 hours or tirilazad mesylate for 48 hours in the treatment of acute spinal cord injury: Results of the third National Acute Spinal Cord Injury randomized controlled trial. *Journal of the American Medical Association* 277(20): 1597-1604.

Catz A, Itzkovich M, Agranov E, Ring H, Tamir A. 1997. SCIM—Spinal Cord Independence Measure: A new disability scale for patients with spinal cord lesions. *Spinal Cord* 35(12): 850-856.

Clifton GL, Knudson P, McDonald M. 2002. Waiver of consent in studies of acute brain injury. *Journal of Neurotrauma* 19(10): 1121-1126.

Creasey GH, Grill JH, Korsten M, Sang H, Betz R, Anderson R, Walter J, Implanted Neuroprosthesis Research Group. 2001. An implantable neuroprosthesis for restoring bladder and bowel control to patients with spinal cord injuries: A multicenter trial. *Archives of Physical Medicine and Rehabilitation* 82(11): 1512-1519.

Curt A, Schwab ME, Dietz V. 2004. Providing the clinical basis for new interventional therapies: Refined diagnosis and assessment of recovery after spinal cord injury. *Spinal Cord* 42(1): 1-6.

Dekkers W, Boer G. 2001. Sham neurosurgery in patients with Parkinson's disease: Is it morally acceptable? *Journal of Medical Ethics* 27(3): 151-156.

DHHS (U.S. Department of Health and Human Services). 1996. Protection of human subjects, informed consent and waiver of informed consent requirements in certain emergency research: Final rules (21 CFR Part 50, 45 CFR Part 46). *Federal Register* 61(192): 51500-51533.

Dietrich WD. 2003. Confirming an experimental therapy prior to transfer to humans: What is the ideal? *Journal of Rehabilitation Research & Development* 40(4 Suppl 1): 63-69.

Ditunno JF, Young W, Donovan WH, Creasey G. 1994. The international standards booklet for neurological and functional classification of spinal cord injury. *Paraplegia* 32(2): 70-80.

Ditunno JF Jr, Cohen ME, Hauck WW, Jackson AB, Sipski ML. 2000. Recovery of upper-extremity strength in complete and incomplete tetraplegia: A multicenter study. *Archives of Physical Medicine and Rehabilitation* 81(4): 389-393.

Dobkin BH, Havton LA. 2004. Basic advances and new avenues in therapy of spinal cord injury. *Annual Review of Medicine* 55: 255-282.

Dumont RJ, Verma S, Okonkwo DO, Hurlbert RJ, Boulos PT, Ellegala DB, Dumont AS. 2001. Acute spinal cord injury. Part II. Contemporary pharmacotherapy. *Clinical Neuropharmacology* 24(5): 265-279.

Ellaway PH, Anand P, Bergstrom EMK, Catley M, Davey NJ, Frankel HL, Jamous A, Mathias C, Nicotra A, Savic G, Short D, Theodorou S. 2004. Towards improved clinical and physiological assessments of recovery in spinal cord injury: A clinical initiative. *Spinal Cord* 42(6): 325-337.

Fahn S, Marsden CD, Calne DB, Goldstein M, eds. 1987. *Recent Developments in Parkinson's Disease*. Florham Park, NJ: Macmillan Health Care Information.

FDA (Food and Drug Administration). 2004a. *Office of Orphan Product Development*. [Online]. Available: http://www.fda.gov/orphan/index.htm [accessed December 21, 2004].

FDA. 2004b. *Innovation, Stagnation: Challenge and Opportunity on the Critical Path to New Medical Products*. Washington, DC: U.S. Department of Health and Human Services.

Hanigan WC, Anderson RJ. 1992. Commentary on NASCIS-2. *Journal of Spinal Disorders* 5(1): 125-131.

Harding A. 2004. More compounds failing phase I. *The Scientist* 18(13): 5.

Huang H, Chen L, Wang H, Xiu B, Li B, Wang R, Zhang J, Zhang F, Gu Z, Li Y, Song Y, Hao W, Pang S, Sun J. 2003. Influence of patients' age on functional recovery after transplantation of olfactory ensheathing cells into injured spinal cord injury. *Chinese Medical Journal* 116(10): 1488-1491.

Hurlbert RJ. 2000. Methylprednisolone for acute spinal cord injury: An inappropriate standard of care. *Journal of Neurosurgery: Spine* 93(1 Suppl): 1-7.

ICORD (International Collaboration on Repair Discoveries). 2004. *ICCP Workshops on Spinal Cord Injury: Report on the First Working Group*. [Online]. Available: http://www.icord.org/ICCP/ICCP_SCI_Guidelines1.doc [accessed February 21, 2005].

Ingelfinger JR, Drazen JM. 2004. Registry research and medical privacy. *New England Journal of Medicine* 350(14): 1452-1453.

IOM (Institute of Medicine). 1999. *A Report on the Sponsors of Cancer Treatment Clinical Trials and Their Approval and Monitoring Mechanisms*. Washington, DC: National Academy Press.

IOM. 2001. *Small Clinical Trials: Issues and Challenges*. Washington, DC: National Academy Press.

Kleitman N. 2004. Keeping promises: Translating basic research into new spinal cord injury therapies. *Journal of Spinal Cord Medicine* 27(4): 311-318.

Lev M. 2004, August 27. Fetal-cell surgery raises hopes, fears. A procedure that involves aborted fetuses is drawing spinal-injury patients from the U.S., but a lack of clinical trials concerns researchers. *Chicago Tribune*. p. C4.

Loh ED, Meyer RE. 2004. Medical schools' attitudes and perceptions regarding the use of central institutional review boards. *Academic Medicine* 79(7): 644-651.

Matthew G., 2001. *Neurobiology: Molecules, Cells, and Systems*. 2nd ed. Malden, MA: Blackwell Science.

Maynard FM, Reynolds GG, Fountain S, Wilmot C, Hamilton R. 1979. Neurological prognosis after traumatic quadriplegia. Three-year experience of California regional spinal cord injury care system. *Journal of Neurosurgery* 50(5): 611-616.

Meyers AR, Andresen EM, Hagglund KJ. 2000. A model of outcomes research: Spinal cord injury. *Archives of Physical Medicine and Rehabilitation* 81(12 Suppl 2): S81-90.

Munsat TL. 1995. World Federation of Neurology Research Group on Neuromuscular Diseases Subcommittee on Motor Neuron Disease. Airlie House guidelines—Therapeutic trials in amyotrophic lateral sclerosis. *Journal of the Neurological Sciences* 129(Suppl): 1-10.

NCI (National Cancer Institute). 2004. *The Central Institutional Review Board Initiative*. [Online]. Available: http://www.ncicirb.org/ [accessed August 22, 2004].

NINDS (National Institute of Neurological Disorders and Stroke). 2002. *Facilities of Research in Spinal Cord Injury*. [Online]. Available: http://grants2.nih.gov/grants/guide/notice-files/NOT-NS-02-011.html [accessed October 4, 2004].

NINDS. 2003. *Translating Promising Strategies for Spinal Cord Injury Therapy February 3–4, 2003, Bethesda, Maryland*. [Online]. Available: http://www.ninds.nih.gov/news_and_events/proceedings/sci_translation_workshop.htm?format=printable [accessed August 9, 2004].

Nobunaga AI, Go BK, Karunas RB. 1999. Recent demographic and injury trends in people served by the model spinal cord injury care systems. *Archives of Physical Medicine and Rehabilitation* 80(11): 1372-1382.

Northwest Regional Spinal Cord Injury System. 2000. *SCI Forum—Fampridine (4-AP) Study at UW*. [Online]. Available: http://depts.washington.edu/rehab/sci/fampridine.html [accessed November 11, 2004].

NRC (National Research Council). 1993. *Clinical Trials and Statistics: Proceedings of a Symposium*. Washington, DC: National Academy Press.

Peckham PH, Keith MW, Kilgore KL, Grill JH, Wuolle KS, Thrope GB, Gorman P, Hobby J, Mulcahey MJ, Carroll S, Hentz VR, Wiegner A, Implantable Neuroprosthesis Research Group. 2001. Efficacy of an implanted neuroprosthesis for restoring hand grasp in tetraplegia: A multicenter study. *Archives of Physical Medicine and Rehabilitation* 82(10): 1380-1388.

PhRMA (Pharmaceutical Research and Manufacturers of America). 2004a. *New Drug Approvals in 2003*. [Online]. Available: http://www.phrma.org/newmedicines/resources/2004-01-22.123.pdf [accessed November 22, 2004].

PhRMA. 2004b. *Medicine in Development for Women*. [Online]. Available: http://www.phrma.org/newmedicines/resources/2004-03-02.124.pdf [accessed November 11, 2004].

Pocock SJ, 1983. *Clinical Trials: A Practical Approach*. New York: Wiley, Inc.

Quest for new cures. 2003. *The Pfizer Journal* 7(3): 4-11.

Ramer MS, Harper GP, Bradbury EJ. 2000. Progress in spinal cord research: A refined strategy for the International Spinal Research Trust. *Spinal Cord* 38(8): 449-472.

Redmond DE Jr, Freeman T, American Society for Neural Transplantation and Repair. 2001. The American Society for Neural Transplantation and Repair considerations and guidelines for studies of human subjects. The Practice Committee of the Society. Approved by Council. *Cell Transplantation* 10(8): 661-664.

Roberts I, Yates D, Sandercock P, Farrell B, Wasserberg J, Lomas G, Cottingham R, Svoboda P, Brayley N, Mazairac G, Laloe V, Munoz-Sanchez A, Arango M, Hartzenberg B, Khamis H, Yutthakasemsunt S, Komolafe E, Olldashi F, Yadav Y, Murillo-Cabezas F, Shakur H, Edwards P, CRASH Trial Collaborators. 2004. Effect of intravenous corticosteroids on death within 14 days in 10008 adults with clinically significant head injury (MRC CRASH trial): Randomised placebo-controlled trial. *Lancet* 364(9442): 1321-1328.

Rosenfeld JV, Gillett GR. 2004. Ethics, stem cells and spinal cord repair. *Medical Journal of Australia* 180(12): 637-639.

Sauerland S, Maegele M. 2004. A crash landing in severe head injury. *Lancet* 364(9442): 1291-1292.

Smithline HA, Gerstle ML. 1998. Waiver of informed consent: A survey of emergency medicine patients. *American Journal of Emergency Medicine* 16(1): 90-91.

Sugarman J. 1999. Ethical considerations in leaping from bench to bedside. *Science* 285(5436): 2071-2072.

Sugarman J, McKenna WG. 2003. Ethical hurdles for translational research. *Radiation Research* 160(1): 1-4.

Tu JV, Willison DJ, Silver FL, Fang J, Richards JA, Laupacis A, Kapral MK, Investigators in the Registry of the Canadian Stroke Network. 2004. Impracticability of informed consent in the registry of the Canadian Stroke Network. *New England Journal of Medicine* 350(14): 1414-1421.

Tufts Center for the Study of Drug Development. 2001. *Backgrounder: A Methodology for Counting Costs for Pharmaceutical R&D*. [Online]. Available: http://csdd.tufts.edu/NewsEvents/RecentNews.asp?newsid=5 [accessed November 11, 2004].

VA (U.S. Department of Veterans Affairs). 2002. *Spinal Cord Dysfunction Registry*. [Online]. Available: http://www.sci-queri.research.med.va.gov/Registry.htm [accessed August 10, 2004].

World Medical Association. 2004. *World Medical Association Declaration of Helsinki Ethical Principles for Medical Research Involving Human Subjects*. [Online]. Available: http://www.wma.net/e/policy/pdf/17c.pdf [accessed November 11, 2004].

Young W. 2002. *Spinal Cord Injury Levels & Classification*. [Online]. Available: http://www.sci-info-pages.com/levels.html [accessed September 30, 2003].

7

RESEARCH ORGANIZATION: CREATING AN ENVIRONMENT TO ACCELERATE PROGRESS

What we need to do is create organizational structures that allow us to mine what is an incredibly rich field of basic science discovery.

—Oswald Steward[1]

Although much progress has been made in understanding the basic mechanisms of neuronal injury and repair, the field is grappling with how to translate these discoveries into effective therapeutic interventions. As the field is currently configured, it cannot quickly capitalize on research leads because there are few centers for collaborative translational research on spinal cord injuries.

Progress in spinal cord injury research will require adequate research funding; well-trained and innovative investigators with career development opportunities; translational efforts that move preclinical findings to clinical trials with humans, insofar as it is safe and appropriate; and an environment that promotes and encourages interdisciplinary collaboration. There are currently efforts by foundations and other nonprofit organizations, health care systems, state and federal governments, academic institutions, and others to fund and conduct spinal cord injury research. The pressing issue is how best to improve the current organization of basic and clinical research—the research infrastructure—to nurture and accelerate progress. This chapter examines the current status of the infrastructure supporting

---

[1]Presentation to IOM Committee on Spinal Cord Injury, February 24, 2004.

spinal cord injury research and presents the committee's recommendations for the next steps needed to accelerate progress.

WHO IS CURRENTLY FUNDING AND SUPPORTING SPINAL CORD INJURY RESEARCH?

Neuroscience research into the basic mechanisms of nerve conduction, plasticity, and regeneration has enormous implications for many neurological disorders and disease entities (e.g., multiple sclerosis, Alzheimer's disease, amyotrophic lateral sclerosis [ALS], and Parkinson's disease), including spinal cord injuries. For example, what is learned about remyelination in research on multiple sclerosis is likely to be of benefit in examining nerve conduction in individuals with spinal cord injuries. Therefore, it is difficult to draw distinct boundaries for funding or to define the precise parameters for research exclusively on spinal cord injuries.

One of the challenges in examining research infrastructure issues is the lack of quantitative measures targeted to a specific field of research, in this case, spinal cord injuries. Most often, the measures highlight the bigger picture and can provide broader sets of statistics (such as the number of Ph.D. candidates in neuroscience), but the data on the specific infrastructure for spinal cord injury research (such as the number of doctoral candidates who pursue research careers focused on spinal cord injuries) are not available.

The following discussion provides a brief overview of the current funding and support for spinal cord injury research. Researchers and research centers often receive funding from multiple sources; and research centers leverage federal, state, and private sector funding to make the best use of the resources.

Federal Funding

National Institutes of Health

As the major federal funder of biomedical research in the United States, the National Institutes of Health (NIH) supports extensive preclinical and clinical research, training opportunities, and collaborative ventures that are relevant to spinal cord injury research. In fiscal year (FY) 2003, $89.2 million in NIH funding was designated for spinal cord injury research; the funding estimate for FY 2005 is $93 million. This funding level is comparable to that for research on multiple sclerosis ($99.2 million in 2003 and an estimated $102.8 million in 2005) and epilepsy ($94.3 million in 2003 and an estimated $99.5 million in 2005) (Personal communication, A. Howard, NIH, August 4, 2004). NIH funding for research on Parkinson's disease in FY 2005 is estimated to be $240 million, and research on

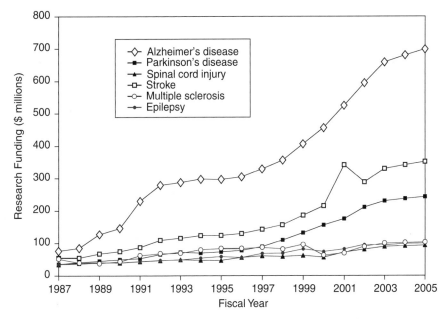

FIGURE 7-1 NIH research funding for specific diseases and conditions, 1987 to 2005.

NOTE: Funding levels are in actual, not constant, dollars. Funding for 2004 and 2005 are estimates. The data point for stroke in 2001 reflects, in part, an additional $70 million distributed by NINDS.

SOURCE: NIH, 2004c; Personal communication, A. Howard, NIH, August 3, 2004.

Alzheimer's disease is estimated to be funded for approximately $700 million (NIH, 2004c; Personal communication, A. Howard, NIH, August 4, 2004). The levels of NIH funding for spinal cord injury research have shown steady but modest increases since 1987 (Figure 7-1). Data from the Computer Retrieval of Information on Scientific Projects (CRISP) database[2] indicate that the number of NIH investigator-initiated research

---

[2]CRISP is a searchable database, maintained by NIH, of federally funded biomedical research projects funded by NIH, the Substance Abuse and Mental Health Services, the Health Resources and Services Administration, the Food and Drug Administration, the Centers for Disease Control and Prevention, the Agency for Health Care Research and Quality, and the Office of the Assistant Secretary of Health. To determine the number of grants, fellowships, training grants, and career development awards, among others, the CRISP database was searched by using the following search terms found in the CRISP thesaurus: "spinal cord injury," "multiple sclerosis," "Parkinson's disease," "Alzheimer's disease," "stroke," and "epilepsy."

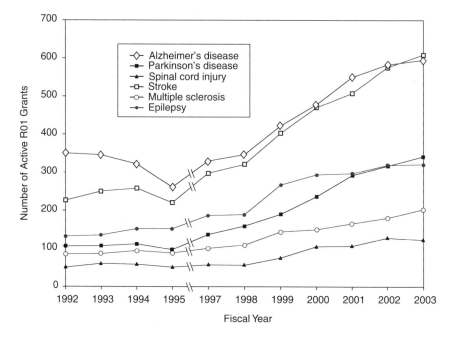

FIGURE 7-2 NIH support for research projects (R01 grants), 1992 to 2003.
NOTE: The 1996 data from the CRISP database were not used to compile this
figure, as NINDS and CRISP staff indicated that the significant decreases in R01
grants reported in the 1996 CRISP database are not accurate.
SOURCE: CRISP database: http://www.crisp.cit.nih.gov (accessed November 10,
2004).

projects (R01 grants) focused on spinal cord injuries showed a modest
increase over the 10-year period, 1992 to 2003 (Figure 7-2). R01 grants are
the major mechanism used to fund basic biomedical research. Although the
data on funding for spinal cord injury research indicate that the funding is
steady, additional resources have not been forthcoming, including funding
for the research infrastructure needed to accelerate research progress. NIH
sponsors a number of fellowships that provide additional education and
training to predoctoral and postdoctoral students. In 2002, NIH awarded
nearly 2,700 fellowships in all fields of research, with more than 60 percent
given to individuals who had completed their doctoral training (NIH, 2003).
Additionally, NIH supports predoctoral fellowships, which provide funds
to doctoral students who will be performing dissertation research and training (NIH, 2000). From 2001 to 2003, NIH awarded 11 predoctoral fellowships specifically related to spinal cord injury research. This compares with

17 predoctoral fellowships for multiple sclerosis research. From 2001 to 2003, NIH awarded 13 postdoctoral fellowships in spinal cord injury research, an increase of 5 such awards from 1998 to 2000; this compares with 9 postdoctoral fellowships in multiple sclerosis, 30 in Parkinson's disease, and 64 in Alzheimer's disease awarded to individuals from 2001 to 2003. These fellowships provide a means of attracting new investigators to the field and, as noted later in this chapter, offer an opportunity for furthering the field of spinal cord injury research. However, the current number of fellowships is inadequate to expand and build the research base needed for progress in spinal cord injury research.

National Institute of Neurological Disorders and Stroke. The majority of NIH-supported spinal cord injury research is funded by the National Institute of Neurological Disorders and Stroke (NINDS), which was created in 1950 to further research and treatment for more than 200 different neurological diseases. The extensive research portfolio of NINDS includes considerable support for preclinical neurological research that has relevance for multiple neurological conditions in key research areas, including neural circuits, neural degeneration, neurogenetics, repair and plasticity, and neural prostheses. NINDS supports an extensive extramural research program in spinal cord injuries and should continue to devote resources to both extramural and intramural research programs to build on these efforts.

In FY 2003, the NINDS budget for spinal cord injury research was approximately $60 million. Of this amount, $42.6 million was for single- and multiple-investigator research projects (e.g., R01, R21, R03, and P01 grants) (see glossary for description); $2.8 million for P50 research centers; and $14.3 million for other funding mechanisms, including training, intramural research, contracts, and small-business grants (Personal communication, NINDS Budget Office, November 10, 2004). A recent NINDS announcement of note established contracts for Facilities of Research Excellence in Spinal Cord Injury (FOR-SCI). These contracts, first funded in 2002, have been used to create a course in spinal cord injury research methods, provide resources for established researchers and postdoctoral trainees to work together in studying animal models of spinal cord injuries, support a series of replication studies of promising therapeutic strategies by using models of acute and chronic injuries, and enable the development of new functional outcome evaluations (NINDS, 2002).

NINDS has also sponsored a number of relevant workshops on spinal cord injury research, including the Role of the Immune System in Spinal Cord Injury (April 5-6, 2000) (NINDS, 2004b), Functional and Dysfunctional Spinal Circuitry: Role for Rehabilitation and Neural Prostheses (June 14-15, 2000) (NINDS, 2004a), and Translating Promising Strategies for Spinal Cord Injury Therapy (February 3-4, 2003) (NINDS, 2003).

Several different NIH grant mechanisms are used to fund the infrastructure for research involving multiple investigators in research centers. The primary mechanisms are the P30 Center Core Grants, which fund shared resources and facilities, and the P01 and P50 Program Project and Specialized Center Grants, which fund multidisciplinary research. NINDS funds four ongoing P30 Center Core Grants that provide support to laboratories studying spinal cord injuries. These centers conduct research into a range of neurological disorders, including spinal cord injuries; and as mentioned in Chapter 3, the Ohio State University program also has an extensive training program in spinal cord injury research methods and techniques. NINDS also currently funds two P50 Center Grants for research (at Yale University and Medical College of Pennsylvania Hahnemann University) that focus on strategies for the repair of spinal cord injuries and the restoration of function.[3]

National Center for Medical Rehabilitation Research. The National Center for Medical Rehabilitation Research (NCMRR), housed within the National Institute of Child Health and Human Development, funds research on spinal cord injuries that is related to medical rehabilitation. NCMRR was established in 1990 to improve the health and quality of life for individuals living with physical disabilities. NCMRR's research portfolio focuses on improving functional mobility, developing adaptive technologies, understanding the body's responses to impairments, and improving the tools used to assess improvements in functional outcomes. From 1990 to 2000, NCMRR provide funding of $20.4 million for research and training related to spinal cord injuries (NICHD, 2004). Recently, NCMRR established four regional rehabilitation research networks to facilitate collaborations through multidisciplinary and multicenter research. The recent recognition of the benefits of maintaining the nervous system (activity-dependent plasticity) for functional improvement provides a greater priority for collaborative efforts between basic research, including that funded by NINDS, and rehabilitative research, including research funded by NCMRR.

Centers for Disease Control and Prevention

The Centers for Disease Control and Prevention's (CDC's) National Center for Injury Prevention and Control provided funding and technical

---

[3]Additionally, the National Institute of Dental and Craniofacial Research funds a P50 Center Grant at Ohio State University for research on behavioral and neuroendocrine modulation in individuals with spinal cord injuries.

support for spinal cord injury surveillance efforts in four to seven states from 2000 to 2004; however, this program is no longer funded. CDC continues to provide technical support through its *Guidelines for the Surveillance of Central Nervous System Injury*. Relevant extramural research funded by CDC focuses on preventing the secondary conditions of spinal cord injuries, including research on chronic pain prevention and on long-term renal function (National Center for Injury Prevention and Control, 2001).

U.S. Department of Veterans Affairs

The U.S. Department of Veterans Affairs (VA) provides health care and rehabilitation services to approximately 15,000 veterans with spinal cord injuries and specialty care to 9,000 of these veterans (VA, 2002). The care is provided through the VA's 23 spinal cord injury centers, with additional support clinics and primary care teams (Hammond, 2002). The VA system also provides care for newly injured active-duty personnel through an agreement with the U.S. Department of Defense.

The spinal cord injury research funded by VA focuses primarily on rehabilitation and engineering approaches, but also includes some basic research on the restoration of nerve function. In FY 2000, VA provided $9.7 million in funding for 84 research projects on spinal cord injuries; additionally, VA researchers conducted another 95 related projects with $7.7 million in grants from other sources (VA, 2002). Four of the VA's research centers focus on spinal cord injuries. The Center for Functional Recovery in Chronic Spinal Cord Injury in Miami examines spasticity, pain management, and functional recovery. Its research endeavors are enhanced by its affiliation with the Miami Project to Cure Paralysis. The Center for Functional Restoration in Multiple Sclerosis and Spinal Cord Injury in West Haven, Connecticut, examines molecular and cellular approaches to protecting and repairing the injured spinal cord. The Center for Medical Consequences of Spinal Cord Injury at the Bronx VA Medical Center, Bronx, New York, examines a range of treatment approaches. The Functional Electrical Stimulation Center of Excellence in Cleveland, Ohio, focuses on research in neural plasticity and neuroprotheses, with much of this activity focused on spinal cord injuries. In addition to research grants, VA funds training efforts, including career development and fellowship grants.

U.S. Department of Education, National Institute on Disability and Rehabilitation Research

Created in 1978, the National Institute on Disability and Rehabilitation Research (NIDRR) works to conduct rehabilitative research in several areas relevant to spinal cord injuries, including rehabilitative technology, health and function, and independent living and community integration (NIDRR, 2004). From 2000 to 2004, NIDRR provided funding of approximately $12 million annually for research on rehabilitation from spinal cord injuries (Personal communication, R. Melia, NIDRR, November 10, 2004). NIDRR uses a variety of funding mechanisms, including individual grants, fellowships, and centers of excellence.

The Model Spinal Cord Injury Care Systems, which are funded and administered by NIDRR, were designed in the 1970s to develop a comprehensive integrated system of care for individuals with spinal cord injuries (Tulsky, 2002). Sixteen centers throughout the country are currently designated model systems. This program focuses on providing a multidisciplinary system of rehabilitation services and on collaborative approaches to rehabilitation research (DeVivo, 2002). The level of funding designated for the Model Systems has varied widely over the past 30 years, with current funding being at fairly minimal levels. In the past 5 years, each of the 16 centers has received an average of $340,000 (Personal communication, R. Brannon, NIDRR, January 26, 2005). For FY 2005, an additional $2 million has been designated to develop a multicenter clinical trials network.

Each of the centers contributes data on patient demographics, treatment, and costs of care as well as follow-up data to the National Spinal Cord Injury Model Systems Database, which is run by the National Spinal Cord Injury Statistical Center at the University of Alabama in Birmingham. The Model Systems centers have conducted a number of clinical trials, including studies examining treatments for urinary tract infections and pain therapies. Studies examining the effects of body weight support and treadmill training are under way (Tate and Forchheimer, 2002). Although this program offers the potential to coordinate multicenter trials, it has been minimally funded in recent years. Increased funding is urged to bolster this program and to use its resources to conduct multicenter clinical trials. Furthermore, collaborative efforts between the "care" and "cure" communities and resources are critically important for the development of therapeutic interventions for spinal cord injuries (see Chapter 6).

State Funding

Spinal cord injury research is also supported by funds provided by individual states. Currently, 14 states have enacted legislation to provide funds totaling more than $27 million for spinal cord injury research (see Chapter 8 and Appendix H). Many of the states that fund spinal cord injury research do so through surcharges on fines for traffic violations. For example, New York State collects approximately $8 million each year from a surcharge of $5 for traffic violations,[4] whereas New Jersey adds a $1 surcharge to any motor vehicle or traffic violation to provide an estimated $3.5 million per year for research and prevention efforts (Personal communication, C. Traynor, New Jersey Commission on Spinal Cord Research, January 28, 2005).

Some state programs, such as those in Florida, Indiana, and Kentucky, provide funding to specific universities to conduct research on spinal cord injuries. Several states have developed or have contributed to funding extensive research centers in the state, including the Miami Project to Cure Paralysis and the Kentucky Spinal Cord Injury Research Center (see Chapter 8). Other states diversify their funding, as in the case of South Carolina, which supports young investigator grants, career development awards, and clinician-scientist recruitment awards, and Maryland, which supports fellowships and research at private and public facilities. Chapter 8 provides greater detail on these programs.

Nonprofit Organizations

A number of foundations and other nonprofit organizations explicitly support spinal cord injury research or fund training opportunities and collaborative conferences. Private funds have the advantage of being able to be quickly targeted to specific research efforts and generally have more flexibility than government funding in terms of the types of research and the resources that can be funded.

For example, the Minnesota-based Spinal Cord Society has distributed more than $10 million to spinal cord injury research efforts since 1979 (Spinal Cord Society, 2004); the Wisconsin-based Bryon Riesch Paralysis Foundation, established in 2001, has provided more than $400,000 to spinal cord injury research, with particular emphases on remyelination, axon regeneration, and drug therapies (Bryon Riesch Paralysis Foundation, 2002, 2004); and the Paralysis Project of America, established in 1987, provides research support to postdoctoral fellows and senior investigators investigating the pathophysiology of spinal cord injuries and the development of treatments for spinal cord injuries (Paralysis Project of America, 2004). Many other foundations, including the Buoniconti Fund to Cure Paralysis and the Geoffrey Lance Foundation for Spinal Cord Injury Research and Support, also actively support spinal cord injury research. The American Spinal Injury Association works to promote standards of excel-

---

[4]New York State Senate Introducer's Memorandum in Support of S7287C (1998).

lence in health care for individuals with spinal cord injuries and provides seed grant funds to researchers through its G. Heiner Sell Research and Education Fund and Erica Nader Award.

A number of organizations are also active in education and prevention efforts. These include the Think First National Injury Prevention Foundation, founded by the American Association of Neurological Surgeons and the Congress of Neurological Surgeons. This program is dedicated to injury prevention policy and public education efforts. The next section highlights the efforts of a few nonprofit organizations dedicated to furthering spinal cord injury research.

American Paraplegia Society

Established in 1954, the American Paraplegia Society (APS) uses several mechanisms to disseminate research findings to clinicians and basic scientists. For example, since 1994, APS has provided seed grants to relatively new investigators who use the funds to develop preliminary data to secure future funding (APS, 2004c). APS, which "fosters a multi-specialty approach to prevention, clinical care, basic science, and technology research in the management of [spinal cord injuries]" (APS, 2004b), holds annual conferences to foster communication between clinicians and researchers, provides awards for practitioners who have made significant contributions in the spinal cord injury field, and publishes the *Journal of Spinal Cord Medicine* (APS, 2004a).

Christopher Reeve Paralysis Foundation

The American Paralysis Association, established in 1982, merged with the Christopher Reeve Foundation to form the Christopher Reeve Paralysis Foundation (CRPF) in 1999 to support groundbreaking research in spinal cord injuries. Since the organization's founding 22 years ago, it has distributed more than $40 million in research grants (CRPF, 2003) in the form of individual research grants, center grants, and quality-of-life grants (CRPF, 2004b). Since 1997, CRPF has funded 260 individual research grants and has provided a total of nearly $20 million in research funding (CRPF, 2004a). CRPF established the Research Consortium on Spinal Cord Injury in 1995 to bring together international experts to develop and discuss research priorities and interlaboratory studies. CRPF is active in advocating for spinal cord injury research, hosting meetings to increase research collaborations, and improving patient knowledge and awareness of research resources.

Paralyzed Veterans of America

Congressionally mandated in 1946, the Paralyzed Veterans of America (PVA) was established to provide a range of services to veterans who sustained spinal cord injuries or dysfunction. PVA represents 38,000 veterans and advocates on behalf of veterans, develops clinical practice guidelines, and funds research (PVA, 2003). In 1975, PVA created the PVA Spinal Cord Research Foundation to fund research to improve treatment and care for those who have sustained spinal cord injuries. The Foundation funds 1- or 2-year basic and clinical research grants, research on assistive device development, fellowships, and conferences and symposia (PVA, 2004). In addition to funding research, PVA also established the Consortium for Spinal Cord Medicine in 1995. The Consortium, which is composed of 20 international health professional organizations that focus on spinal cord injuries, develops evidence-based clinical practice guidelines for health care professionals and consumer guides.

United Spinal Association

The recently expanded mission of the United Spinal Association involves outreach, research, and advocacy for veterans and other individuals with spinal cord and related injuries. Begun in 1947 as the Eastern Paralyzed Veterans Association, the organization became the United Spinal Association in January 2004. The Research and Education Department of the United Spinal Association works to promote research partnerships and facilitate the dissemination of research findings. The association funds clinical fellowships at several universities and VA hospitals and has worked to establish three professional associations, the American Paraplegia Society, the American Association of Spinal Cord Injury Psychologists and Social Workers, and the American Association of Spinal Cord Injury Nurses, each of which has a program that provides seed grants for research.

International Efforts

Many international efforts are focused on research on spinal cord injuries and collaborative initiatives. A few of these are described below.

The International Campaign for Cures of Spinal Cord Injury Paralysis (ICCP) consists of eight affiliates[5] that distributed more than $23 million

---

[5]The eight affiliates are Spinal Cure Australia, Christopher Reeve Paralysis Foundation, French Institute for Spinal Cord Research, International Spinal Research Trust, the Miami Project to Cure Paralysis, Paralyzed Veterans of America, Rick Hansen Man in Motion Foundation, and Spinal Research Fund of Australia, Inc.

for 150 basic and clinical research projects in 2001 (Adams and Cavanagh, 2004). ICCP supports funding for new investigators; hosts forums to bring together researchers from many countries; develops clinical trial guidelines; and seeks to enhance various neurotrauma initiatives at the local, state, federal, and international levels (Adams and Cavanagh, 2004; ICCP, 2004b). For example, it offers the Outstanding Young Investigator Award, which provides $10,000 for novice postdoctoral investigators seeking monies to travel to other laboratories and learn techniques and procedures for spinal cord injuries (ICCP, 2004a). ICCP recently conducted a workshop focused on the translation of relevant research on spinal cord injuries to clinical trials (Steeves et al., 2004).

International Collaboration on Repair Discoveries (ICORD) is a recently initiated interdisciplinary research effort in Vancouver, British Columbia, Canada, with the mission of facilitating and accelerating collaborative research on promoting functional recovery and improving quality of life after a spinal cord injury (ICORD, 2004). Bringing together ICORD's 45 principal investigators and approximately 300 researchers and staff members in one research center is the goal of a current building construction effort. This effort, primarily funded by foundations, works in partnership with the Rick Hansen Institute, the University of British Columbia, and the Vancouver Coastal Health Authority.

The International Spinal Research Trust (ISRT), based in the United Kingdom, funds basic and clinical research on spinal cord injuries as well as Nathalie Rose Barr Ph.D. Studentships, which support doctoral students through 3- to 4-year fellowships. ISRT has developed a strategic and targeted approach to its research funding (Harper et al., 1996; Ramer et al., 2000).

NEXT STEPS IN ACCELERATING PROGRESS

Given the multiple and varied sources of funding and support for spinal cord injury research and the numerous potential therapeutic approaches and interventions at various stages of the research process (Chapters 4 and 5), the challenge is to develop a coordinated, collaborative, and focused approach to translational research with a strong research infrastructure. An extensive effort is needed to bolster basic research efforts, catalyze collaborative research efforts, and attract the breadth of talented researchers who will be able to move this field of research forward to achieve the therapeutic solutions needed by the community of individuals with spinal cord injuries.

Bolstering Basic Research

Clinical advances in treatments for spinal cord injuries and other nervous system disorders depend on the quality and extent of fundamental knowledge on neuronal injury and repair. Basic research on the plasticity of the injured nervous system has implications for multiple diseases and outcomes (e.g., central nervous system development, brain trauma, ALS, multiple sclerosis, Parkinson's disease, and spinal cord injuries) and builds the knowledge base on which therapeutic interventions can be developed. One important element of accelerating progress in treating spinal cord injuries will be sustaining research advances in the basic mechanisms of the biological processes that inhibit, promote, sustain, and target the growth of axons and neurons. A fully funded and active research program on neuronal injury and repair not only stands to benefit the thousands of people with spinal cord injuries but also will likely shed new light on other related disorders facing millions of Americans.

Neuronal injury and repair is an issue that is of interest to a number of NIH institutes, including NINDS, the National Institute on Aging, the National Institute of Mental Health, the National Institute of Dental and Craniofacial Research, and the National Institute of Child Health and Human Development. The recently announced *NIH Blueprint for Neuroscience Research* has the potential to facilitate trans-NIH initiatives and increase research collaborations (NIH, 2004a). This initiative will include a focus on neurodegeneration and on the plasticity of the nervous system, both of which are of critical importance in spinal cord injury research. The active involvement of all relevant institutes and support from institute management are critical to ensuring the sustainability of such an initiative.

Enhancing Research Collaborations

Although a number of funding sources are interested in spinal cord injury research, no concerted national effort is in place to push toward the cures that are needed for spinal cord injuries. What is needed is a strengthened research infrastructure that will feature the development of research centers of excellence focused on spinal cord injuries and a structured network to facilitate and ensure collaborative multidisciplinary approaches.

Research centers of excellence are needed to establish and enhance research on spinal cord injuries. These centers should foster collaborations between basic and clinical researchers and promote the interdisciplinary research that is needed to explore the translation of effective laboratory therapies into the clinical setting. The research network is needed to integrate the efforts of the broad array of researchers (investigators both at centers of excellence and from other institutions) who study issues involved in neuronal injury and repair and other relevant avenues of therapeutic intervention for spinal cord injury.

Establishing Research Centers of Excellence

The committee urges a strong commitment by the federal government to designate and support Spinal Cord Injury Research Centers of Excellence. These centers would provide the interdisciplinary research environment that is needed to accelerate the development of future advances in treating spinal cord injuries. The centers would bring together and support investigators from multiple fields, including, but not limited to, neuroscience, cellular and molecular biology, systems biology, immunology, engineering, bioengineering, biostatistics, epidemiology, and clinical medicine.

This would involve both the establishment of new centers and the designation of several current spinal cord injury research programs as centers of excellence. Several multidisciplinary spinal cord injury research programs already exist, including the Miami Project to Cure Paralysis, the Kentucky Spinal Cord Injury Research Center, the Reeve-Irvine Research Center, and NIH-funded research centers (discussed earlier in this chapter and in Chapter 8).

Comprehensive research centers of excellence would offer expansive laboratory facilities; focused interactions between preclinical researchers, clinical researchers, and patients; and central sites for clinical trial design. This investment would likely draw new senior-level researchers into spinal cord injury research and would heighten the interest of young investigators in devoting their research interests to spinal cord injury treatment.

These centers should be supported with the infrastructure needed to promote and enhance the institutional development of spinal cord injury research and treatment capabilities. This includes core research laboratory equipment, tools, and facilities; an emphasis on training programs; strong basic and clinical research components; and a structured plan for research priorities. For example, the 38 comprehensive cancer centers funded primarily by the National Cancer Institute incorporate a requirement for the centers to perform basic research, clinical research, cancer prevention and control activities, and population-based research (NCI, 2004a,b). The centers should also have the capacity to facilitate clinical trials; educate the community; screen and counsel individuals with spinal cord injuries; and educate health professionals about state-of-the-art diagnostic, preventive, and treatment techniques. The centers can serve as a resource for individuals with spinal cord injuries by facilitating patient input to researchers and by maintaining a clinical registry to allow for prompt dissemination of information regarding conferences, upcoming clinical trials, and research findings.

The centers of excellence should be developed regionally to facilitate the development of clinical trial networks. It is important that the centers interface not only with state research programs and nonprofit organizations but also with the VA spinal cord injury centers and the Model Spinal Cord Injury Care System clinics and patient care centers to broaden the potential research base for clinical trials. A national effort to prioritize translational research on spinal cord injuries would expand the capacity to explore and develop therapeutic approaches.

Although it is difficult for the committee to recommend precisely the number of centers of excellence that should be established, the committee believes that creating and sustaining two to three new centers and designating three to four of the existing programs as Spinal Cord Injury Research Centers of Excellence will allow the accelerated progress needed to explore all potential therapeutic pathways. Additionally, the committee urges the NIH Clinical Center to play an active role in translational spinal cord injury research, as it offers extensive expertise and resources. The centers of excellence should serve as the cornerstone of a National Spinal Cord Injury Research Network designed to coordinate and support spinal cord injury research efforts.

Developing a National Spinal Cord Injury Research Network

Key to accelerating progress in the treatment of spinal cord injuries is the development of a coordinated, focused, and centralized network that connects individual investigators, research programs, and research centers; facilitates collaborative and replicative projects; encompasses relevant research from diverse fields; and builds on the unique strengths of each research effort to move toward effective therapies. A research network is of particular importance in spinal cord injury research because of the need for interdisciplinary research and an organized and systematic approach to examining potential combination therapies. The Spinal Cord Injury Research Centers of Excellence discussed above would spearhead this dedicated focus on translational research and would promote collaborations among all sites conducting research relevant to spinal cord injuries. Although online technologies greatly enhance the nearly instantaneous sharing of ideas across the nation and globally, the research network envisioned by the committee would involve not only a strong virtual component but also a structured plan for periodic and regular meetings and workshops to set priorities and strengthen interactions.

The process of developing a national research network for spinal cord injury research can draw on the experiences of several such networks that already exist. The Robert Packard Center for ALS Research is an example of a focused research network that takes a strong collaborative approach. Although the center is physically based at Johns Hopkins University in Baltimore, Maryland, more than 40 percent of the investigators are from other institutions. Self-described as an aggressive approach to developing successful effective therapies for ALS (Johns Hopkins University, 2004), the focus is on translational research with an emphasis on both basic and clinical research. The researchers meet each month to discuss promising research approaches and evaluate each other's progress. This interaction is a structural part of the center, as each researcher's contract specifies that principal investigators and postdoctoral staff based at Johns Hopkins University will attend 9 of the 12 monthly meetings and that outside researchers will attend 4 of the 12 meetings. Researchers are also expected to attend the annual retreat and minisymposium. Several foundations fund the center, with additional support from private donors, federal research grants, and industry.

A coordinated approach to spinal cord injury research is being implemented in Canada through the Rick Hansen Spinal Cord Injury Network (RH SCI Network). Begun in 2003, the RH SCI Network is establishing two subnetworks—the Spinal Cord Injury Translational Research Network and the Spinal Cord Injury Service Network—to integrate the spinal cord injury community across Canada (Rick Hansen Man in Motion Foundation, 2004). The Spinal Cord Injury Translational Research Network connects researchers and facilitates research collaborations. One of the initial efforts is a pilot program aimed at developing a national registry with data on outcome measures for Canadians with spinal cord injuries. The Spinal Cord Injury Service Network connects patients, researchers, and health care professionals. The Canadian government has invested $15 million in the network over 7 years, and private-sector sources also provide funding (Rick Hansen Man in Motion Foundation, 2004).

The committee envisions a sustained network for spinal cord injury research in the United States that would facilitate translational research and the implementation of multicenter clinical trials. Because of the rapid pace with which research on neuronal injury and repair and other aspects of spinal cord injury research is moving forward, it is critical that researchers have access to the most up-to-date research tools and that they be given opportunities to share information and build on new research findings. Further, it will be important for the network to draw on international expertise and for extensive collaborations to be developed with researchers in the Canadian network and across the globe.

The National Spinal Cord Injury Research Network envisioned by the committee should begin its work by convening a consensus conference to prioritize and promote the pre-clinical and translational efforts needed to bring experimental therapies to the clinic; this includes treatments to improve functional deficits and reduce pain and spasticity as well as those focused on neuronal injury and repair. The conference should explore incentives to encourage the pre-clinical studies that are needed to move initial promising discoveries to the point of a clinical trial. Leaders of the spinal cord injury research community, including basic researchers, neurologists, neurosurgeons, physiatrists, radiologists, urologists, pain researchers, emergency physicians, and clinical trial specialists, should develop a set of research and funding priorities that encourage focused, coordinated, and collaborative research projects and that recognize the funding opportunities provided by the states and private foundations, in addition to the federal government. This initial meeting would be followed by regular (perhaps quarterly) meetings of researchers to communicate progress, discuss next steps, prioritize research strategies, and facilitate multicenter clinical trials and other collaborative efforts. The research network would be structured so that the active involvement of the participants and substantive interactions between basic and clinical researchers are expected as part of their participation.

In summary the National Spinal Cord Injury Research Network should:

- convene an initial consensus conference to identify research and funding priorities and continue on a periodic basis to convene researchers and clinicians to update progress, prioritize research strategies, facilitate multicenter clinical trials, and engage in other collaborative efforts;
- facilitate research on the range of outcomes and complications (including sensory, motor, bowel, bladder, autonomic, and sexual function and pain) that individuals with spinal cord injuries face;
- enhance career development opportunities for young researchers by providing transitional support and other career-path opportunities, including participation in laboratory-based spinal cord injury training courses;
- create and support virtual networking centers to facilitate the sharing of resources online and enhance collaborations with researchers not working in research centers and foster international collaborations;
- convene annual or semiannual colloquia that particularly focus on research outside the traditional areas of spinal cord injury research to examine the approaches being used to address other complex health problems and to address the utility of that research to the treatment of spinal cord injuries; and
- develop standardized protocols for patient registry systems so that registries can be coordinated and used to assist in identifying candidates for clinical trials and provide information on upcoming clinical trials to individuals with spinal cord injuries.

Efforts to develop a Spinal Cord Injury Research Network are consistent with many of the goals of the NIH Roadmap (NIH, 2004b), including an emphasis on translational research that results in clinically useful therapies and a need for multidisciplinary efforts to be used to address this complex medical condition.

Expansion of Training and Career Opportunities

An integral part of accelerating progress in research on spinal cord injuries is an emphasis on training and career opportunities to attract and retain top-notch spinal cord injury researchers. There are few measures of the number of graduate students and postdoctoral researchers who are interested in focusing on spinal cord injury research. What is known is that the number of doctoral theses focused on spinal cord injuries has increased in recent years, from 54 from 1990 to 1992 to 83 from 1999 to 2001, as indicated by a search of the Dissertations Abstracts database (see Appendix A for details on search strategy). The number of predoctoral fellowships for research focused on spinal cord injuries awarded by NIH has increased in the past 10 years but is less than the numbers awarded for other neurological conditions. For example, from 2001 to 2003, 11 predoctoral NIH fellowships (F30 and F31 awards) were awarded for work on spinal cord injuries, according to the CRISP database, whereas 15 were awarded for epilepsy, 17 were awarded for multiple sclerosis, 26 were awarded for stroke, 32 were awarded for Parkinson's disease, and 38 were awarded for Alzheimer's disease. The trends for postdoctoral fellowships are similar. The number of fellowships for research on spinal cord injuries is modest and is insufficient to take maximum advantage of the opportunities for furthering research on spinal cord injuries and attracting new investigators to the field.

Enhancing career opportunities for researchers at all points in their careers is vital to accelerating progress in spinal cord injury research. The committee believes that strengthening the research infrastructure through the development of new comprehensive research centers will be the impetus needed to attract and retain midcareer and senior-level researchers. At these centers they will have the opportunity to fully engage in their own research initiatives, in addition to having the resources to develop and nurture trainees and sustain a full research effort.

The committee believes that additional steps need to be taken to attract graduate students, medical students, and postdoctoral researchers to spinal cord injury research. Raising the awareness of research opportunities in this field is a critical step in attracting graduate and medical students to the field, and efforts such as the development of a training module that describes the unique biology of the spinal cord could be an important mode for ensuring that the information reaches students. In addition to increasing the fellowship opportunities offered by NIH, the committee also encourages the development of privately funded competitive graduate fellowships in spinal cord injury research. Competitive fellowships attract top students to the field, raise the profile of spinal cord injury research, and become sought-after mechanisms for engaging talented young investigators in a specific research focus.

RECOMMENDATIONS

Recommendation 7.1: *Bolster and Coordinate Research on Neuronal Injury and Repair*
The National Institutes of Health should increase the funding for mechanisms that encourage research coordination in neuronal injury and repair and should actively develop and support cross-institute and cross-disciplinary working groups, as outlined in the *NIH Blueprint for Neuroscience Research.*

Recommendation 7.2: *Establish Spinal Cord Injury Research Centers of Excellence*
The National Institutes of Health should designate and support five to seven Spinal Cord Injury Research Centers of Excellence with adequate resources to sustain multidisciplinary basic, translational, and clinical research on spinal cord injuries. This would involve establishing two to three new Centers of Excellence and designating three to four current spinal cord injury research programs as Centers of Excellence.

Recommendation 7.3: *Establish a National Spinal Cord Injury Research Network*
The National Institutes of Health should be appropriately funded to establish a National Spinal Cord Injury Research Network that would coordinate and support the work of an expanded cadre of researchers.

Recommendation 7.4: *Increase Training and Career Development Opportunities*
Resources should be designated to strengthen education programs for pre- and postdoctoral training in spinal cord injury research.

• The National Institutes of Health Office of Science Education and the National Institute of Neurological Disorders and Stroke should enhance training and develop a training module on the functional complexity of the spinal cord for neuroscience Ph.D. and medical students.

• The National Institutes of Health, state programs, and other research organizations should increase funding for training and career development opportunities for graduate and postdoctoral researchers interested in spinal cord injury research, including individual graduate student and postdoctoral fellowships, transitional fellowships for postdoctoral researchers, and competitive fellowships sponsored by private-sector funders with links to ongoing research centers and networks.

REFERENCES

Adams M, Cavanagh JF. 2004. International Campaign for Cures of Spinal Cord Injury Paralysis (ICCP): Another step forward for spinal cord injury research. *Spinal Cord* 42(5): 273-280.

APS (American Paraplegia Society). 2004a. *American Paraplegia Society.* [Online]. Available: http://www.apssci.org/pages.php?catid=1&pageid=1 [accessed August 30, 2004].

APS. 2004b. *American Paraplegia Society 50th Annual Conference Program.* [Online]. Available: http://www.apssci.org/documents/DownLoad/2004APSProgram.pdf [accessed August 30, 2004].

APS. 2004c. *Seed Grant Program Guidelines.* [Online]. Available: http://www.apssci.org/pages.php?catid=32&pageid=19 [accessed August 30, 2004].

Bryon Riesch Paralysis Foundation. 2002. *Bryon Riesch Paralysis Foundation—Instructions for Research Grant Applications.* [Online]. Available: http://www.brpf.org/Grant%20Instructions.doc [accessed August 30, 2004].

Bryon Riesch Paralysis Foundation. 2004. *Bryon Riesch Paralysis Foundation.* [Online]. Available: http://www.brpf.org/index.htm [accessed August 30, 2004].

CRPF (Christopher Reeve Paralysis Foundation). 2003. *Research—Introduction.* [Online]. Available: http://www.christopherreeve.org/Research/ResearchList.cfm?c=61 [accessed August 11, 2004].

CRPF. 2004a. *Research Grant History.* [Online]. Available: http://www.christopherreeve.org/Research/ResearchList.cfm?c=26 [accessed August 11, 2004].

CRPF. 2004b. *Individual Grant Application.* [Online]. Available: http://www.guidelinespacket-igam and meeting121504.pdf [accessed August 11, 2004].

DeVivo MJ. 2002. Model spinal cord systems of care. In: Lin V, Cardenas DD, Cutter NC, Frost FS, Hammond MC, Lindblom LB, Perkash I, Waters R, eds. *Spinal Cord Medicine: Principles and Practice.* New York: Demos Medical Publishing. Pp. 955-958.

Hammond MC. 2002. VA spinal cord injury system of care. In: Lin V, Cardenas DD, Cutter NC, Frost FS, Hammond MC, Lindblom LB, Perkash I, Waters R, eds. *Spinal Cord Medicine: Principles and Practice.* New York: Demos Medical Publishing. Pp. 959-960.

Harper GP, Banyard PJ, Sharpe PC. 1996. The International Spinal Research Trust's strategic approach to the development of treatments for the repair of spinal cord injury. *Spinal Cord* 34(8): 449-459.

ICCP (International Campaign for Cures of Spinal Cord Injury Paralysis). 2004a. *ICCP Outstanding Young Investigator Award.* [Online]. Available: http://www.campaignforcure.org/Young%20Investigator%20Award.htm [accessed August 30, 2004].

ICCP. 2004b. *Research Grants Funded by ICCP Member Organisations.* [Online]. Available: http://www.campaignforcure.org/funding.htm [accessed August 30, 2004].

ICORD (International Collaboration On Repair Discoveries). 2004. *About ICORD.* [Online]. Available: http://www.icord.org/about.html [accessed November 21, 2004].

Johns Hopkins University. 2004. *The Robert Packard Center for ALS Research at Johns Hopkins.* [Online]. Available: http://www.alscenter.org/ [accessed November 11, 2004].

National Center for Injury Prevention and Control. 2001. *Injury Fact Book, 2001-2002.* Atlanta: Centers for Disease Control and Prevention.

NCI (National Cancer Institute). 2004a. *Description of the Cancer Centers Program.* [Online]. Available: http://www3.cancer.gov/cancercenters/description.html [accessed November 11, 2004].

NCI. 2004b. *NCI-Designated Cancer Centers (P30).* [Online]. Available: http://www3.cancer.gov/cancercenters/centerslist.html [accessed November 11, 2004].

NICHD (National Institute of Child Health and Human Development). 2004. *NCMRR Research Priorities*. [Online]. Available: http://www.nichd.nih.gov/publications/pubs/counncmrr/sub4.htm [accessed October 4, 2004].

NIDRR (National Institute on Disability and Rehabilitation Research). 2004. *NIDRR's Core Areas of Research*. [Online]. Available: http://www.ed.gov/rschstat/research/pubs/core-area.html [accessed August 28, 2004].

NIH (National Institutes of Health). 2000. *National Research Service Award for Individual Predoctoral Fellows*. [Online]. Available: http://grants1.nih.gov/grants/guide/pa-files/PA-00-125.html [accessed June 21, 2004].

NIH. 2003. *Trends in Training and Fellowships—Fiscal Years 1976-2002*. [Online]. Available: http://grants.nih.gov/training/data/tf_trends/index.htm [accessed June 25, 2004].

NIH. 2004a. *NIH Blueprint for Neuroscience Research*. [Online]. Available: http://neuroscienceblueprint.nih.gov [accessed December 22, 2004].

NIH. 2004b. *Overview of the NIH Roadmap*. [Online]. Available: http://nihroadmap.nih.gov/overview.asp [accessed January 7, 2005].

NIH. 2004c. *Estimates of Funding for Various Diseases, Conditions, Research Areas*. [Online]. Available: http://www.nih.gov/news/fundingresearchareas.htm [accessed September 3, 2004].

NINDS (National Institute of Neurological Disorders and Stroke). 2002. *Facilities of Research in Spinal Cord Injury*. [Online]. Available: http://grants2.nih.gov/grants/guide/notice-files/NOT-NS-02-011.html [accessed October 4, 2004].

NINDS. 2003. *Translating Promising Strategies for Spinal Cord Injury Therapy February 3-4, 2003, Bethesda, Maryland*. [Online]. Available: http://www.ninds.nih.gov/news_and_events/proceedings/sci_translation_workshop.htm?format=printable [accessed August 9, 2004].

NINDS. 2004a. *Functional and Dysfunctional Spinal Circuitry: Role for Rehabilitation and Neural Prostheses*. [Online]. Available: http://www.ninds.nih.gov/news_and_events/proceedings/spinalcircuitrywkshp_pr.htm [accessed November 11, 2004].

NINDS. 2004b. *Role of the Immune System in Spinal Cord Injury*. [Online]. Available: http://www.ninds.nih.gov/news_and_events/proceedings/immunesciwkshp_pr.htm [accessed November 11, 2004].

Paralysis Project of America. 2004. *Paralysis Project of America Spinal Cord Injury, Rehabilitation and Neuroplasticity Research—Request for Applications*. [Online]. Available: http://www.paralysisproject.org/PPA_Grant_Guidelines_2004.pdf [accessed August 30, 2004].

PVA (Paralyzed Veterans of America). 2003. *Paralyzed Veterans of America 2003 Annual Report*. Washington, DC: Paralyzed Veterans of America.

PVA. 2004. *Paralyzed Veterans of America's Spinal Cord Research Foundation Policies and Procedures, FY2005*. [Online]. Available: http://www.pva.org/res/pdf/res_policy_05.PDF [accessed August 9, 2004].

Ramer MS, Harper GP, Bradbury EJ. 2000. Progress in spinal cord research: A refined strategy for the International Spinal Research Trust. *Spinal Cord* 38(8): 449-472.

Rick Hansen Man in Motion Foundation. 2004. *Rick Hansen Spinal Cord Injury Network Executive Summary Year One Report May, 2004*. [Online]. Available: http://www.rickhansen.com/SCINetwork/Documents/RH%20SCI%20Network%20Year%20One%20Exec%20Summary.pdf [accessed November 11, 2004].

Spinal Cord Society. 2004. *Spinal Cord Society Research Support*. [Online]. Available: http://members.aol.com/scsweb/private/support.htm [accessed August 30, 2004].

Steeves J, Fawcett J, Tuszynski M. 2004. Report of International Clinical Trials Workshop on Spinal Cord Injury February 20-21, 2004, Vancouver, Canada. *Spinal Cord* 42: 591-597.

Tate DG, Forchheimer M. 2002. Contributions from the Model Systems Programs to spinal cord injury research. *Journal of Spinal Cord Medicine* 25(4): 316-330.
Tulsky DS. 2002. The impacts of the Model SCI System: Historical perspective. *Journal of Spinal Cord Medicine* 25(4): 310-315.
VA (U.S. Department of Veterans Affairs). 2002. *Fact Sheet: VA and Spinal Cord Injury*. [Online]. Available: http://www1.va.gov/opa/fact/spinalcfs.html [accessed November 11, 2004].

8

STATE PROGRAMS IN
SPINAL CORD INJURY

More than one-quarter of the states in the United States have passed legislation creating programs expressly devoted to spinal cord injury research. Most state programs, launched in the late 1990s, represent an important new trend in which state legislatures channel funds to a particular area of health research. However, there is nothing new about states investing in research.

For more than three decades, state governments have carved out a role for themselves in supporting research within their borders. States' total research and development spending for all areas of science and health was approximately $88 million in the mid-1960s. By 1995 that spending had surged to $3 billion nationwide (Jankowski, 1999). The prime motivations behind state investments in research have been to propel economic growth and to improve the health of their citizenries (SSTI, 1997, 1999a; Jankowski, 1999).

This chapter examines state programs for spinal cord injury research to determine how they are structured and how states—as well as researchers—stand to benefit from their creation. It then looks in depth at three spinal cord injury programs that have successfully leveraged the funds received from their own states to draw in much larger sums in federal research funding. The goal is to set the stage for the chapter's final section on New York State. That section examines the unique strengths of New York State's institutions and researchers in neurological, basic, clinical, and translational research on spinal cord injuries and offers recommendations on what distinctive contributions New York's spinal cord injury research program can make to accelerate the search for improving the outcome after a spinal cord injury. Many of the chapter's recommendations for New York State are also applicable to other states interested in setting or revising strategic directions for their spinal cord injury research programs. The states can learn much from one another to develop and strengthen their spinal cord injury research programs.

STATE PROGRAMS AND LEGISLATION

Since 1988, 14 states have passed legislation that has resulted in annual funding for spinal cord injury research of about $27 million (Table 8-1).

TABLE 8-1 State Legislation Relevant to Spinal Cord Injury Research

State	Year Legislation Enacted	Year Legislation Proposed but Not Enacted
California	2000[a]	
Colorado		2004[a]
Connecticut	1999	
Florida	1988	
Illinois	2000[a]	
Indiana	1998	
Iowa		2004[a]
Kansas		2001
Kentucky	1994	
Maryland	2000	
Massachusetts	2004[a]	
Michigan		1989
Minnesota		2000[a]
Missouri	2001	
New Jersey	1999[a]	
New York	1998[a]	
Ohio		2000[a]
Oregon	1999[a]	
Pennsylvania		2000
South Carolina	2000	
South Dakota		2003
Texas		1999[a]
Virginia	1997	
Washington		2004[a]

[a]The legislation specifically notes that research is conducted to cure spinal cord injuries.
NOTE: The data were compiled in October 2004 and are based on a review of state legislature websites, searches on Lexis-Nexis, and telephone interviews. The table includes the year that the legislation was first enacted or considered (i.e., data on later years when the legislation was revised or considered are not included). Enacted legislation supersedes proposed legislation (e.g., legislation considered in 1996 but approved in 1998 is listed as enacted in 1998 and does not appear in the proposed legislation column).

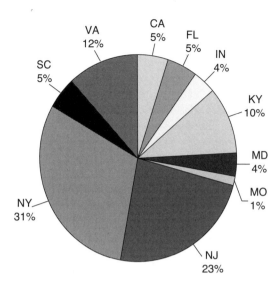

FIGURE 8-1 Percentage of total state spinal cord injury research funding for states with dedicated spinal cord injury research programs. Data for only 10 states are listed. Oregon, Illinois, and Connecticut do not have budgets for their programs. The Massachusetts program was approved in August 2004, and the budget amounts have not yet been specified.

Another 10 states have proposed but have not yet enacted similar legislation. The surge in state legislation, which occurred from the late 1990s to 2001, reflects growing acceptance and awareness that motor vehicle crashes are the leading cause of spinal cord injuries. The concept behind most state legislation can be traced back to a pioneering 1988 Florida law that designated a set percentage of revenues from fines for unsafe driving for spinal cord injury care and research. Today, the amounts and the percentages vary, but the majority of the 14 states each spend at least $1 million each year for spinal cord injury research. New York State supports the program with the largest amount of state funding, $8.5 million per year (Figure 8-1).

The structures and sources of funding vary among the state programs (see Appendix H). New York, for example, collects funds from a surcharge of $5[1] for traffic violations, whereas New Jersey adds an additional $1 to each motor vehicle or traffic violation fine. Some state programs, such as those in Florida, Indiana, and Kentucky, designate that the funds obtained

---

[1]New York State Senate Introducer's Memorandum in Support of S7287C (1998).

from surcharges go to support specific university programs. Other states diversify the types of awards that they grant and allow any university-based researcher in the state to apply. South Carolina, for example, provides an estimated $1 million every 2 years for individual and small pilot research grants, career development awards, and faculty recruitment initiatives. Maryland also distributes $1 million annually for spinal cord injury research through a tax on health insurers. Several states have developed or contribute funding to extensive research centers, including the Miami Project to Cure Paralysis and the Kentucky Spinal Cord Injury Research Center (see below). Some states use their funds for patient care, in addition to research.

The largest and most innovative state programs (see below) have used state funds as seed money to expand their programs' sizes, scopes, and impacts by using their funds to support pilot projects that generate enough data to help them garner more state, federal, and private financing.

BENEFITS TO STATES FROM THEIR INVESTMENTS

In the aggregate, states invest billions of dollars each year on research and development across all fields of science and technology. Those state expenditures represent a consistent trend that began more than three decades ago. The earliest statistics, gathered in 1965, revealed that states collectively spent about $88 million annually on research and development. That amount rose to $3 billion in 1995 (Jankowski, 1999). These data were reported by the National Science Foundation, based on a 1995 survey of 1,000 state agencies and universities. The total is likely to be significantly higher today, almost a decade later, but no recent surveys have been conducted.

What is known about state spending for research and development in general and biomedical research in particular? What motivates this investment? And what is the return on the investment? These questions are addressed in the next section.

OVERVIEW OF STATE
RESEARCH AND DEVELOPMENT SPENDING

The 1995 survey found that the vast majority of the $3 billion in state research and development spending (73 percent, or $2 billion) went to academic institutions in each state. Most of the remainder went to state agencies (14 percent, or $408 million). Of the 73 percent distributed to academic institutions, the majority (67 percent) went to public universities, while the remainder was directed to private universities within the state (Jankowski, 1999).

An overwhelming proportion of the $3 billion in state research and development spending was for research, as opposed to the physical plant infrastructure ($228 million). States typically financed their research and development expenditures from one of four sources: general revenues, lottery proceeds, revenue bonds, and specially designated tax funds. Another source, which accounted for about 9 percent of state spending, was from federal research dollars passed through state agencies (e.g., funding for state health department research from the Centers for Disease Control and Prevention). Revenue bonds floated by a state are commonly used to finance the research infrastructure, such as new construction and equipment (Personal communication, M. Skinner, State Science & Technology Institute [SSTI], November 11, 2004).

These amounts are likely to be relevant to biomedical research because biomedical research accounts for a large share of the spending on research. Although the 1995 survey did not compile actual amounts by field of research, it did report that biological and medical sciences received the highest proportion of state funds, regardless of whether they were directed to academic institutions or to state agencies (Figure 8-2). Engineering and environmental sciences were ranked second and third, respectively. Since 1995, when the survey was conducted, a huge infusion of state funds to life sciences research has been obtained from a new source: state tobacco settle-

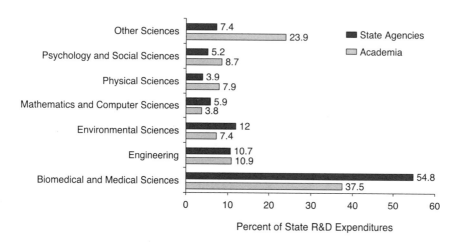

FIGURE 8-2 State government research and development expenditures, by performer of the research and field, 1995.
SOURCES: Battelle Memorial Institute/SSTI, 1998; Jankowski, 1999; National Science Foundation, 2004.

ments (SSTI, 1999b). The tobacco industry agreed to pay $250 billion over the next 25 years to resolve Medicaid lawsuits filed by the states to cover their tobacco-related health care expenditures (Center for Social Gerontology, 2004). Many state legislatures have allocated their settlements to fund life sciences research more generally rather than smoking-related research per se.

Motivation for State Spending on Research and Development

State spending on research and development is largely driven by the quest for economic growth. The recognition of research and development as a growth engine became more apparent during the 1990s, when states increasingly began to incorporate expansion of their research and development capacities into their economic development plans (SSTI, 1997). An analysis of governors' state of the state speeches, inaugural addresses, and budget speeches signaled a consistently high level of interest in expanding the state's research and development capacity to promote economic development (Jankowski, 1999). In New York State, for example, Governor George Pataki spearheaded several research and development initiatives worth more than $500 million, including the formation of the New York State Office of Science, Technology, and Academic Research (NYSTAR). NYSTAR issued a report that attributes its creation as "reflect[ing] the recognition that New York's world-class public and private research universities and academic centers are powerful economic development engines that can help create high-tech jobs and opportunity in New York" (NYSTAR, 2001). The following are some of the specific economic objectives that motivate most states to invest in research (SSTI, 1997, 1999a; Attorney General of California, 2004; Battelle Technology Partnership Practice/SSTI, 2004):

- to propel a state's economic growth by strengthening the capacity of the state's public and private universities;
- to attract additional investment from federal and private sources;
- to attract or retain home-grown businesses, investment capital, and high-paying jobs;
- to expand access to high-quality education and to cultivate an educated workforce;
- to encourage academia-industry collaborations to commercialize the goods and services that result from research; and
- to obtain revenues from patents, royalties, and licenses (Jankowski, 1999).

During the past 10 or more years, states have increasingly begun to focus more specifically on biomedical research. In addition to the economic benefits listed above, states view the biosciences as a rapidly growing industry sector and as a means to improve the health of its citizens (Battelle Technology Partnership Practice/SSTI, 2004). In contrast to earlier efforts, which were more broad based, states are now targeting specific niches within biomedical research, such as spinal cord injury research. The motivation comes from several considerations:

- to accelerate research to improve health care services and quality of life;
- to reduce the high cost of care for recipients of assistance from state health programs (e.g., Medicaid) and state employees;
- to prevent injuries and improve motor vehicle safety; and
- to improve the health and productivity of the state's entire workforce.

Returns on the Investment

Several high-profile studies have sought to quantify the economic and health benefits of state support for biomedical research and development in terms of job creation, the health care costs saved (e.g., the hospitalizations avoided), the value of an increased life span, and reduced morbidity and disability (Silverstein et al., 1995; Lasker Foundation, 2000). The overall cost savings derived from the economic and health benefits of support for biomedical research are estimated to be $69 billion annually (Silverstein et al., 1995). Although evaluation of these estimates is important and demanding, they are national in focus and do not specify the economic and health benefits to a given investor, such as a state or a local government.

Several smaller studies, cited by Silverstein and colleagues (1995), have been conducted to assess the economic returns to states that invest in biotechnology. A Bank of Boston study found that 25.5 jobs were created for every $1 million spent on biotechnology research (Bank of Boston Economics Department, 1991; Silverstein et al., 1995). Similar benefits were estimated in California and Maryland (California Health Care Institute, 1993; Maryland Department of Economic and Employment Development, 1994).

The most relevant study for the purposes of this report was conducted by a team of New York State-based university economists who, at the request of the New York Academy of Medicine, quantified the returns to New York State from investments in biomedical research (Sclar and Aries, 2000). The researchers surveyed 20 biomedical institutions within the state, covering 86 percent of the state's population. They asked the institutions about the grants that they receive, grant-related expenditures, and institutional expenditures. They assessed the economic impact by applying an

---

BOX 8-1
Economic Benefits to State or Local Governments
Investing in Research

For every $1 million invested, a state or local government can expect:

• 20 full-time jobs (including, directly, 12 jobs in research and, indirectly, 8 jobs induced by spending);
• about $50,000 to $100,000 in additional tax revenues to the state, mostly through income taxes; and
• additional research grants from the National Institutes of Health that reap additional jobs and tax revenues (the case studies in this chapter show at least a 200 percent return on investment).

SOURCES: Aries and Sclar, 1998; Sclar and Aries, 2000.

---

input-output economic model that can trace the effects of research spending on the economy (industries and households) of the region where the research took place. Apart from the direct effects of research funding (e.g., employee compensation and the purchase of goods and services), ripple effects came in two forms: the secondary expenditures of vendors whose businesses were stimulated by the institutional spending (i.e., indirect effects) and induced spending effects resulting from the increased household incomes that the cumulative chain of spending creates. The study found that research investment led to high payoffs in terms of well-paying jobs (an average compensation package of $115,000 per employee) and additional tax revenues from businesses, including excise taxes, property taxes, fees, licenses, and sales taxes, as well as income taxes to the state and federal governments. The magnitude of the effect is presented in Box 8-1.

Advantages of State Programs for Studying Spinal Cord Injuries

Testimony to the committee and interviews with scientific directors of state programs showed that state-sponsored spinal cord injury research programs offer several advantages to researchers: flexibility; the capacity to leverage more funding, especially for renovation or new construction; a steady form of financing (e.g., from motor vehicle surcharges); and a strong investment in the regional economy.

Flexibility

Flexibility is a major reason that researchers and institutions obtain funding from states. Grantees often use state funding for pilot studies that give them an edge to compete successfully for grants from the National Institutes of Health (NIH), which are highly competitive, lucrative, and prestigious. In each model program described in this chapter, funds from state or local grants were parlayed into the receipt of NIH grants of double or triple the value of the state or local grant. State funds have also been used to fill the gaps left unfilled by NIH grants. Examples include endowed faculty chairs (see the description below of the Kentucky Spinal Cord Injury Research Center), lecture series, and special fellowships. Flexibility in state funding enables researchers to pursue high-risk research or to capitalize on new and unexpected research directions. In sum, state funds not only are used to establish a program but also can be used as a building block.

New Construction or Renovation

State funding has been used, directly or indirectly, for renovation and new construction. Physical infrastructure not only is important for research in its own right but also is key to attracting new talent. The Miami Project to Cure Paralysis was able to build a $36 million building with partial state funding. The project obtained $10 million from the state as a one-time line item in the state budget that matched the funds that the project had raised from a private donor. The receipt of state funds for construction helped the program secure even more private funding. In this instance, state funds for construction were separate from the state's annual fund for research and treatment for spinal cord injuries.

States can finance construction by floating bonds. That was the preferred vehicle of financing listed in a survey reported by the National Science Foundation (see above). State-issued bonds will also be used by the state of California to finance the building of new facilities under its stem cell research initiative that was approved by voters in 2004.[2]

NIH rarely funds new construction through its extramural research program, although it does fund new construction for public health priorities, such as, most recently, biological defense. NIH construction grants also impose restrictions. They are normally capped at $4 million. In recent years the annual congressional appropriations for these grants, which represent funding for the Research and Facilities Improvement Program, has been approximately $110 million to $120 million (U.S. Senate Committee on Appropriations, 2003). A portion of NIH's Centers of Biomedical Research Excellence[3] grants ($500,000) can also be used for renovation. How-

---

[2]California Codes Health and Safety. §125290.70(a)(4) (2004).

[3]Centers of Biomedical Research Excellence grants are awarded through NIH's National Center for Research Resources, which is authorized under Sections 481A and 481B of the Public Health Service Act, as amended by Sections 303 and 304 of P.L. 106-505, to "make grants or contracts to public and nonprofit private entities to expand, remodel, renovate, or alter existing research facilities or construct new research facilities."

ever, these grants are generally awarded only to those states that have historically been unsuccessful in competing for NIH grants. Furthermore, NIH infrastructure grants often require matching funds.

Reliability

State funding also provides a reliable and steady stream of resources if the funding comes from a dedicated revenue generator, such as fines for surcharges on motor vehicle violations. Stable funding enables multiyear planning, which is important for research continuity. Program directors in states that have yearly line-item appropriations rather than dedicated funding sources for spinal cord injury research emphasized the limitations of the year-to-year variability and the need to expend scarce resources to lobby state legislators. It is imperative that a certain level of funding be ensured each year for long-term organization and planning, the continuity of personnel, and more rapid progress in research.

Investment in Regional Impact

State governments, in contrast to the federal government, have a more direct and enduring investment in the success of their spinal cord injury research and development programs. As discussed earlier, states have increasingly come to view their research and development programs as part of their economic development plans or as a means to improve health care services for their populations. Even without a direct financial investment in a spinal cord injury research and development program, states can help to build a program by, for example, fostering linkages to local governments or to biopharmaceutical firms in the region. New York City, for example, set up an important program to help young biomedical investigators (Box 8-2). Furthermore, states can also help to steer patients to clinical trials for acute spinal cord injuries by virtue of their direct management of regional trauma systems.

MODELS OF STATE-SPONSORED
SPINAL CORD INJURY RESEARCH PROGRAMS

The following sections profile the efforts of three states to support state spinal cord injury research programs (Kentucky, Florida, and California). The material in this section was gathered by interviewing the director or the scientific director of the state's major spinal cord injury research center. These programs offer three different models that have all been extremely successful in making a significant research contribution and in stimulating

BOX 8-2
Municipal Support of Biomedical Research:
Case Study of New York City

What began as a municipal program to enhance the recruitment of young bio-medical investigators to institutions in New York City turned out to be a case study of the high economic returns—in both human (scientific talent) and funding terms—that can be obtained by investing in biomedical research.

The New York City Council launched the program in 1997 by allocating $15 million over 5 years to the New York Academy of Medicine. The program was confined to grant support for new assistant professors or postdoctoral fellows in eight research-intensive New York City institutions, six of which were academic medical centers. Each year, each institution was allowed to submit up to four pro-posals selected by the dean. The grants provided $100,000 annually for 3 years for each awardee, with renewal for the second and third years dependent on the results of a scientific review of progress reports. Funds could be used for the inves-tigator's salary and equipment and laboratory supplies, but the institutional over-head was limited to 8 percent. The program was intended to promote any type of research on diseases of importance to urban populations, whether it was clinical, translational, or basic research.

A committee whose members were the deans or presidents of the eight institu-tions oversaw the program, and the president of the New York Academy of Medi-cine chaired the committee. Proposals mirrored the general format of R01 grants at the National Institutes of Health (NIH). Experts selected by the president of the Institute of Medicine of the National Academy of Sciences, which oversaw the review process, reviewed the proposals for scientific quality. Ten grants were awarded annually, usually for the proposals achieving the 10 highest review scores.

Evaluation of the program revealed that the first 3 years of funding had enabled grantees to amass an additional $18 million in direct and indirect grant awards, largely from NIH. Additional funding was received by 70 percent of the grantees. This $18 million represented a return of about 200 percent on the $9 million in grants awarded to the first 30 young investigators that the program funded.

A standard input-output economic model was used to calculate the return on the investment (Aries and Sclar, 1998) The inputs were $27 million (the original $9 million awarded during the first 3 years of the program plus the $18 million in additional extramural grants) plus the standard multiplier effects that incorporate direct, indirect, and induced spending effects. The model suggested that each million dollars of research funding to these research-intensive institutions generat-ed approximately 20 full-time equivalent jobs. On this basis, the level of research funding in the program at that time could be expected to generate approximately 540 new full-time equivalent positions, with employee compensation totaling $32.1 million, as well as approximately $1.1 million in indirect business taxes and $9.7 million in state and federal taxes, primarily income taxes (Barondess, 2002).

the state's economy by creating high-paying jobs and increasing state and local tax revenues.

Kentucky

History and Role of State Funding

In 1994, Kentucky passed legislation creating the Kentucky Spinal Cord and Head Injury Trust, which directed traffic violation surcharges to spinal cord and head injury research. A state senator, Tim Shaughnessy, whose niece had a spinal cord injury, spearheaded the legislation. Christopher Shields of the University of Louisville was instrumental in establishing the Kentucky Spinal Cord Injury Research Center.

The enabling legislation targeted trust fund revenues to two Kentucky universities, the University of Louisville and the University of Kentucky (Box 8-3). From 1995 to 2004, the trust paid out $0.725 to $2.15 million annually for individual research grants (depending on the amount of surcharges collected). These funds were competitively awarded to researchers

---

BOX 8-3
Kentucky

Type of Program: Centralized program in two universities

State Trust Fund Revenues: $1.5 million to $3 million per year from vehicle surcharges

Trust Fund Use: Research, endowed chairs, graduate student and postdoctoral support, and a visiting lecture series

Estimated Annual Research Budget: $3.5 million plus salaries from endowed chairs for faculty at the Kentucky Spinal Cord Injury Research Center (see Figure 8-3)

Growth Indicators Since the Program's Inception:
  NIH research grants: $0 to $2.5 million per year
  Principal investigators: 2 to 16 (8 in the center plus 8 affiliated faculty at the universities)
  Personnel: 6 to 60 FTEs (plus 30 full-time equivalents at affiliated laboratories)
  Space: 700 to 11,000 square feet

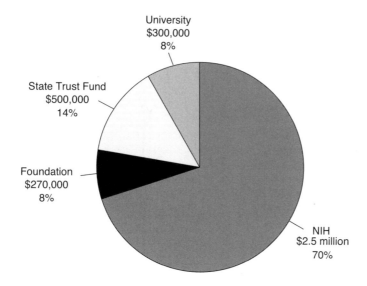

FIGURE 8-3 Kentucky Spinal Cord Injury Research Center funding at the University of Louisville: Estimated sources of yearly research budget.
SOURCE: Personal communication, Scott R. Whittemore, Kentucky Spinal Cord Injury Research Center, February 27, 2005.

from the two universities after review by an external study section. In the early years, the majority of these funds went to University of Kentucky researchers, but over the past few years they have been equally divided between the two institutions. The remainder of this section focuses on the University of Louisville because its program is exclusively devoted to spinal cord injury, whereas the University of Kentucky's emphasis is on head injury research.

The University of Louisville's program expanded over time to become the Kentucky Spinal Cord Injury Research Center. Today, the center has both a scientific and clinical director, attesting to its broad research focus. Its mission is to "develop successful spinal cord repair strategies in the laboratory that can be taken to the clinic in a timely and responsible fashion" (KSCIRC, 2004).

Kentucky Spinal Cord Injury Research Center

Over the past decade, the trust fund has been used to transform a small laboratory at the University of Louisville into a nationally recognized program of research in spinal cord injuries. The trust fund's annual investment of about $1.5 million has been strategically used as seed money to attract large amounts of private and public investments. Since 1998, the program gained momentum by accumulating more than $20 million in federal research funds. The university designated the program a center in 2002, and the center expects sustained growth.

The program is highly centralized around four senior and four junior investigators and state-of-the-art core facilities for animal surgery, electrophysiology, behavioral analysis, gene therapy, and microscopic analyses. Its clinical research focuses on the use of novel imaging methods to assess the acutely injured human spinal cord. The center has set its sights on expanding its faculty in the area of clinical rehabilitation research. Much of its operating research budget, around 67 percent, is from NIH grants; the second largest source of revenues is from the state trust fund (Figure 8-3). The remainder is split between university and foundation funds. The center uses trust fund revenues in several ways, most commonly to fund competitively awarded research proposals and to endow faculty chairs. Driven by a commitment to collaboration the center has a research agenda that encourages translational research and that seeks out collaborations to extend the impact of the center (see below).

The state's trust fund revenues have been instrumental in building the center. The trust fund is a stable and flexible source of funding. A board of directors oversees the fund. The board of directors has seven members: two from each university and other members appointed by the state medical society or governor. Although the trust funds were largely steered toward individual research grants at first, the University of Louisville program shifted its expenditures to launch significant growth. Starting in 1997, trust funds began to be used as a nucleus for garnering private, state, and federal funds. The key step was the awarding of $500,000 to each university for faculty development. The University of Louisville used those funds for newly endowed faculty chairs that required matching funds. The $500,000 was matched by a private donation; and the total, $1 million, was matched again by a novel state program set up by the Kentucky governor, known as *Bucks for Brains*.[4] Over time, $10 million has been raised and has been used to endow five chairs of $2 million each. The funds are invested, with salaries produced from the interest on the principal. All of the private donations thus far have come from Norton Healthcare, which supports the

---

[4]The *Bucks for Brains* program is funded through the Research Challenge Trust Fund, which directs surplus state budget revenues for research and education. Started in 1997, it is guided by the belief that increased economic growth is fueled by quality education. The fund is no longer available because the state has no surplus from which to draw.

BOX 8-4
Timeline for the Kentucky
Spinal Cord Injury Research Center

1988	Formation of small laboratory for spinal cord injury research
1994	Creation of the Kentucky Spinal Cord and Head Injury Trust
1995	Receipt of a $2.6 million grant (over 5 years) from the National Science Foundation Experimental Program to Stimulate Competitive Research
1997-2004	Receipt of matching funds from Norton Healthcare and the Commonwealth of Kentucky's Bucks for Brains Program
2001	Receipt of an $8.5 million grant (over 5 years) from the NIH Centers of Biomedical Research Excellence
2002	Designation as the Kentucky Spinal Cord Injury Research Center

Department of Neurological Surgery at the University of Louisville. The endowed chairs have been used to recruit four senior investigators to the Kentucky Spinal Cord Injury Research Center or to endow laboratories to which outstanding junior faculty are recruited. More recently, each university has received $150,000 per year for graduate student and postdoctoral fellow support.

Another key to growth has involved the efforts of the Kentucky Spinal Cord Injury Research Center faculty in generating new federal research dollars from NIH and the National Science Foundation (Box 8-4). In addition to individual research grants, several large infrastructure grants, as well as program project grants, have been awarded for core resources and program projects. Thus far, none of the funds has been used for new construction, but that is the goal of current fund-raising efforts being done in the community.

Florida

History and Role of State Funding

In 1988, the state of Florida allocated $250,000 to the Miami Project to Cure Paralysis (further detail below) as a result of the efforts of advocates for spinal cord research. Legislation was passed in 1992 to designate a percentage of state revenues from traffic violations for research at the University of Miami and the University of Florida. Distributions from the fund are approximately $500,000 annually for each university and support brain and spinal cord injury research. In some years these distributions are supplemented by general revenues in the state's annual budget directed to the Miami Project to Cure Paralysis. Because the amount of general revenues depends heavily on lobbying, the total amount of state funding varies from year to year. Over the last 4 years, state funding for the Miami Project to Cure Paralysis oscillated between a total of $750,000 and $1.4 million annually (Box 8-5). This uncertainty in state funding, however, affects its capacity for multiyear planning.

Although the state funds for the project vary from year to year, the programs that receive the funding have flexibility over its use. The Evelyn F. and William L. McKnight Brain Institute at the University of Florida, College of Medicine has used the moneys it receives for many different projects designed to improve programmatic development. State funds have been used as seed money to support preliminary research required to obtain NIH research project, program, and training grants. Individual researchers, including senior researchers, received funds ($400,000 over 2 years) to develop sustainable research programs allowing them to successfully compete for NIH grants. The University of Florida program also used some of the state allocations to help support a human clinical trial, which investigated the feasibility and safety of neural tissue transplantation in patients with syringomyelia.

The Miami Project to Cure Paralysis has historically used state funding

---

BOX 8-5
Miami Project to Cure Paralysis

Type of Program: Centralized in one facility

State Funding: Variable, but ranges from $750,000 to $1.4 million each year (2000 to 2004)

Use of State Funds: Primarily salaries and equipment for new faculty to perform the pilot research needed to obtain federal grants

Estimated 2005 Budget: $15.8 million (see Figure 8-4)

Growth Indicators Since the Program's Inception:
NIH grants and contracts: $100,000 (1987 and 1988) to $5.9 million (2005)
Principal investigators: 7 to 26
Personnel: 15 to 212 (including fundraisers and administrators)
Space: 800 square feet (1986) to 118,000 square feet in the new building (new building cost, $36 million)

BOX 8-6
Timeline for the Miami Project to Cure Paralysis

1986	Allotment of 800 square feet of laboratory space in medical science building
1987	Expansion to seven principal investigators and 1,000 square feet
1990-1992	Expansion to 13 principal investigators and 22,000 square feet
1991	Recognition as a center of excellence by the University of Miami
2000	Opening of new building, the Lois Pope Life Center

---

to attract young investigators and give them the tools that they need to successfully compete for NIH grants. With input from a senior advisory committee, the project's scientific director allocates the state funding after each new faculty member submits a research proposal. The funds are spent on salary and equipment for individual projects; but core facilities, which are funded by NIH program project grants and other sources, are available in the same building. All of the young faculty recruited in the past 7 years have later successfully competed for NIH grants.

For its new $36 million building, the Miami Project to Cure Paralysis received a large, one-time infusion of $10 million in state matching funds, after it had raised $10 million from a private benefactor, Lois Pope, after whom the building is named. The remaining funds were collected from a variety of private sources. Thus, in addition to the yearly appropriation, the state made a sizable contribution to new construction (Box 8-6).

The Miami Project to Cure Paralysis

The Miami Project to Cure Paralysis was founded in 1985, and is the nation's largest single program devoted to spinal cord injury research. It traces its origins to the combined vision of a neurosurgeon and three families with firsthand exposure to spinal cord injuries. What began as a $300,000 private gift in 1985 has blossomed into a broad-based research center at the University of Miami School of Medicine, with 26 researchers and annual funding of about $16 million.

The stunning growth of the project is driven by the philosophy of its founding neurosurgeon, Barth Green, who wrote about "gather[ing] a critical mass of scientists . . . in one center under one roof with a mutual committed goal of curing paralysis" (Kleitman, 2001). Significant segments of the funding for the Miami Project to Cure Paralysis come from private philanthropy and active fundraising and from NIH grants (Figure 8-4). The funds from the state of Florida are mainly directed to new faculty to help

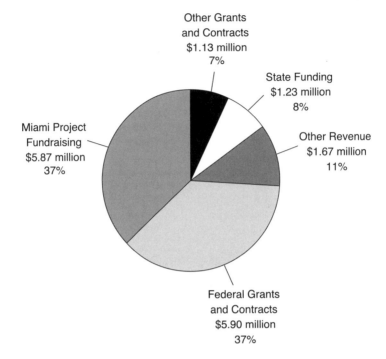

FIGURE 8-4 Fiscal year 2005 budgeted income for the Miami Project to Cure Paralysis.
SOURCE: Adapted from a presentation by Mary Bunge to the Institute of Medicine Committee on Spinal Cord Injury, September 27, 2004.

them generate results from pilot studies, which are highly advantageous in gaining NIH grant funding. The state funding for new faculty has been the engine behind garnering more NIH grants.

The project's scope is comprehensive and multidisciplinary. Although the majority of research resources (70 percent) are spent on basic research, the project's overall perspective is that basic research should be geared so that the research findings can be translated to clinical research. Consequently, the project has core resources for animal models, including the establishment of spinal cord lesions, postsurgery care, behavioral testing, image analysis, histology, electron microscopy, and viral vector preparation. Those core resources allow the rapid translation of the basic research, particularly because the uniformity of the lesions and analysis of their effects are paramount. The project also receives funding from NIH contracts for studies to replicate important findings from other laboratories, training of students and fellows, and support for university scholars (see the description of the Facilities of Research Excellence in Spinal Cord Injury [FOR-SCI] in Chapter 6). Replication studies are necessary to translate the findings from basic research into clinical practice, but they are rarely done because researchers in all scientific fields are rewarded for innovation, not replication.

The project also sponsors or participates in clinical trials, including clinical trials of drugs and rehabilitation devices. The project maintains a database with information on more than 2,000 chronically injured individuals who wish to participate in clinical research. This is easily accomplished because the university's hospital is a regional trauma center that treats approximately 100 cases of acute spinal cord injury per year.

The Miami Project to Cure Paralysis also has a fertility program that has helped nearly 75 men with spinal cord injuries father children. It is one of two institutions in North America that collects spinal cord tissue from individuals with spinal cord injuries. It has amassed a bank with more than 200 samples from individuals with spinal cord injuries that researchers and clinicians use to investigate the etiology, mechanisms of complications, and potential avenues of treatment.

Recently, the project has begun to work with the Food and Drug Administration (FDA) to explore the process of obtaining approval for combination therapeutic interventions involving several drugs or other modes of therapeutic intervention. Investigators have found that the drug rolipram, a type IV-specific phosphodiesterase inhibitor that has FDA approval for use for another indication, is neuroprotective and growth promoting because it prevents cyclic AMP hydrolysis. When rolipram and additional cyclic AMP are combined with Schwann cell grafts, they promote axonal growth in an animal model of spinal cord injury (Pearse et al., 2004). Combination therapies, particularly those that combine cell-based therapies with drugs, will have far more complex regulatory requirements than single therapeutic approaches.

An external advisory committee evaluates the Miami Project to Cure Paralysis every 3 to 4 years. This form of evaluation is supplemented by the standard peer-review process involved in obtaining NIH grants.

California

History and Role of State Funding

In 2000, California Governor Gray Davis signed The Roman Reed Spinal Cord Injury Research Act of 1999, which is devoted to finding treatments for spinal cord injuries. The Act is named for Roman Reed, who sustained a spinal cord injury while playing college football. Reed's family, along with many others, pressed for the legislation under the auspices of

Californians for a Cure. Their efforts galvanized the legislature to authorize up to $2 million annually, which is appropriated as a line item in the state budget. The state funds provided by the legislature are allocated to the University of California Office of the President, which in turn allocates the funds to the Reeve-Irvine Research Center to administer. After the first 5 years, the Roman Reed Research Program has grown to a consortium of 150 researchers across 10 California universities and institutions. Its decentralized structure is similar to that of the center to receive the first grant from the New York State Spinal Cord Injury Research Program (see below).

Reeve-Irvine Research Center

The Reeve-Irvine Research Center named for actor Christopher Reeve and philanthropist Joan Irvine Smith, was established in 1998 through a lead gift from Joan Irvine Smith that endowed a chair in spinal cord injury research at the University of California at Irvine and established a research endowment. The mission of the center is to carry out research on injuries to and diseases of the spinal cord that result in paralysis or other loss of neurological function, with the goal of finding treatments.

In addition to the center's three core faculty whose labs are physically located in the Reeve-Irvine Research Center, scientists and physician scientists at the University of California at Irvine have been recruited to participate in the center's research and training activities. Currently, there are 15 "center associates" carrying out research on nervous system injury, stroke, and neurodegenerative disorders as well as on basic processes that underlie nervous system development, regeneration, and plasticity. Several center associates are active clinicians as well as scientists, and bring a unique clinical perspective to the Reeve-Irvine Research Center.

Roman Reed Research Grants Program

The Roman Reed Research Program consists of a state-of-the-art core laboratory facility (with a budget of $400,000 per year) and a research grants program, both of which are open to any California-based researcher. The core laboratory, situated in the Reeve-Irvine Research Center, is equipped with animal facilities, dedicated laboratory space, and trained technical personnel who can readily produce uniform and standardized types of spinal cord injuries in rodent models. Most research conducted by the program is basic, but to be funded, it must lend itself to the legislation's intent: ready translation to finding treatments for spinal cord injuries.

The concept behind the core laboratory is to attract new researchers to the field by making it relatively easy for them to turn their ideas into

---

BOX 8-7
Roman Reed Research Program

Type of Program: Decentralized in multiple universities and institutions

State Funding: Up to $2 million annually under the Roman Reed Spinal Cord Injury Research Act; funding varies from year to year but ranges from $1 million to $2 million (2000 to 2004)

Use of State Funds: $400,000 per year for an open core laboratory; the remainder is used for grants to California-based researchers in public or private institutions

Growth Indicators Since the Program's Inception:
 Roman Reed grants: 57 new research projects funded throughout the state (2000 to 2004); 9 are for investigators new to the spinal cord injury research field
 NIH and foundation grants: $3.7 million in Roman Reed Research Program funding to state researchers (the total over the first 3 years) has led to $18 million in other grants and 24 new jobs in California
 Researchers: between 2001 and 2004, more than 180 California researchers have participated in 57 Roman Reed Research Program research projects

---

experiments that can be performed with animals. In fact, about one-quarter of the projects from the program's inception have been conducted by researchers who are new to the field (Box 8-7).

The grant program, which funds about 20 projects each year (about $100,000 each), encourages use of the funds as seed money to obtain larger amounts of federal and private funding. That goal has been realized, considering that $3.7 million in Roman Reed Research Program funding to state researchers (over the first 3 years) has led to $18 million in other grants and 24 new jobs in California.

The program's concept and structure were established in 2001 by a town meeting of interested researchers from the University of California system, NIH specialists, and members of the External Advisory Board representing leaders from public, private, and non-profit entities. Attendees refined and elaborated a plan suggested by the Scientific Steering Committee. The final plan calls for the allocation of approximately $400,000 of the state's yearly appropriation to run the core laboratory; the remainder is directed to research grants, a small number of fellowships, and other training opportunities. The appropriation varies from year to year but has a ceiling of $2 million, as authorized under the Act.

Grant proposals undergo a two-tier review process. An external advisory committee first reviews the proposals and assigns priority scores on the basis of the merit and the appropriateness of the proposal to the program's goals. Using those rankings, the Scientific Steering Committee decides on the distribution of funds. Grants are administered through the Reeve-Irvine Research Center at the University of California at Irvine. Except for its core facility, which serves the Roman Reed Research Program, the Reeve-Irvine Research Center is funded separately. The 3 principal investigators located at the Reeve-Irvine Research Center and the 15 research associates on the campus apply for Roman Reed Research Program funds just as other California-based researchers do. The center also receives NIH contract funding, totaling $2.6 million for 2003 through 2008, for training and research facilities for spinal cord injury research. This center also holds an NIH FOR-SCI contract to replicate the findings from other laboratories.

A key goal of the program is to foster collaboration and communication, both for scientists and for the lay public. Beginning in 2002 the program has sponsored an annual Roman Reed Research Meeting, which includes presentations by grant recipients, a poster session for graduate students and postdoctoral fellows that allows sharing of preliminary research findings, and a Meet the Scientists Forum for scientists and the lay public. The purpose of the meeting is to bring investigators together as they launch projects to promote collaborations and devise experiments that take advantage of economies of scale (Box 8-8).

Impact of New Stem Cell Research Initiative in California

In November 2004 California voters approved Proposition 71, which provides a fresh infusion of about $295 million annually for stem cell research in California (approximately $3 billion over 10 years).[5] The financing for the research comes from state-issued long-term bonds. A substantial portion of the funds allocated during the first years of the program will go to the establishment of research facilities. The goal of Proposition 71 is to circumvent specific restrictions on NIH funding of stem cell research projects involving human embryos. Although it gives priority to embryonic stem cell research, the proposition broadly covers stem cells of all types, whether they come from an embryo, a fetus, or an adult or from humans or animals. The proposition explicitly prohibits human reproductive cloning research.

Proposition 71 is likely to benefit spinal cord injury research, one of the commonly named conditions identified to benefit from stem cell research.

---

[5]California Proposition 71. §3 (2004).

BOX 8-8
Roman Reed Research Program and
Reeve-Irvine Research Center Timeline

1998	Establishment of the Reeve-Irvine Research Center at the University of California at Irvine
1999-2000	Introduction and passage of The Roman Reed Spinal Cord Injury Research Act.
	Reeve-Irvine Research Center designated by the University of California Office of the President as the coordinator of the Roman Reed Program.
2001	A town meeting of researchers from the University of California system, the External Advisory Board, and NIH staff recommends the use of Roman Reed Research Program funds for grants and core laboratory
2001	Allocation of first round of funds for researchers in California
2002	Dedication of Roman Reed Spinal Cord Injury Core Laboratory at the University of California at Irvine and designation of the Reeve-Irvine Research Center as FOR-SCI Center as a result of the award of two FOR-SCI contracts
2003	Funding of fellowships, in addition to research projects
2004	Passage of legislation to extend the Roman Reed Research Program's authorization until 2011 (the original legislation had a sunset date of 5 years)

Some 10 percent of current applications for funding under the Roman Reed Research Program propose the use of stem cells. The sheer magnitude of new funds is likely to stimulate more research on spinal cord injuries in California. Additionally, Proposition 71 requires the establishment of a 29-member Independent Citizen's Oversight Committee and stipulates that this committee must include an advocate for spinal cord injury research who is to be appointed by the governor.

The impact of Proposition 71 is likely to extend beyond California's borders. Other states may find that some of their finest researchers, lured by the availability of new resources, may move their laboratories to California. Some may be spinal cord injury researchers. Other state governments, including those in New Jersey, Wisconsin, Illinois, and Minnesota, are responding by enacting or debating stem cell research legislation to help to retain senior investigators and attract young researchers (Garvey, 2004).

NEW YORK STATE SPINAL CORD INJURY RESEARCH PROGRAM

In 1998, New York State passed legislation to establish a new program whose ambitious mission is to support research "towards a cure for [spinal cord] injuries and their effects."[6] Funding for the program comes from a surcharge on fines for traffic violations, which is directed to the newly created Spinal Cord Injury Research Trust Fund. With a ceiling of $8.5 million in annual appropriations, the funding level is the largest of any of those for state programs (Figure 8-1). Its size and scope give the program the potential to become a major force in spinal cord injury research.

The program possesses several strong features, all of which are discussed here:

- a sophisticated grant review structure (two tiered) and scientific board;
- a strong translational component through its legislative mission and through its first center grant award;
- multiple types of grants; and
- an expansion capacity obtained by drawing on the unique strengths of New York's biomedical research and clinical research programs.

Legislation to establish the spinal cord injury research program was originally proposed by Senator Vincent Leibell and Assemblyman Edward Griffith and was signed into law by Governor George Pataki on July 14, 1998.[6] This legislation is often referred to as the Paul Richter Bill, after a New York state trooper who was shot while on duty in 1973. Christopher Reeve was also a strong advocate.

The legislation mandated the formation of a 13-member panel, the Spinal Cord Injury Research Board, to solicit, receive, and review research proposals and to make recommendations to the Commissioner of Health for approval of funding. The individuals chosen to serve on the Spinal Cord Injury Research Board have expertise in neuroscience, neurology, neurosurgery, neuropharmacology, rehabilitative medicine, and advocacy and are appointed by the governor and senior legislative officers, as shown in Table 8-2.[7] Board members serve for 4 years and may serve no more than two consecutive terms. The governor appoints one board member to serve as the chair.

In addition to reviewing grant applications, the Spinal Cord Injury Research Board is required to submit progress reports to the governor and the legislature on January 31 of each year to describe the previous year's funded research and the board's accomplishments. Unlike the Miami Project to Cure Paralysis, beyond the yearly submission of progress reports and the

---

[6]Chapter 338, Laws of New York; amended by A194C, later substituted by S.5328.
[7]S.B. 7287.

TABLE 8-2 Spinal Cord Injury Research Board Appointments

Person Appointing Board Member	Number of Appointees
Governor	7
Senate President	2
Assembly Speaker	2
Senate Minority Leader	1
Assembly Minority Leader	1
Total number of board members	13

sponsorship of this Institute of Medicine report, the New York State Spinal Cord Injury program has no periodic mechanism for the independent evaluation of its overall performance in meeting its strategic objectives.

Research proposals are reviewed by using a two-tiered process: an initial review for scientific merit and a review for programmatic relevance. Initially, a scientific advisory committee reviews the research proposals. The state of New York contracts with a company to select members of the Scientific Advisory Committee and to manage the peer review process. Members of the Scientific Advisory Committee are researchers who are not affiliated with New York State research institutions and who are experts in fields relevant to spinal cord injuries.

The Scientific Advisory Committee reviews the proposals for their scientific merit and then ranks them. Using the Scientific Advisory Committee's recommendations as a starting point, board members review the proposals and rank the applications according to their consistency with the Spinal Cord Injury Research Board mission, potential impact, and scientific feasibility. Applications that meet these criteria are forwarded to the commissioner of health for review and approval.

Types of Grants

Although New York State has not specified research topics for funding, it has targeted projects that involve tissue repair, regeneration, and restored function.[8] It uses several types of granting mechanisms to support these research efforts and has three different funding mechanisms: the Collaborations to Accelerate Research Translation; the Innovative, Developmental, or Exploratory Activities; and the Center of Research Excellence grants.

---

[8] Projects focusing on rehabilitation are not eligible for research funding.

The lead recipient institution for each of these grants must be located in New York State, but collaborative institutions may be located outside the state. A brief description of each type of funding mechanism follows.

- **Collaborations to Accelerate Research Translation (CART).** CART comprises a 4-year grant that provides a maximum of $300,000 each year to direct costs for cross-disciplinary, translational research. This grant does not support "program projects, research centers, or large scale clinical trials" (New York State Spinal Cord Injury Research Board, 2002). Principal investigators are required to commit more than 10 percent full-time equivalent time toward research.
- **Innovative, Developmental, or Exploratory Activities (IDEA).** IDEA is a 2-year grant that provides a total of $300,000 in program costs. According to the request for proposals, these grants support research projects that "hold out significant likelihood of leading to breakthroughs or new avenues of investigation" (New York State Spinal Cord Injury Research Board, 2002). The grant supports preliminary research with the expectation that principal investigators will later pursue additional, larger-scale funding elsewhere.
- **Center of Research Excellence (CORE).** CORE is a 5-year grant that provides up to $3 million in total costs each year for multi-institutional, collaborative research projects. Funds are used for three to six interrelated research projects, one of which must be a treatment study. Awardees must partner with a patient care facility, in this case, the Helen Hayes Hospital, the New York State Department of Health's rehabilitation facility, which also conducts clinical trials. Those projects most likely to be funded are at institutions that have already demonstrated a high level of expertise. This is a one-time-only grant (New York State Spinal Cord Injury Research Board, 2003). The first CORE grant was awarded for an integrated translational program that linked together 11 research institutions within New York and other states (see Box 8-9).

Funding History and Focus

The legislation sets a ceiling of allocating $8.5 million annually for research. During the program's first year of awarding grants, $3.6 million was awarded. In the next year, 2001, nearly $7 million was distributed to nine research projects (CRPF, 2000; Times Newsweekly, 2001). Table 8-3 lists the number of awards and the total amounts distributed since 2000.

The grants awarded in 2000 focused largely on basic research, including axonal guidance, plasticity, growth factors, regeneration, calcium channels, and adhesion molecules (New York State Spinal Cord Injury Research

---

BOX 8-9
An Integrated Translational Program to
Treat Spinal Cord Injury

Spinal Cord Injury Center of Research Excellence (CORE)

The New York State Spinal Cord Injury Research Program's first center grant, which was for $15 million over 5 years, was awarded to a unique network of researchers from 11 institutions. The major goal is to translate basic science into safe and effective treatments for the acute or chronic phase of a spinal cord injury. Through a decentralized yet highly coordinated effort, the research team has set as its primary objective the development of drugs in combination with other therapies (e.g., cell replacement therapies) that can be moved safely and rapidly to human clinical trials at the seven medical schools within its network, among other clinical sites.

The centerpiece of the grant is an in vitro screening program that uses eight cell-based or organelle-based assays to test 2,000 drugs previously approved by the Food and Drug Administration and marketed for other conditions. Restriction of the screening to Food and Drug Administration-approved drugs has the advantage that the drugs have already been shown to be safe. "Toxicity often defeats new compounds," says Rajiv Ratan of Burke Medical Institute, one of the principal investigators funded by the grant.

The screening program is designed to find drugs with the capacity to overcome three major complications of spinal cord injuries: glial cell inhibition, cell death, and demyelination. A drug found to overcome all three complications then progresses to detailed physiological assessment with animal models, including real-time imaging, to ensure penetration into the central nervous system and to establish therapeutic efficacy. Some of the physiological testing will be done with grant funds at a nearby pharmaceutical firm. If a compound is successful in studies with the animal model, it will be tested in studies with humans through the center's evolving clinical trials network, which will have a centralized data management and analysis structure. Grant funds and the findings that they generate will be key to building the program by obtaining grants from the National Institutes of Health and partnerships with drug or biotechnology companies.

Board, 2002). The year 2001 grants were also awarded for basic research, including research on neuron regulation, axonal guidance, myelination, repair and protection, and glial cells (New York State Spinal Cord Injury Research Board, 2002). Year 2002 grants focused on axon regeneration, cellular mechanisms after an injury, injury diagnostics, and treatment (New York State Spinal Cord Injury Research Program, 2003). The large center award, made in 2003, was for translational research.

TABLE 8-3 New York State Spinal Cord Injury Research Program's Grant Award History

Year	Number of Awards	Total Funds Awarded (in millions)
2000	10[a]	$ 3.6
2001	9	$ 7
2002	15[b]	$ 8.4
2003	1	$15

[a]Of 45 applications submitted (22 percent success rate).
[b]Five researchers received CART awards, and 10 received IDEA awards.
SOURCES: CRPF, 2000; Times Newsweekly, 2001; New York State Spinal Cord Injury Research Board, 2004.

Challenges Facing New York State's Program

Expanding the Number of Spinal Cord Injury Researchers in New York

In 2003, only six principal investigators in New York State received NIH grants (R01 grants) for projects specifically designated to be related to research on spinal cord injuries (Table 8-4), and there were no program project grants or center grant recipients in the state in this specifically designated research area. For the years 1998 to 2003, New York ranked

TABLE 8-4 NIH R01 Grants for Spinal Cord Injury Research in New York State, 1998 to 2003

Year	Number of R01 Grants
1998	5
1999	6
2000	4
2001	3
2002	5
2003	6

NOTE: The number of R01 grants for each year was derived by searching the NIH CRISP database (see Appendix A for more details). The search was restricted to the term "spinal cord injury," and the activity was restricted to research projects, specifically those supported by R01 grants.
SOURCE: NIH, 1999.

third in the nation in grants for spinal cord injury-related research (Table 8-5) as well as third in the nation for overall NIH grants (NIH, 2004a) (Figure 8-5).

These data suggest that New York State has too few spinal cord injury researchers to accomplish its legislatively mandated mission: to cure spinal cord injuries or their effects. The greatest challenge for the New York State program will be to attract new researchers to the spinal cord injury research field, either by collaboration with or recruitment from researchers in related fields of neuroscience or neurology and bioengineering. It is hoped that over the next 3 years the number of researchers in New York focused on fundamental and translational studies related to spinal cord injuries will at least double.

TABLE 8-5 NIH Research Grants Related to Spinal Cord Injuries in States with State-Funded Spinal Cord Injury Research Programs, 1998 to 2003

State	Fellowships[a]	Training Grants	Career Development Awards	R01 Awards
California	5	1	2	31
Connecticut	1	0	0	4
Florida	0	1	2	13
Illinois	3	0	0	7
Indiana	0	0	0	1
Kentucky	2	0	1	7
Maryland	0	1	1	5
Massachusetts	0	0	0	6
Missouri	1	0	2	6
New Jersey	0	0	0	0
New York	3	1	4	11
Oregon	0	0	0	0
South Carolina	0	0	0	2
Virginia	0	0	1	4
Total for 14 states	15	4	13	97
Total for 50 states	27	4	21	194

[a]Fellowships include predoctoral, postdoctoral, and senior fellowships.
NOTE: Duplicate awards were removed. The number of awards was based on narrow searches of the NIH CRISP database. The database was searched with the term "spinal cord injury" for each of the types of grants and awards.
SOURCE: NIH, 1999.

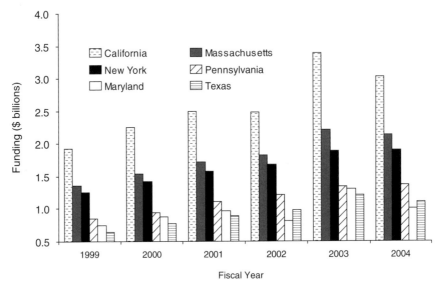

FIGURE 8-5 Overall NIH support for research in top six states, 1999 to 2004.
NOTE: NIH support for 1999 through 2004 was based on reviews of the levels of
funding for extramural awards (by state).
SOURCE: NIH, 2004a.

Funding and Administrative Issues

There are several indications that an overly burdensome bureaucracy
has resulted in funding delays for research grants. Several individuals testi-
fied to the committee that the New York State program has been slow to
allocate and deliver grant funds after a project's approval, with the lag time
generally being almost 1 year from the grant award announcement to the
receipt of funding (see Appendix A; IOM Committee on Spinal Cord Injury
Workshop, September 27, 2004). The program's centerpiece, its CORE
grant for translational research involving 11 institutions, has experienced a
1-year funding delay. Delays are highly disruptive and discourage investigators from getting involved in spinal cord injury research with the New York
State program, which is exactly the opposite of the program's intent.

Furthermore, issues regarding board members' appointments and at-
tendance remain. The legislation behind the New York State program specifies a 13-member board; 7 of these members must be appointed by the
governor, and the others are appointed by leaders of the state legislature.
Several slots on the board have been unfilled, which has presented difficulty
in fulfilling the work of the board.

Unique Strengths of New York State's Research Infrastructure

New York State has an unquestionably strong biomedical research infrastructure that could be drawn upon to build a strong program of research on spinal cord injuries. As mentioned above, New York State ranks third among the states in terms of total NIH grant funding, based on an analysis of data published by NIH. Key indicators of New York State's strengths are summarized in Table 8-6.

This section highlights the strengths of the biomedical research infrastructure and sets the context for understanding current state efforts in spinal cord injury research.

Unique Concentration of Researchers and Institutions

New York State stands out by its confluence of researchers, medical schools, universities, and numbers of individuals with spinal cord injuries.

TABLE 8-6 Indicators of New York State's Biomedical and Neuroscience Research Infrastructure

Indicator	Number or Amount	Year(s)	Rank Among 50 States
Total NIH grant funds, all types	$1.9 billion	2004	3
Total NIH grants to medical schools	$943 million	2002	2
Total NIH grants (R01 grants) specific to spinal cord injury research	11	1998–2003	6
Society for Neuroscience members	1,854	2004	2
Number of medical schools in the state	12	2004	1
State funds for spinal cord injury research	$8.5 million	Annual	1[a]
Nearby states with spinal cord injury research programs	4[b]	NA[c]	NA

[a]Rank among 14 other states with spinal cord injury research programs.
[b]New Jersey, Connecticut, Maryland, Massachusetts.
[c]NA = not applicable.
SOURCES: NIH, 1999; New York State Spinal Cord Injury Research Board, 2002; AAMC, 2004; NIH 2004a,b; Personal communication, F. Johnson, Society for Neuroscience, November 19, 2004.

No other state has, in such a close geographic proximity, as many resources vital to building a formidable research capacity in spinal cord injuries. In 2004, the state received nearly $2 billion from NIH (Figure 8-5), ranking only behind California and Massachusetts. New York has sustained its third-place ranking over the past 5 years (Figure 8-5), but the state faces increasingly stiff competition from other states. Although New York was the leading recipient of NIH funds in the 1980s, from 1981 to 1995 New York's share of total NIH research funding gradually eroded, from a high of 15 percent in 1981 to 11 percent in 1995 (Sturman et al., 1997, 2000).

Apart from NIH, grant funding for biomedical research comes from a variety of other sources (e.g., the U.S. Department of Veterans Affairs, state and local governments, and private sources). In a 1998 survey of the 20 largest New York State-based biomedical research institutions, NIH funding accounted for about 51 percent of research revenues from all sources, defined as federal, state, and local governments; industry; and foundations (Sclar and Aries, 2000). Thus, the total biomedical research funding from all sources in New York State is estimated to be nearly $4 billion.

Capacity for Clinical Research and Clinical Trials

New York has more medical schools than any other state. Of the nation's 125 medical schools, New York has 12; the state with the next highest number, California, has 8 (AAMC, 2004). In addition to hospital and outpatient facilities, New York is also home to several centers of rehabilitation medicine, including the Mount Sinai Spinal Cord Injury Model System center, Burke Rehabilitation Hospital, Rusk Institute of Rehabilitation, Helen Hayes Hospital, the Bronx Veterans Affairs Medical Center, and several other U.S. Department of Veterans Affairs hospitals. The most research-intensive areas within the state are the New York City metropolitan area[9] and the Buffalo-Rochester area (Sclar and Aries, 2000).

Beyond its borders, New York is strategically situated in a populous region with a high density of major medical centers and medical schools. Its neighboring states—New Jersey, Connecticut, Pennsylvania, and Maryland—also have strong research and clinical capacities (Brookings Institution, 2002). These states rank high in terms of NIH research dollars (Table 8-5). All of the states except Pennsylvania have state spinal cord injury programs (Table 8-1). More than 4,700 life scientists work in the New York City metropolitan area, which includes New York City, Long Island, and northern New Jersey. This region has 20 institutions that grant Ph.D.'s in the life sciences (Brookings Institution, 2002).

---

[9]Includes Long Island and Westchester County.

These features make New York State situated to forge regional networks of clinical, basic, and translational research on spinal cord injuries. A regional clinical trials center could facilitate efforts to link the many resources in the New York region. The proximity of multiple trauma centers in and near New York City offers the opportunity to coordinate efforts on acute phase clinical trials. Further, pilot studies examining the impact of health care delivery such as the immediate triage and rapid transport of spinal cord injured patients to specialized centers could be conducted.

Concentration of Expertise in Neuroscience, Neurosurgery, and Neurology

New York also has a rich concentration of researchers with expertise in neuroscience, including several Nobel Prize winners. Of the 36,000 basic scientists and clinicians who are members of the Society for Neuroscience, 1,854 (about 5 percent) are from New York State (Personal communication, F. Johnson, Society for Neuroscience, November 19, 2004). New York's neuroscience or neurology research programs at Columbia University, New York University, Cornell University, Rockefeller University, and the State University system are world renowned. The abundance of researchers in fields that overlap the spinal cord injury research field makes it possible for the New York State Spinal Cord Injury Research Program to expand by cultivating collaborations and by sharing core facilities, equipment, and other resources. Opportunities to increase the focus on spinal cord injury research and draw talented researchers to New York could be enhanced through the funding of two to four endowed chairs in spinal cord injury research at New York universities.

Potential for Private and Public Linkages

Another major strength of New York is its rich potential for institutional linkages with pharmaceutical firms, foundations, and patient advocacy organizations. Helping to forge such linkages is the Biomedical Research Alliance of New York, a for-profit alliance of 138 affiliates, including large New York State-based university medical centers. This alliance largely focuses on aiding the organization and start-up of clinical research, including the preparation of regulatory documents and submissions to institutional review boards. Public and private research organizations stand to gain by creating local and regional consortia for clinical trials and other collaborations that are key to greater access by individuals with spinal cord injuries and research efficiency.

Apart from clinical trials, core facilities for animal research are an important shared resource. Just as the Miami Project to Cure Paralysis and the Reeve-Irvine Research Center in California have created core facilities for production and analysis of the findings from studies with animal models, a New York-based institution could also create the same types of facilities through various cost-sharing agreements between payers. The Christopher Reeve Paralysis Foundation, which has distributed more than $40 million in research grants over the past two decades, is headquartered in nearby New Jersey.

New York and neighboring states are headquarters to numerous pharmaceutical companies. A new economic analysis by the pharmaceutical industry attempted to measure the relative intensities of their activities by state by formulating a new measure, the biopharmaceutical innovation pipeline index. By this new index, New York State ranked 10th in the nation; most of its neighboring states ranked higher. The index captures measures in four areas: biopharmaceutical research funding, biopharmaceutical risk capital funding, biopharmaceutical industry human capital and workforce, and biopharmaceutical innovation output (DeVol et al., 2004). A separate analysis found that since 1995 biopharmaceutical firms in the New York City metropolitan area have attracted more than $639 million in venture capital (Brookings Institution, 2002).

Finally, the state of New York is another potential source of help in forming public and private partnerships. In 1999, the New York State legislature passed a comprehensive law to fund a $522 million economic development stimulus by providing support for science and academic research. The New York State Office of Science, Technology, and Academic Research is the administrative locus. This 1999 law enhanced what was already a strong state investment. A survey in 1995 found that New York ranks fourth in the nation in total state investment in research and development (Jankowski, 1999).

Strengthening the Research Infrastructure in New York State

As demonstrated in this chapter, state spinal cord injury research programs can make a significant contribution to the research endeavor to find a cure for spinal cord injuries. Several model spinal cord injury research programs, working with fewer resources than those available in New York State, used funding from their states as seed money to build programs of far greater magnitude and scientific impact than those in New York State. New York State, with the highest level of state funding for spinal cord injury research of any state program, has the potential to assume a leadership role in spinal cord injury research. However, for it to do so, its program must have a sustainable research infrastructure. New York has an impressive concentration of researchers who could be working on spinal cord injury research. Continued efforts to support and strengthen the program will attract these scientists into the field. To maximize its efforts and build its program, the New York State program should continue to enter into collaborations that draw on the unique strengths of New York's biomedical expertise, clinical caseload, and infrastructure, as well as the strengths of the region beyond New York's borders.

RECOMMENDATIONS

Further development of the New York State Spinal Cord Injury Research Board should build on the recommendations presented in this report, with additional focus on the following recommendations.

Recommendation 8.1: *Build and Strengthen New York State's Research Infrastructure*
The New York State Spinal Cord Injury Research Board should increase its research infrastructure to meet the program's mission. The Board should

• develop and sustain a vigorous recruitment and training effort for fundamental and translational research; the number of investigators should be increased progressively over the next 3 years with the goal of at least doubling the number of researchers focused on fundamental and translational studies of spinal cord injuries;
• establish a coordinated statewide research network that encourages collaborations among individual investigators and interinstitutional research efforts; the Board should convene a statewide meeting of investigators and relevant stakeholders to plan a research strategy and coordinate research efforts;
• cultivate formal linkages with researchers, programs, and biopharmaceutical companies in the region to forge partnerships for basic, translational, and clinical research; and
• establish regional core laboratory facilities.

Recommendation 8.2: *Develop a Regional Clinical Trials Center*
The state of New York should use its unique strengths to establish a regional clinical trials center. This center should

• develop and coordinate multicenter clinical trials to examine therapies for the treatment of spinal cord injuries;
• sponsor a clinical trial of decompression as an early intervention and clinical trials of other therapies to be used during the acute phase of a spinal cord injury by using the special opportunities offered by New York City's geographic location and the unique resources of its trauma centers; and
• manage a clinical trials clearinghouse.

Recommendation 8.3: *Restructure Research Funding and Oversight Processes*
The New York State Spinal Cord Injury Research Board should work with the state of New York to reduce administrative burdens, improve the approval and grant distribution processes, and establish a rapid-response funding mechanism to capitalize on new research ideas.

Recommendation 8.4: *Ensure Independent Evaluation*
The New York State Spinal Cord Injury Research Board should establish an independent external review panel that meets periodically to rigorously assess the program's efforts toward its stated mission to cure spinal cord injuries.

REFERENCES

AAMC (Association of American Medical Colleges). 2004. *Medical Schools of the U.S. and Canada—Alphabetical Listing.* [Online]. Available: http://www.aamc.org/members/listings/msalphaae.htm [accessed November 11, 2004].

Aries NR, Sclar ED. 1998. The economic impact of biomedical research: A case study of voluntary institutions in the New York metropolitan region. *Journal of Health Politics, Policy & Law* 23(1): 175-193.

Attorney General of California. 2004. *Proposition 71—Stem Cell Research.* [Online]. Available: http://www.voterguide.ss.ca.gov/propositions/prop71-title.htm [accessed November 11, 2004].

Bank of Boston Economics Department. 1991. *The Job-Related Impacts of the Biotechnology Industry in Massachusetts.* Boston: Bank of Boston.

Barondess JA. 2002. Municipal support of biomedical research. *Academic Medicine* 77(1): 31-33.

Battelle Memorial Institute/SSTI. 1998. *Survey of State Research and Development Expenditures: Fiscal Year 1995.* Westerville, OH: Battelle Memorial Institute.

Battelle Technology Partnership Practice/SSTI. 2004. *Laboratories of Innovation: State Bioscience Initiatives 2004.* Washington, DC: Biotechnology Industry Organization.

Brookings Institution. 2002. *Profile of Biomedical Research and Biotechnology Commercialization: New York–Northern New Jersey–Long Island Consolidated Metropolitan Statistical Area.* [Online]. Available: http://www.brookings.edu/dybdocroot/es/urban/publications/biotechnewyork.pdf [accessed November 4, 2004].

California Health Care Institute. 1993. *The Health Care Technology Industry: What's Growing in California.* La Jolla, CA: California Health Care Institute.

Center for Social Gerontology. 2004. *Tobacco Settlement Funds Daily Updates.* [Online]. Available: http://www.tcsg.org/tobacco/settlement/updates.htm [accessed November 11, 2004].

CRPF (Christopher Reeve Paralysis Foundation). 2000. *New York State Spinal Cord Research Trust Fund Awards $3.6 Million in Grants.* [Online]. Available: http://www.charitywire.com/charity44/01180.html [accessed October 3, 2003].

DeVol R, Wong P, Bedroussian A, Wallace L, Ki J, Murphy D, Koepp R. 2004. *Biopharmaceutical Industry Contributions to State and U.S. Economies.* Santa Monica, CA: Milken Institute.

Garvey M. 2004, November 22. California stem cell project energizes other states to act. *Los Angeles Times*. p. A1.

Jankowski JE. 1999. *What Is the State Government Role in the R&D Enterprise?* NSF Report 99-348. Arlington, VA: National Science Foundation.

Kleitman N. 2001. Under one roof: The Miami Project to Cure Paralysis model for spinal cord injury research. *Neuroscientist* 7(3): 192-201.

KSCIRC (Kentucky Spinal Cord Injury Research Center). 2004. *Overview*. [Online]. Available: http://www.kscirc.org/overview.htm [accessed December 29, 2004].

Lasker Foundation. 2000. *Exceptional Returns: The Economic Value of America's Investment in Medical Research*. New York: Lasker Foundation.

Maryland Department of Economic and Employment Development. 1994. *The Impact of the National Institutes of Health in Maryland and the U.S.* Baltimore, MD: Maryland Office of Research.

National Science Foundation. 2004. *Science and Engineering Indicators 2004*. Arlington, VA: National Science Foundation.

New York State Spinal Cord Injury Research Board. 2002. *Request for Proposal: Guidelines and Instructions for CART and IDEA Grants (FY2002)*. [Online]. Available: http://www.wadsworth.org/new/rfp/scirb/finalrfp.pdf [accessed June 6, 2003].

New York State Spinal Cord Injury Research Board. 2003a. *Center of Research Excellence*. [Online]. Available: http://www.wadsworth.org/new/rfa/spinal/rfa.doc [accessed June 6, 2003].

New York State Spinal Cord Injury Research Board. 2003b. *Program Profile*. Albany: New York Department of Health.

New York State Spinal Cord Injury Research Board. 2004. *$15 Million Award for Research to Find Treatment and Cure for Spinal Cord Injury and Paralysis Announced*. [Online]. Available: http://www.wadsworth.org/new/rfa/spinalaward.htm [accessed January 7, 2005].

NIH (National Institutes of Health). 1999. *Computer Retrieval of Information on Scientific Projects*. [Online]. Available: http://crisp.cit.nih.gov/ [accessed January 8, 2004].

NIH. 2004a. *NIH Extramural Awards by State and Foreign Site*. [Online]. Available: http://grants.nih.gov/grants/award/state/state.htm [accessed January 7, 2005].

NIH. 2004b. *NIH Extramural Awards Ranking Tables Medical Schools Long-Term Trends and Historical Data*. [Online]. Available: http://grants1.nih.gov/grants/award/trends/medschl.htm [accessed January 7, 2005].

NYSTAR (New York State Office of Science, Technology, and Academic Research). 2001. *Discovery Drives Progress in New York*. [Online]. Available: http://www.nystar.state.ny.us/pa/papers120501.htm [accessed November 3, 2004].

Pearse DD, Pereira FC, Marcillo AE, Bates ML, Berrocal YA, Filbin MT, Bunge MB. 2004. cAMP and Schwann cells promote axonal growth and functional recovery after spinal cord injury. *Nature Medicine* 10(6): 610-616.

Sclar E, Aries N. 2000. *Biomedical Research and the New York State Economy*. New York: Council on Biomedical Research and Development, New York Academy of Medicine.

Silverstein SC, Garrison HH, Heinig SJ. 1995. A few basic economic facts about research in the medical and related life sciences. *FASEB Journal* 9(10): 833-840.

SSTI (State Science & Technology Institute). 1997. *State Science and Technology Strategic Planning: Creating Economic Opportunity*. Westerville, OH: State Science & Technology Institute.

SSTI. 1999a. *Governors Talk Technology*. [Online]. Available: http://www.ssti.org/Digest/1999/042399.htm [accessed November 11, 2004].

SSTI. 1999b. *S&T Programs Funded through Tobacco Settlements*. [Online]. Available: http://www.ssti.org/Digest/1999/111299.htm [accessed November 11, 2004].

Sturman LS, Sorin MD, Larkins E, Cavanagh KA, DeBuono BA. 1997. Losing ground: NIH funding to New York State researchers. *Bulletin of the New York Academy of Medicine* 74(1): 6-19.

Sturman LS, Sorin MD, Hannum RJ. 2000. Opportunities lost: NIH research funding to New York's medical schools. *Journal of Urban Health* 77(1): 86-95.

Times Newsweekly. 2001. *Research of Spinal Cord Injury Gets State Funds.* [Online]. Available: http://www.timesnewsweekly.com/OldSite/092001/NewFiles/SPINAL.html [accessed October 3, 2003].

U.S. Congress, Senate Committee on Appropriations. 2003. *Departments of Labor, Health and Human Services, and Education, and Related Agencies Appropriation Bill, 2004.* 108th Cong., 1st Sess. June 23, 2003.

A

STUDY PROCESS

The committee reviewed and considered a broad array of information in its work on issues involving spinal cord injury research. Information sources included the primary scientific literature; books and scientific reviews; and presentations from researchers, representatives from federal agencies and nonprofit organizations, and individuals with spinal cord injuries.

LITERATURE REVIEW

Extensive bibliographic searches were conducted and resulted in a reference database of more than 2,000 entries. Searches of the primary biomedical bibliographic databases, Medline and EMBASE,[1] were supplemented with searches of Dissertation Abstracts, Lexis-Nexis, and THOMAS (a federal legislative database). The Dissertation Abstracts database provided information on the current level of Ph.D. thesis production in the field of neurological diseases.[2] Additionally, a specific Medline search for clinical trials of therapeutic interventions for spinal cord injuries performed from 1998 to 2003 was conducted (see Appendix G).

---

[1]Excerpta Medica.

[2]IOM staff searched the Dissertation Abstracts database using the search terms "spinal cord injur?," "multiple sclerosis," "brain AND (ischemia OR stroke)," "Parkinson? (within two spaces) disease," and "Alzheimer? (within three spaces) disease." The question mark is used to search for terms with multiple endings. For example, the search term "spinal cord injur?" resulted in hits that included "spinal cord injury" and "spinal cord injuries."

To identify information on funding mechanisms and trends from the National Institutes of Health (NIH), Institute of Medicine (IOM) staff queried the Computer Retrieval of Information on Scientific Projects (CRISP) database. This database collects information on the number of federally funded biomedical research projects. Data from the CRISP database were used to assess the number of fellowships (F grants), career grants (K grants), research grants (e.g., R01 grants), project grants (P grants), and Small Business Innovation Research and Small Business Technology Transfer awards funded by NIH. To discern the number of NIH grants directed toward various neurological disorders, IOM staff used appropriate keywords (which appeared in a 9,000-word thesaurus) for various neurological conditions. Projects that addressed more than one neurological condition were counted separately for each condition. Additional information on general funding trends at NIH was located in published documents and was provided by NIH staff.

PUBLIC WORKSHOPS

The committee held four meetings over the course of the study to address the study charge, review the data collected, and develop the report. Three of those meetings included public workshops: February 23-24, 2004; May 24-25, 2004; and September 27-28, 2004.

The first workshop (Box A-1) included three sessions that covered basic and clinical research needs, clinical trials in industry, and translational research.

The committee held the second public workshop (Box A-2) on May 24-25, 2004, in Washington, D.C. In that workshop the committee heard from 13 speakers who had expertise in emerging therapies for spinal cord injuries, stem and olfactory ensheathing cells, neuropathic pain, robotics and physical therapy, clinical research methods, and federal program management.

The third meeting took place on September 27-28, 2004, in Washington, D.C. The public workshop (Box A-3) consisted of three sessions that included a review of state-sponsored spinal cord injury research programs, a discussion of how the Food and Drug Administration (FDA) deals with the complexities associated with spinal cord injuries, and a community perspectives session in which nonprofit organizations and individuals with spinal cord injuries provided input on future research priorities.

BOX A-1

Institute of Medicine
Committee on Spinal Cord Injury Workshop
Tuesday, February 24, 2004

8:30   **Welcome to the Workshop**
Richard T. Johnson, Johns Hopkins University

Session I: Basic and Clinical Research Needs

8:40   **What Do Basic Scientists Most Need to Apply Their Knowledge About Neural Injury and Repair to Clinical Use?**
Moses V. Chao, New York University

9:00   **What Do Clinicians Need Most to Improve Treatment of Spinal Cord Injuries?**
John A. Jane, University of Virginia

Session II: Clinical Trials in Industry

9:35   **Challenges of Developing New Treatments from the Context of Current Industry Models**
Dennis W. Choi, Merck & Company, Inc.

9:55   **Challenges of Conducting Clinical Trials on Spinal Cord Injury in Industry**
Andrew R. Blight, Acorda Therapeutics, Inc.

Session III: Translational Research

10:45   **The Reeve-Irvine Research Center for Spinal Cord Injury**
Oswald Steward, University of California, Irvine

11:05   **Translational and Clinical Research in a Related Disorder (Amyotrophic Lateral Sclerosis)**
Jeffrey D. Rothstein, Johns Hopkins University

11:40   **General Discussion**

BOX A-2

Institute of Medicine
Committee on Spinal Cord Injury Workshop

May 24, 2004

8:25   **Welcome and Introductions**
        Richard T. Johnson, Johns Hopkins University

Session I: Emerging Therapies and Evaluation of Their Potential

8:30   **Cell Death and Plasticity: Identifying Therapeutic
        Targets for the Treatment of Spinal Cord Injuries**
        Alan Faden, Georgetown University

8:55   **Oxidative Stress and Cell Death: An Overview of
        Stroke Research and Lessons for Spinal Cord Injuries**
        Pak Chan, Stanford University

9:20   **Developing Animal Models for Spinal Cord Injuries**
        Michael Beattie, Ohio State University

Session II: Stem and Olfactory Ensheathing Cells

10:20   **Potentials and Pitfalls of Stem Cell Therapies:
        Lessons Learned from the Treatment of Cancer**
        Irving Weissman, Stanford University

10:45   **Is There a Role for Stem Cell Treatments for Patients
        with Spinal Cord Injuries?**
        Evan Snyder, Burnham Institute, San Diego

11:10   **Olfactory Ensheathing Cell Transplants as a Treatment
        for Spinal Cord Injuries**
        Geoff Raisman, National Institute for Medical Research,
        London, United Kingdom

Session III: Neuropathic Pain

1:00   **Potential Therapies to Treat Pain Syndromes in Spinal Cord Injuries**
Claire Hulsebosch, University of Texas Medical Branch

Session IV: Robotics and Physical Therapy

1:35   **Developing Neural Prostheses**
William Heetderks, National Institute of Biomedical Imaging and Bioengineering

2:00   **Physical Therapies and Electrical Stimulation as Treatments for Spinal Cord Injuries**
V. Reggie Edgerton, University of California, Los Angeles

Session V: Clinical Research Methods

2:55   **Statistical Methods and Patient Registries as Tools for Clinical Spinal Cord Injury Research**
Ralph Frankowski, University of Texas at Houston

3:20   **Registries as Clinical Research Tools: A Case Study of the Bone Marrow Transplant Registries**
Fausto Loberiza, Jr., Medical College of Wisconsin

3:45   **Alternatives to Large-Scale, Randomized Controlled Trials**
Curtis Meinert, Johns Hopkins University

Session VI: Discussion of Overarching Themes

4:30   General Discussion

5:00   Adjourn

Tuesday, May 25, 2004

10:45   **NIH Programs That Facilitate Clinical Research on Spinal Cord Injuries**
Naomi Kleitman, Program Director, Repair and Plasticity, National Institute of Neurological Disorders and Stroke

BOX A-3

Institute of Medicine
Committee on Spinal Cord Injury Workshop

September 27, 2004

9:30   **Welcome and Introductions**
        Richard T. Johnson, Johns Hopkins University

        Review of State-Sponsored Spinal Cord Injury
        Research Programs
        Mary Bunge, Miami Project to Cure Paralysis
        Marie Filbin, Hunter College of the City University of New York
        Rajiv Ratan, Burke/Cornell Medical Research Institute
        Christopher Shields, Kentucky Spinal Cord Injury
        Research Center

10:00   **Discussion: How Can State-Run Programs Maximize**
        Their Impact?

11:00   **Spinal Cord Injury Therapeutics—Regulatory Challenges**
        Cynthia Rask, Director, Division of Clinical Evaluation
        and Pharmacology/Toxicology, Food and Drug
        Administration

11:20   **Discussion: How to Overcome the Challenges in Getting**
        Drug Therapies and Devices Approved by the FDA?

September 28, 2004

Community Perspectives

11:00   **Welcome and Introductions**
        Richard T. Johnson, Johns Hopkins University

        Community Perspectives Session
        John Bollinger, Paralyzed Veterans of America
        Paul J. Tobin, United Spinal Association
        Z. Alexander Gentle, an individual with arachnoiditis

11:30   **Discussion of Community Needs and Priorities**

2:30   **Community Perspectives (continued)**
        Congressman James Langevin,
        2nd Congressional District, Rhode Island

B

ACRONYMS

AANS/CNS	American Association of Neurological Surgeons and the Congress of Neurological Surgeons
ADL	activities of daily living
ALS	amyotrophic lateral sclerosis
ALSFRS	Amyotrophic Lateral Sclerosis Functional Rating Scale
AMP	adenosine monophosphate
APS	American Paraplegia Society
ASIA	American Spinal Injury Association
BBB scale	Basso, Beattie, and Bresnahan scale
BDNF	brain-derived neurotrophic factor
BMS	Basso mouse scale
CART	Collaborations to Accelerate Research Translation
CDC	Centers for Disease Control and Prevention
CIRB	Central Institutional Review Board (National Cancer Institute)
CNS	central nervous system
CORE	Center of Research Excellence
COX2	cyclooxygenase 2
CPG	central pattern generator
CRASH	Corticosteroid Randomization After Significant Head Injury
CRISP	Computer Retrieval of Information on Scientific Projects
CRPF	Christopher Reeve Paralysis Foundation

CSPG	chondroitin sulfate proteoglycan
CT (or CAT)	computed tomography (or computer-assisted tomography)
DNA	deoxyribonucleic acid
DVT	deep vein thrombosis
EDRN	Early Detection Research Network
EMG	electromyogram
EMS	emergency medical services
FAM	functional assessment measure
FDA	Food and Drug Administration
FES	functional electrical stimulation
FGF	fibroblast growth factor
FIM	functional independence measure
fMRI	functional magnetic resonance imaging
FMS	functional magnetic stimulation
FOR-SCI	Facilities of Research Excellence in Spinal Cord Injury
FY	fiscal year
GABA	γ-aminobutyric acid
GDNF	glial cell-derived neurotrophic factor
HIV-AIDS	human immunodeficiency virus-acquired immunodeficiency syndrome
HL7	Health Level Seven
ICCP	International Campaign for Cures of Spinal Cord Injury Paralysis
ICIDH	International Classification of Impairment, Disabilities, and Handicaps
ICMIC	In Vivo Cellular and Molecular Imaging Centers
ICORD	International Collaboration on Repair Discoveries
IDEA	Innovative, Developmental, or Exploratory Activities
IND	investigational new drug
IOM	Institute of Medicine
IRB	institutional review board
ISRT	International Spinal Research Trust
MASCIS	Multicenter Animal Spinal Cord Injury Study
MR	magnetic resonance
MRI	magnetic resonance imaging
mRNA	messenger ribonucleic acid

MS	multiple sclerosis
NARCOMS	North American Research Consortium on Multiple Sclerosis
NASCIS	National Acute Spinal Cord Injury Study
NCI	National Cancer Institute
NCMRR	National Center for Medical Rehabilitation Research
NGF	nerve growth factor
NIDRR	National Institute on Disability and Rehabilitation Research
NIH	National Institutes of Health
NINDS	National Institute of Neurological Disorders and Stroke
NMDA	N-methyl-D-asparate
NSAID	nonsteroidal anti-inflammatory drug
NSCISC	National Spinal Cord Injury Statistical Center
NT-3	neurotrophic factor-3
NYSTAR	New York State Office of Science, Technology, and Academic Research
OEC	olfactory ensheathing cell
OSU	Ohio State University
PET	positron emission tomography
PKC	protein kinase C
PVA	Paralyzed Veterans of America
RH SCI	Rick Hansen Spinal Cord Injury Network
RNA	ribonucleic acid
ROCK	Rho-associated kinase
SAIRP	Small Animal Imaging Resources Program
SEER	Surveillance, Epidemiology, and End Results
SF	Short Form
SSTI	State Science & Technology Institute
TRH	thyrotropin-releasing hormone
UPDRS	Unified Parkinson's Disease Rating Scale
VA	U.S. Department of Veterans Affairs

C

GLOSSARY OF MAJOR TERMS

Action potential Electrical impulses that result from the influx and efflux of ions across the plasma membrane of neurons.

Antioxidants Natural body chemicals or drugs that reduce oxidative damage, such as that caused by free radicals.

Apoptosis Programmed cell death, a form of cell death in which a controlled sequence of events (or program) leads to the elimination of cells, minimizing the release of harmful substances into the surrounding area. Many types of cell damage can trigger apoptosis, and it also occurs normally during the development of the nervous system and other parts of the body. Strictly speaking, the term apoptosis refers only to the structural changes that cells go through, and programmed cell death refers to the complete underlying process, but the terms are often used synonymously.

Ascending pathways Nerve pathways that carry sensory information from the body up the spinal cord toward the brain.

Astrocytes The largest and most numerous of the supporting, or glial, cells in the brain and spinal cord. Astrocytes (meaning "star cells," because of their shape) contribute to the blood-brain barrier, help regulate the chemical environment around cells, respond to injury, and release regulatory and trophic substances that influence nerve cells.

Autonomic dysreflexia A potentially life-threatening increase in blood pressure, sweating, and other autonomic reflexes in reaction to bowel impaction or some other stimulus.

Autonomic nervous system The portion of the nervous system that governs involuntary actions and innervates smooth and cardiac muscles and glandular tissues.

Axon Long nerve cell fibers that arise from a neuron's cell body and that conduct electrical impulses to the target cell. Axons contact other nerve, muscle, and gland cells at synapses and release neurotransmitters that influence those cells.

Axonal transport The process by which nerve cells move substances from the cell body down the axon and from the end of the axon back to the cell body. Transport down the axon is necessary because axons cannot synthesize many substances, such as proteins, that they need. Transport back to the cell body recycles substances and also carries signals taken up by axon terminals, such as trophic factors, to the cell body, where they can affect cellular processes.

Blood-brain barrier Tight junctions are formed by endothelial cells that line blood vessels and regulate the entry of circulating substances and immune cells into the brain and spinal cord. Trauma may compromise these barriers and contribute to further damage in the brain and spinal cord. These barriers also prevent the entry of some potentially therapeutic drugs.

Brain-derived neurotrophic factor (BDNF) Exogenous neurotrophic factor.

Cell adhesion molecules Molecules on the outside surfaces of cells that bind to other cells or to the extracellular matrix (the material surrounding cells). Cell adhesion molecules influence many important functions, such as the entry of immune cells into the damaged spinal cord and the path finding of growing axons.

Central nervous system (CNS) The portion of the nervous system that consists of the brain and spinal cord. The CNS coordinates the entire nervous system and is responsible for receiving sensory information from the environment and responding using motor impulses.

Central pattern generator (CPG) A complex circuit of neurons responsible for coordinated rhythmic muscle activity, such as locomotion.

Clinical trials Systematic studies with human patients aimed at determining the safety and effectiveness of new or unproven therapies. Systematic testing in clinical trials has four phases. Phase I trials determine both the safety of a drug or intervention and the appropriate dosage. Phase II trials, which are performed with relatively small groups of patients, establish efficacy and evaluate reported side effects. Phase III trials, which usually require much larger numbers of patients, compare the new therapies to established therapies or a placebo, or both, and continue to monitor the participants for adverse side effects. Phase IV trials are required by the FDA for additional analysis of postmarking, long-term risks, and benefits.

Computed tomography (CT) or computer-assisted tomography (CAT) Diagnostic imaging method in which X-ray measurements obtained from many angles are combined into a single image. CT scans help physicians evaluate bone structures and bleeding within the skull and spine.

Contusion A bruising injury. Spinal cord contusions result in a cavity or hole in the center of the spinal cord. Myelinated axons typically survive around the perimeter of the spinal cord, and the dura may even remain unbroken by the injury.

Corticospinal tracts The nerve fibers that carry signals from the motor control areas of the brain's cerebral cortex to the spinal cord.

Cyclic AMP (cAMP) An adenosine-based mononucleotide that mediates hormonal effects and that acts as a second messenger.

Cytokines Chemical messenger molecules by which immune cells communicate with one another and with other cells. Some nerve cells also use cytokines as messenger molecules.

Cytoskeleton The internal scaffolding of cells. The cytoskeleton determines the cell shape, organizes structures within cells, and helps cells and growth cones of developing axons move.

Dendrites The tree-like branches from nerve cell bodies that receive and integrate signals from other nerve cells at synapses.

Deoxyribonucleic acid (DNA) Basic unit of heredity. DNA consists of a double helix containing ribose sugars, nucleic acids, phosphate groups, and hydrogen bonds.

Dermatome Predefined regions of the skin that are innervated by nerve fibers and tested (via a pinprick or light touch) to determine sensory response.

Descending pathways Nerve pathways that go down the spinal cord and that allow the brain to control the movement of the body below the head and autonomic function.

Dorsal Relating to the back or posterior of an animal.

Excitotoxicity Excessive release of neurotransmitters causing damage to nerve and glial cells. Excitotoxicity probably contributes to damage following nervous system trauma and stroke and may also contribute to some neurodegenerative diseases. Glutamate, the most prevalent neurotransmitter by which nerve cells excite (activate) one another, is often involved in excitotoxicity.

Extracellular matrix The material that surrounds cells. Important regulatory molecules in the extracelluar matrix promote, inhibit, or guide the growth of axons.

F30 fellowship Federally supported fellowship sponsored by the National Institutes of Health and given to predoctoral students seeking combined M.D. and Ph.D. degrees. These fellowships were created to increase the number of physician-researchers in the field of mental health, substance abuse, and environmental sciences. The fellowships, which are limited to no more than 6 years, subsidize the cost of tuition and associated fees, stipends, and certain allowable costs.

F31 fellowship Federally supported fellowship sponsored by the National Institutes of Health for predoctoral students that require a dissertation research project and training program. Fellowships are typically limited to no more than 5 years and support tuition and fees, stipends, and other costs. Specific F31 fellowships are available for ethnic and racial minorities and individuals with disabilities.

Fibroblast growth factor (FGF) Exogenous neurotrophic factor.

Free radicals Highly reactive chemicals that attack molecules crucial for cell function by capturing electrons and thus modifying chemical structures.

Gamma-aminobutyric acid (GABA) A neurotransmitter that typically inhibits subsequent neurons from being excited.

Gap junction Site of communication between adjacent cells and exchange of low-molecular-weight substances.

Gene expression Term used to describe those genes that are transcribed into proteins and that are active in or influence a biological process.

Glia Supporting cells of the nervous system. Glial cells in the brain and spinal cord far outnumber nerve cells. They not only provide physical support but also respond to injury, regulate the chemical composition surrounding cells, participate in the blood-brain and blood-spinal cord barriers, form the myelin insulation of nerve pathways, help guide neuronal migration during development, and exchange metabolites with neurons. They may also produce substances that help and hinder regeneration in the spinal cord. The major types of glial cells in the central nervous system are astrocytes, oligodendrocytes, and microglia.

Glia-derived neurotrophic factor (GDNF) Exogenous neurotrophic factor.

Glutamate A neurotransmitter that elicits subsequent neurons to fire an action potential.

Gray matter The parts of the brain and spinal cord composed mainly of neuronal cell bodies and dendrites and not myelinated (white) axons. The gray matter of the spinal cord lies in a butterfly-shaped region in the center of the cord.

Growth cones Specialized structures at the tips of growing axons. Growth cones detect guidance signals in their environment and "steer" growing axons.

Immediate-early genes Genes that respond quickly to many types of stimuli and that control the activities of other genes. They participate in the cellular programs that control regeneration and apoptosis.

Interneurons Neurons in the spinal cord that primarily communicate between neurons over short distances (compare interneurons with sensory and motor neurons, whose axons project outside the cord). Spinal cord interneurons help integrate sensory information and generate co-ordinated muscle commands.

Ischemia Inadequate blood flow. The brain and spinal cord are easily damaged by ischemia because of a decreased oxygen supply.

Knockouts Genetically engineered animals (usually mice) in which a particular gene has been removed from the animal's DNA.

Lipid peroxidation Breakdown of membrane lipids that eventually destroy the cell. This reaction is typically caused by free-radical formation, usually from oxygen atoms, which gives rise to a series of pathological reactions inside cells.

Magnetic resonance imaging (MRI) A type of diagnostic imaging technique that relies on the interactions of magnetic fields and radio-frequency radiation with body tissues. MRI is better than computed tomography scans for viewing soft tissue.

Methylprednisolone A corticosteroid, similar to a natural hormone produced by the human adrenal glands. It is used to relieve inflammation and to treat certain forms of arthritis; skin, blood, kidney, eye, thyroid, and intestinal disorders (e.g., colitis); severe allergies; and asthma.

Microarray Biochemical application that allows the rapid reproducibility of gene fragments of known sequence and that can be used to assess gene expression.

Microglia Small cells located throughout the central nervous system that act as phagocytes and that typically engulf and destroy particulate matter.

Motor neurons Nerve cells whose axons pass from the central nervous system to a muscle to regulate the muscle's activity.

Myelin The electrically insulating coating around axons that gives white matter its whitish appearance. Myelin increases the speed and reliability of signal transmission along nerve fibers. In the central nervous system, oligodendrocytes generate myelin; in the peripheral nervous system, Schwann cells generate myelin.

Myelin-associated glycoprotein (MAG) An inhibitory molecule present in myelin. The response of neurons to MAG is modulated by a cyclic AMP-dependent pathway. If cyclic AMP levels increase, protein kinase A is activated and inhibition by MAG is blocked.

Necrosis A type of cell death in which cells swell and break open and release their contents. The contents can damage neighboring cells and provoke inflammation.

Nerve growth factor (NGF) Exogenous neurotrophic factor.

Neural prosthesis An electronic or mechanical device, or both, that connects with the nervous system and supplements or replaces functions lost by disease or injury.

Neuron A nerve cell that is responsible for transmitting and receiving information from other cells. Most neurons comprise dendrites, a cell body, and an axon.

Neurotransmitter Chemicals that are released by nerve cells at synapses and that influence the activities of other cells. Neurotransmitters may excite, inhibit, or otherwise influence the activities of cells.

Neurotrophic-3 (NT-3) Exogenous neurotrophic factor.

Neurotrophic factor Any of a group of neuropeptides (such as nerve growth factor) that regulate the growth, differentiation, and survival of certain neurons in the peripheral and central nervous systems.

Nogo A protein that is expressed only by mature oligodendrocytes and that may be responsible for some of the inhibitory activity of myelin. Different fragments of Nogo cause growth cone collapse in a classic in vitro test of motility-inhibiting effects.

Oligodendrocyte A type of glial cell in the brain and spinal cord. Oligodendrocytes wrap axons with myelin, which improves the speed and reliability of impulse conduction. These cells also produce substances that inhibit the regeneration of axons in the adult central nervous system.

Oxidative damage Damage to cells caused by oxidants, or chemicals that capture electrons from other substances. The production of these substances increases during certain diseases and after a trauma or stroke and contributes to the secondary damage that follows these events.

P01 grant Federally supported research program project grant that is sponsored by the National Institutes of Health and that funds as many as three separate, multidisciplinary research projects that are based on a central research theme. Funding is limited to about $1 million each year in direct costs.

P30 grant Federally supported center core grant that is sponsored by the National Institutes of Health and that provides funds to develop an infrastructure that supports centralized research, facilities, and resources. Core grants provide resources to investigators to help them achieve a higher level of productivity. Awards are limited to 5 years and about $500,000 in direct costs per year.

P50 grant Federally supported specialized center grant that is sponsored by the National Institutes of Health and that provides funds for multi-investigator, multidisciplinary research. The purpose of the grant is to provide a higher level of integration that might not be achieved with individual research projects. Funding is limited to about $1 million each year in direct costs.

Paraplegia Paralysis of the lower half of the body with involvement of legs.

Peripheral nervous system (PNS) The network of nerves outside the brain and spinal cord. Unlike nerves in the central nervous system, peripheral nerves can regrow after an injury.

Placebo An inert substance or inactive treatment given instead of a therapy that is being evaluated in a clinical trial.

Plasticity The ability of neurons to modify the physical connections, thus changing the property of a neuronal circuit.

Progenitor cell Any type of cell that spawns other cells.

Programmed cell death Apoptosis (see above).

Proprioception The unconscious perception relating to position, posture, equilibrium, or internal condition.

Proteases Enzymes that degrade proteins. Proteases are important regulators of cell function, but the inappropriate activation of proteases resulting from trauma can be harmful.

Protein Any of numerous naturally occurring, extremely complex substances (such as an enzyme or antibody) that consist of amino acid residues joined by peptide bonds. They are essential constituents of all living cells that are translated from the organism's RNA.

Proteoglycans Proteins on the extracellular side of the cell membrane to which sugar moieties are attached.

Quadriplegia Paralysis of all four limbs, also called tetraplegia.

R01 grant Federal research project grant that supports specific health-based research for 1 to 5 years. It can be investigator initiated or submitted in response to a request for application or program announcement.

R03 grant Federal grant that supports small research projects for a limited period of time and with limited resources. Grants are awarded for up to 2 years with direct costs limited to $50,000 per year.

R21 grant Federally supported exploratory or developmental research grant that supports the early development of an innovative project. Grants are awarded for up to 2 years, with total direct costs not to exceed $275,000 for the length of the project.

Receptors Protein molecules, usually found on the surfaces of cells, that enable cells to respond to neurotransmitters, hormones, and other messenger molecules. Receptors may act directly by opening in the cell membrane ion channels that are part of the same receptor molecule, or they may indirectly by activating second messenger systems that go on to affect various processes in the cell. The term "receptor" also refers to specialized neuronal cells that receive sensory information, such as pain receptors and light receptors in the eye.

Ribonucleic acid (RNA) Carries the code for a particular protein from DNA. Messenger RNA (mRNA) is translated by specialized proteins and ribosomes to form proteins.

Schwann cells Glial cells in the peripheral nervous system that are primarily responsible for wrapping nerve fibers with myelin.

Second messenger system Biochemical pathway within cells that is regulated by hormones or neurotransmitters, which bind to receptors on the cell surface. Second messengers diffuse within the cell and alter cell behavior. They amplify signals, allow a single first messenger to control several cellular processes, and help integrate the many signals that cells receive.

Spasticity A state of increased muscular tone in which abnormal stretch reflexes intensify muscle resistance to passive movements.

Spinal cord segments Divisions of the spinal cord along its length. Each spinal cord segment sends a pair of motor and sensory nerves to the body. Higher segments control movement and sensation in upper parts of the body, whereas lower segments control movement and sensation in lower parts of the body.

Synapse The functional connection between a nerve cell axon and target cells, which may be other nerve cells, muscle cells, or gland cells. At the synapse the axon releases a chemical neurotransmitter that diffuses across a tiny gap and binds to receptors (molecules on the surface of the target cell) that then change the target cell's behavior. Synapses may be excitatory (which increases the probability that the target cell will be activated) or inhibitory (which reduces the probability that the target cell will be activated) or may have more complex influences (such as adjusting the sensitivity of cells to other signals).

Tight junction A junction formed between adjacent cells, which prevents the passage of large molecules.

Transcription Molecular process by which the genetic material deoxyribonucleic acid (DNA) is used as a template to become messenger ribonucleic acid (mRNA), which is subsequently used as a template for protein production.

Translation Molecular process by which messenger ribonucleic acid (mRNA), in conjunction with ribosomes, forms proteins.

Trophic factor A natural cell growth and survival molecule. Neurotrophic factors are trophic factors that affect nerve cells.

Ventral Relating to the belly or front of the body.

White matter Areas of the brain and spinal cord that primarily contain myelinated axons. White matter is located in the outer portion of the spinal cord and surrounds the gray matter.

D

TOOLS TO ASSESS
SPINAL CORD INJURY OUTCOMES

A number of tools can be used to assess the outcomes of spinal cord injuries. Many of these are already being used to assess the outcomes of spinal cord injuries, while others are used in related fields and could be modified for use with spinal cord injury. The following table lists outcome measures and their potential shortcomings and can be divided into the following categories: (1) recovery measures in animals, (2) recovery measures in humans, and (3) measures of quality of life.

Tools to Assess Spinal Cord Injury Outcomes
_____

Animal

Functional recovery
Basso, Beattie, and Bresnahan (BBB) scale, an open-field locomotor test for rats
- Is based on 5-point Tarlov scale
- Analyzes hind-limb movements of a rat in an open field
- Is a 21-point scale used to assess locomotor coordination
- Rates parameters such as joint movements, the ability for weight support, limb coordination, foot placement, and gait stability
- Small changes in tissue correlate to large changes on the scale
- Assesses walking, not other movements requiring coordinated spinal cord activity
- Does not assess pain, bowel, bladder, or sexual function

Basso Mouse Scale (BMS), an open-field locomotor test for mice
- Is an adaptation of rat BBB scale to examine the recovery of hind-limb locomotor function

Tools to Assess Spinal Cord Injury Outcomes

- Assesses walking, not other movements requiring coordinated spinal cord activity
- Does not assess pain, bowel, bladder, or sexual function

Tarlov scale
- 5-point scale to assess upper and lower limb locomotion
- Uses scores ranging from 0 (paraplegia) to 4 (animal can run and has a normal motor system with no other weaknesses); uses MEPs and SSEP (see below)
- Looks at action potentials in muscle and nerves
- Hard to assess minor but significant changes in locomotion
- Does not assess pain, bowel, bladder, or sexual function

Durham scale
- Includes Tarlov scale, as well as functional task, bowel hygiene, and neck position
- Is better than Tarlov scale at predicting spinal cord disorders
- Hard to assess minor but significant changes in locomotion
- Better suited for assessment of incomplete injuries
- Does not assess pain, bowel, bladder, or sexual function

Neuronal activity assessment by electrophysiology
- Assesses MEPs or SSEP
- Stimulates corresponding cortical areas of the brain and records response in target nerves to see if connections are still functional
- Correlates to impairment of locomotor activity
- Is noninvasive
- Neuronal activity may not correlate with functional changes
- Hard to assess subtle but critical improvements to circuitry
- Does not directly assess pain, bowel, bladder, or sexual function

Directed forepaw reaching
- Looks at coordinated limb and muscle movement
- Requires rats to reach under a barrier and pick up food with forepaws
- Limited scale for assessment
- Does not assess pain, bowel, bladder, or sexual function

Grooming response
- A little water is sprinkled on the head of a rat to elicit grooming with the rat's forelimbs and measure forelimb function
- Is a brain stem-mediated spontaneous reflex sensitive to the level and severity of the injury
- Looks only at forelimb response
- Difficult to discriminate between loss of communication with brain stem or damage to other part of the nervous system

Rearing
- A rat is placed in a cylinder and is scored on how often it rears and simultaneously touches the walls of the cylinder with its forelimbs
- Looks only at forelimb response

Tools to Assess Spinal Cord Injury Outcomes

Walking speed
- Is used to assess locomotor training techniques
- Does not assess sensory modalities influenced by muscle strength
- Does not assess pain, bowel, bladder, or sexual function

Rotor rod
- Is used to examine sensory feedback, coordination, and muscle strength required for locomotion
- Is performed by placing the animal on a rotating bar and timing how long it takes for animal to lose balance
- Only measures recovery of locomotion and does not assess restoration of fine motor control or other complications associated with spinal cord injury

Inclined plane
- Is used to examine sensory feedback, coordination, and muscle strength required for locomotion
- Is performed by placing animal on a ramp of a preset incline
- Only measures recovery of locomotion and does not assess restoration of fine motor control or other complications associated with spinal cord injury

Footprint
- Examines an animal's gait by analyzing paw position and toe drags
- Only measures recovery of locomotion and does not assess restoration of fine motor control

Grid walking
- Tests the ability of mice and rats to walk over a wire mesh grid
- Only investigates coordinated walking and not fine motor control

Forepaw withdrawal
- Investigates recovery of heat perception
- The forepaw is placed on a heat block and the time that it takes for the animal to withdraw it is measured
- Forepaw withdrawal requires motor function
- Does not assess pain, bowel, bladder, or sexual function

Assessment of autonomic dysreflexia
- Changes in blood pressure are determined by comparing the animals baseline blood pressure and peak blood pressure during moderate cutaneous pinches to the skin rostral and caudal to the injury
- Autonomic dysreflexia is also characterized in patients by sweating, flushed skin, and piloerection, which are not assessed in mouse model

Morphological assessment of recovery

Histology
- Is used to look at the morphology of axons and assess the degree of tissue sparing, injury, and recovery

Tools to Assess Spinal Cord Injury Outcomes

- Is used for anterograde and retrograde tracing of axons: a substance is injected above or below the location of the injury to determine if the neuron transports it up past the injury location
- Uses electron microscopy to look at the morphology of the spinal cord at very high resolution
- Uses antibody staining to determine the protein distribution in cells
- Assessments cannot be made in real time
- Cannot be performed with living animals

Real-time imaging of the spinal cord
- Uses MRI, CT, and PET, which are safe, noninvasive methods that provide detailed images of hard-to-view areas of the spine
- Resolution is not high enough to detect changes to individual cells

Genetically encoded reporter molecules
- Axon regrowth and formation of functional connections are visualized by use of genetically encoded reporter molecules in intact animal models or in isolated spinal cord preparations
- Requires a correlation to improvements in physiological function

Human

Functional recovery
American Spinal Injury Association (ASIA) International Standards for Neurological Classification
- Analyzes the effect that the injury has on both motor and sensory systems
- Is based on the extent of injury and muscle strength
- Uses an alphabetical score from A (the most severe) to E (the least severe)
- Insensitive to small but significant changes in motor and sensory functions
- May not be sensitive enough to detect even several spinal levels of regeneration in thoracic injuries[a]
- Does not specifically address functions that affect a patient's quality of life
- Does not assess pain, bowel, bladder, or sexual function

Includes:
- ASIA Impairment Scale
  o Is based on the extent of injury and muscle strength
  o Uses an alphabetical score from A (the most severe) to E (the least severe)
  o Insensitive to small but significant changes in motor and sensory functions

Lower-extremity motor scores
- Assess the functions of five key muscle groups of each leg
- Uses scores from 0 (no movement) to 5 (normal resistance)
- Looks only at lower extremities, not at fine hand movements
- Does not assess sensory, pain, bowel, bladder, or sexual function

Tools to Assess Spinal Cord Injury Outcomes

Functional Independence Measure (FIM)
- Is an 18-item, 7-level ordinal scale
- Is designed to assess areas of dysfunction in activities that commonly occur
- The scale has few cognitive, behavioral, and communication-related functional items
- Is not specific for spinal cord injuries but is designed to assess neurological, musculoskeletal, and other disorders

Functional Assessment Measure (FAM)
- Was developed to augment the FIM
- Specifically addresses functional areas that are relatively less emphasized in FIM, including cognitive, behavioral, communication, and community functioning measures
- The scale has few cognitive, behavioral, and communication-related functional items
- Is not specific for spinal cord injuries but is designed to assess neurological, musculoskeletal, and other disorders

Spinal Cord Independence Measure (SCIM)
- Is specifically designed to assess spinal cord injuries and to be sensitive to changes
- Analyzes self-care, respiration, and sphincter management and mobility
- Is more sensitive than FIM for spinal cord injuries

Walking Index for Spinal Cord Injury (WISCI)
- Scale measures functional limitations in walking of individuals after a spinal cord injury
- Grades physical assistance and devices required for walking after paralysis of the lower extremities
- Documents changes in functional capacity in respect to ambulation in a rehabilitation setting
- Limited to assessment of walking

Spinal Cord Injury-Functional Ambulation Inventory
- Analyzes ambulation in individuals with spinal cord injuries relating to gait parameters, assistive device use, and temporal-distance measures
- Limited to assessment of walking

Barthel Index
- Measures individual's independence in mobility
- Assesses many deficits, including those after a stroke
- Is designed to measure three categories of function: self-care, continence of bowel and bladder, and mobility
- Functional ability can be a predictor of discharge from hospital
- Floor and ceiling of scale are not sensitive enough to measure small but significant changes in function

Tools to Assess Spinal Cord Injury Outcomes

Visual Analog Scale (VAS)
- Is a pain assessment test
- Uses a graphic rating scale
- Solely based on self-assessment

Electrophysiology
- Assesses MEPs or SSEP
- Stimulates corresponding cortical areas of the brain and records the response in target nerves to see if connections are still functional
- Is correlated to impairment of locomotor activity
- Is noninvasive
- Electrical activity may not coordinate with function
- Hard to assess subtle but critical improvements to circuitry
- Does not assess pain, bowel, bladder, or sexual function

Ashworth scale for spasticity
- 6-point scale to assess muscle tone
- Too crude for assessment of the daily variability in spasticity

The Stroke Rehabilitation Assessment of Movement (STREAM)
- Measures voluntary movement and basic mobility
- Is designed to be able to assess reemergence of voluntary movement and basic mobility
- Assesses 30 mobility items, including upper and lower extremity mobility, using a 3- or 4-point scale
- Can be used as a predictor of discharge from hospital

Timed "up and go" (TUG)
- Is considered the best test of functional mobility
- The individual sits in a chair and is then required to stand and walk forward 3 meters
- Requires patient to be able to walk

Box and Block test
- Is used to measure unilateral gross manual dexterity
- The individual moves blocks, one by one, from one compartment to another in 60 seconds
- Requires significant muscle strength and control

Quantitative Sensory Testing (QST)
- Was developed for sensory assessment, primarily in individuals with peripheral nerve disorders
- Measures activity in three types of sensory nerve fibers: fast A_b (touch, joint position, mild pressure, vibration), small A_δ (cold sensation, pain), and C fibers (warmth sensation, pain)
- Sensitive to different methodological aspects, including site of testing, pressure of stimulator, subject training, and stimulator size
- Test is time-consuming if many dermatomes are examined

Tools to Assess Spinal Cord Injury Outcomes

Quality of life

NAGI Classification
- Disability is a function of the interaction of the individual with his or her social and physical environments
- Is affected by individual and environmental factors
- Was presented in 1991 by IOM

Activities of Daily Living (ADL)
- Measures basic tasks of everyday living
- Is used as a predictor of admission to nursing homes and hospitals
- Lots of variation, depending on which items are measured and how a disabling condition is classified

SF-12, SF-36, and SF-54
- Measure changes in quality of life, mental health, pain, and social function
- Reflect the individual's perceptions and preferences about physical, emotional, and social well-being
- Hard to detect changes in quality of life over time
- Questions about walking can be construed as offensive to individuals with SCI

Assessment of Life Habits Scale
- Assesses social participation
- Relates accomplishments of daily habits from personal factors and environmental factors

Satisfaction with Life Scale (SWLS)
- Consists of five items that are completed by the patient
- Can assess life satisfaction in a particular domain of life (e.g., work or family) or globally
- Is based on the individual's emotions

International Classification of Impairment, Disabilities, and Handicaps (ICIDH)
- Was designed by the World Health Organization to classify the consequences of disease and their implications on the patient's life
- Defines impairment, disabilities, and handicaps
- ICIDH-2 incorporates disability as a dynamic process and holds that environmental factors can influence the impairment

Craig Handicap Assessment and Reporting Technique (CHART)
- Is based on the World Health Organization model of handicap dimensions
- Uses 27 questions and a 5-point scale to look at physical independence, economic self-sufficiency, social integration, mobility, and occupational functioning

Needs Assessment Checklist (NAC)
- Is used as a rehabilitation outcome measure designed specifically for spinal cord injury population
- Uses a 4-point scale
- Consists of 199 behavioral indicators that assess patient achievement in nine categories required for maintenance of health and quality of living
- Is not subject to floor or ceiling effects

Tools to Assess Spinal Cord Injury Outcomes

Awareness Questionnaire (AQ)
- Was developed as a measure of impaired self-awareness after traumatic brain injury
- Consists of three forms to be filled out by the patient, the patient's family, and a clinician familiar with the patient
- Assesses the ability of the patient to perform tasks before and after the injury using a 5-point scale ranging from "much worse" to "much better"

Community Integration Questionnaire (CIQ)
- Provides a measure of community integration after a traumatic brain injury
- Consists of 15 items relating to home integration, social integration, and productive activities

Craig Hospital Inventory of Environmental Factors (CHIEF)
- Is designed to assess the environmental factors and understand which elements of the environment impede or facilitate the lives of people with disabling conditions
- Respondents use a 5-point scale to quantify the barriers experienced within five domains of environmental factors (policies, physical and structural, work and school, attitudes and support, services and assistance)

Disability Rating Scale (DRS)
- Is intended to measure general functional changes over the course of recovery
- Assesses arousability, awareness, and responsiveness; cognitive ability for self-care activities; dependence on others; and psychosocial adaptability
- Is relatively insensitive at the low end of the scale
- Inability to reflect more subtle but sometimes significant changes

Family Needs Questionnaire (FNQ)
- Provides information about family members' unique needs after a family member has a traumatic brain injury
- Contains 40 items representing diverse needs that may arise during acute rehabilitation, soon after discharge, and in the long term
- Indicates the importance of each perceived need and then rates the degree to which the need has been met

Service Obstacles Scale (SOS)
- Evaluates a patient's and/or caregiver's perceptions of brain injury services in the community with regard to quality and accessibility
- Uses a 7-point Likert-type scale ranging from strongly disagree to strongly agree to assess (1) satisfaction with treatment resources, (2) finances as an obstacle to receiving services, and (3) transportation as an obstacle to receiving services

---

[a]National Institute of Neurological Disorders and Stroke Translating Spinal Cord Injuries workshop, February 3-4, 2003.
NOTE: Abbreviations: MEPs = motor evoked potential; SSEP = somatosensory evoked potential; MRI = magnetic resonance imaging; CT = computed tomography; PET = positron emission tomography; IOM = Institute of Medicine.

E

CLINICAL TRIALS OF
METHYLPREDNISOLONE

The following table summarizes the findings of the American Association of Neurological Surgeons and the Congress of Neurological Surgeons (AANS/CNS, 2002) on studies of methylprednisolone treatment after acute cervical spinal cord injuries.

Continued

Description of Study	Evidence Class (Comments)	Results	Reference
Multicenter, double-blind randomized trial comparing different MP doses (1,000 versus 100 mg/d for 11 d) for treatment of 330 ASCI patients (NASCIS I study)	III (study design, data presentation, interpretation, and analysis flaws)	No treatment effect at 6 wk and 6 mo postinjury, no control group	Bracken et al. (1984)
1-yr follow-up of NASCIS I study	III (study design, data presentation, interpretation, and analysis flaws)	No significant difference in neurological recovery of motor or sensory function at 1 yr postinjury	Bracken et al. (1985)
Multicenter, randomized, double-blind, placebo-controlled trial comparing MP treatment with naloxone and placebo treatment in 487 patients (NASCIS II study)	III (study design, data presentation, interpretation, and analysis flaws)	Significant improvement in motor change scores ($P = 0.03$) and sensation change scores ($P = 0.02$) at 6 mo postinjury for patients treated with MP within 8 h of injury	Bracken et al. (1990)
1-yr follow-up of NASCIS II study	III (study design, data presentation, interpretation, and analysis flaws)	Significant improvement in motor change scores 1 yr postinjury for patients treated with MP within 8 h of injury ($P = 0.03$); administration of MP was detrimental if it was given more than 8 h after injury	Bracken et al. (1992)

Description of Study	Evidence Class (Comments)	Results	Reference
Prospective assessment of 15 patients from 1990 to 1993 with retrospective review of 17 patients from 1987 to 1990 to assess differences in treatment outcomes with MP treatment compared with those with treatment without corticosteroids	III	No difference in neurological outcomes between the two sets of patients; patients treated with MP had immune response alterations, higher rates of pneumonia, and longer hospital stays than patients who did not receive corticosteroids	Galandiuk et al. (1993)
Concurrent cohort comparison study (population based) of 363 ASCI patients managed from 1990 to 1991 and 1993; 188 patients received the NASCIS II MP regimen, whereas 90 patients did not receive MP	III (inadequate statistical power)	No differences in neurological outcomes between MP-treated and non-MP-treated patients by use of the Frankel classification; however, insufficient numbers of patients may have been included to show significant differences	Gerhart et al. (1995)
Retrospective review of 145 ASCI patients: 80 treated with MP and 65 not treated	III	No difference in mortality or neurological outcome between groups, despite the younger age and less severe injuries in MP-treated patients	George et al. (1995)

Continued

Description	Grade	Results	Reference
Retrospective review with historical control of 231 ASCI patients; 91 were excluded; comparison of medical complications among 93 MP-treated patients with those among 47 who received no corticosteroid	III	MP-treated patients had significant increases in pneumonia ($P = 0.02$), acute pneumonia ($P = 0.03$), number of days with ventilation ($P = 0.04$), and lengths of ICU stay ($P = 0.45$); but MP had no adverse effect on long-term outcome	Gerndt et al. (1997)
Case-control analysis of 71 consecutive ASCI admissions; 63 were available for 13 to 57 mo of follow-up; 38 patients were treated with MP, and 25 patients referred >8 h after injury received no MP	III	Multiple factors influenced recovery after SCI; neither MP nor surgery had an effect on the outcome	Poynton et al. (1997)
Multicenter, randomized, double-blind trial comparing MP administered for 24 h with MP administered for 48 h and TM for treatment of 499 ASCI patients (NASCIS III study)	III (study design, data presentation, interpretation, and analysis flaws)	Patients administered MP for 48 h had improved motor recovery at 6 wk and at 6 mo compared with those treated with MP for 24 h and TM for 48 h ($P = $ NS); when treatment was initiated between 3 and 8 h after injury, MP treatment for 48 h resulted in significant improvements in motor scores at 6 wk ($P = 0.04$) and 6 mo ($P = 0.01$); MP administered for 48 h was associated with high rates of sepsis and pneumonia; no control group	Bracken et al. (1997)

Description of Study	Evidence Class (Comments)	Results	Reference
1-yr follow-up of NASCIS III study	III (study design, data presentation, interpretation, and analysis flaws)	Recovery rates were equal in all three groups when treatment was initiated within 8 h; patients treated with MP for 24 h had diminished recovery; patients treated with MP for 48 h had increased motor recovery (P = 0.053)	Bracken et al. (1998)
Multicenter, prospective, randomized clinical trial of 106 ASCI patients treated with MP, nimopidine, neither, or both	III (inadequate statistical power)	No significant difference in neurological outcome between groups at 1 yr of follow-up; patients with incomplete ASCIs had significant improvements below the level of injury compared with that for patients with complete ASCIs (P < 0.0001); higher incidence of infectious complications among patients receiving corticosteroids (P = NS)	Pointillart et al. (2000)
Prospective, randomized, double-blind study comparing incidence of medical complications among 46 ASCI patients: 23 treated with MP and 23 treated with placebo	I	Patients treated with MP had a higher incidence of complications (56.5 and 34.8%, respectively); differences in respiratory complications (P = 0.009) and gastrointestinal bleed (P = 0.036) were most significant between groups; no data on neurological improvement	Matsumoto et al. (2001)

NOTE: Abbreviations: MP = methylprednisolone; ASCI = acute spinal cord injury; SCI = spinal cord injury; h = hour; mo = month; d = day; yr = year; NASCIS = National Acute Spinal Cord Injury Study; NS = not significant; TM = tirilazad mesylate; ICU = intensive care unit.
SOURCE: Reprinted with permission, from AANS/CNS, 2002. Copyright 2002 from Lippincott Williams & Wilkins.

REFERENCES

AANS/CNS (American Association of Neurological Surgeons and the Congress of Neurological Surgeons). 2002. Pharmacological therapy after acute cervical spinal cord injury. *Neurosurgery* 50(3 Suppl): S63-72.

Bracken MB, Collins WF, Freeman DF, Shepard MJ, Wagner FW, Silten RM, Hellenbrand KG, Ransohoff J, Hunt WE, Perot PL Jr, et al. 1984. Efficacy of methylprednisolone in acute spinal cord injury. *Journal of the American Medical Association* 251(1): 45-52.

Bracken MB, Shepard MJ, Hellenbrand KG, Collins WF, Leo LS, Freeman DF, Wagner FC, Flamm ES, Eisenberg HM, Goodman JH, et al. 1985. Methylprednisolone and neurological function 1 year after spinal cord injury. Results of the National Acute Spinal Cord Injury Study. *Journal of Neurosurgery* 63(5): 704-713.

Bracken MB, Shepard MJ, Collins WF, Holford TR, Young W, Baskin DS, Eisenberg HM, Flamm E, Leo-Summers L, Maroon J. 1990. A randomized, controlled trial of methylprednisolone or naloxone in the treatment of acute spinal-cord injury. Results of the second National Acute Spinal Cord Injury Study. *New England Journal of Medicine* 322(20): 1405-1411.

Bracken MB, Shepard MJ, Collins WF Jr, Holford TR, Baskin DS, Eisenberg HM, Flamm E, Leo-Summers L, Maroon JC, Marshall LF, Perot PL Jr, Piepmeier J, Sonntag VKH, Wagner FC Jr, Wilberger JL, Winn HR, Young W. 1992. Methylprednisolone or naloxone treatment after acute spinal cord injury: 1-year follow-up data: Results of the second National Acute Spinal Cord Injury Study. *Journal of Neurosurgery* 76(1): 23-31.

Bracken MB, Shepard MJ, Holford TR, Leo-Summers L, Aldrich EF, Fazl M, Fehlings M, Herr DL, Hitchon PW, Marshall LF, Nockels RP, Pascale V, Perot PL Jr, Piepmeier J, Sonntag VKH, Wagner F, Wilberger JE, Winn HR, Young W. 1997. Administration of methylprednisolone for 24 or 48 hours or tirilazad mesylate for 48 hours in the treatment of acute spinal cord injury: Results of the third National Acute Spinal Cord Injury randomized controlled trial. *Journal of the American Medical Association* 277(20): 1597-1604.

Bracken MB, Shepard MJ, Holford TR, Leo-Summers L, Aldrich EF, Fazl M, Fehlings MG, Herr DL, Hitchon PW, Marshall LF, Nockels RP, Pascale V, Perot PL Jr, Piepmeier J, Sonntag VKH, Wagner F, Wilberger JE, Winn HR, Young W. 1998. Methylprednisolone or tirilazad mesylate administration after acute spinal cord injury: 1-year follow up: Results of the third National Acute Spinal Cord Injury randomized controlled trial. *Journal of Neurosurgery* 89(5): 699-706.

Galandiuk S, Raque G, Appel S, Polk HC Jr, Collins WF Jr, Trunkey D, Hoff JT, Howard J, Lucas CB, Patterson RH. 1993. The two-edged sword of large-dose steroids for spinal cord trauma. *Annals of Surgery* 218(4): 419-427.

George ER, Scholten DJ, Buechler CM, Jordan-Tibbs J, Mattice C, Albrecht RM, Turner W, Edwards M, Jacobs D. 1995. Failure of methylprednisolone to improve the outcome of spinal cord injuries. *American Surgeon* 61(8): 659-664.

Gerhart KA, Johnson RL, Menconi J, Hoffman RE, Lammertse DP. 1995. Utilization and effectiveness of methylprednisolone in a population-based sample of spinal cord injured persons. *Paraplegia* 33(6): 316-321.

Gerndt SJ, Rodriguez JL, Pawlik JW, Taheri PA, Wahl WL, Micheals AJ, Papadopoulos SM, Croce MA, Petersen SR, Hawkins ML. 1997. Consequences of high-dose steroid therapy for acute spinal cord injury. *Journal of Trauma: Injury Infection & Critical Care* 42(2): 279-284.

Matsumoto T, Tamaki T, Kawakami M, Yoshida M, Ando M, Yamada H. 2001. Early complications of high-dose methylprednisolone sodium succinate treatment in the follow-up of acute cervical spinal cord injury. *Spine* 26(4): 426-430.

Pointillart V, Petitjean ME, Wiart L, Vital JM, Lassie P, Thicoipe M, Dabadie P. 2000. Pharmacological therapy of spinal cord injury during the acute phase. *Spinal Cord* 38(2): 71-76.

Poynton AR, O'Farrell DA, Shannon F, Murray P, McManus F, Walsh MG. 1997. An evaluation of the factors affecting neurological recovery following spinal cord injury. *Injury* 28(8): 545-548.

F

Examples of Alternative Therapies

The following alternative therapies have been used in attempts to treat spinal cord injuries. Most of these interventions have not been examined in peer-reviewed randomized clinical trials. Therefore, their safety and efficacy are not known.

Acupuncture	Insertion of fine needles into specific sites of the skin.
Aromatherapy and essential oils therapy	Use of plant essential oils applied through either the nose or the skin.
Ayurvedic medicine	A form of therapy that emphasizes diet and nutrition, exercise, and rest and relaxation, among other treatments, to maintain basic energy.
Blueberry extracts	An extract that contains substances similar to cranberries that may fight urinary tract infections.
Cannabis	Hemp-derived substance with psychoactive properties.
Chiropractic healing	System of therapy that uses manipulation of the muscles and body structures.
Chronologically controlled developmental therapy	System of therapy with a number of traditional physical therapies that includes pressure stimulation and light-touch massage, among other techniques.

Cranberry extract	An extract that contains antibacterial substances, such as proanthocyanidins, that inhibit the bacterium *Escherichia coli* from attaching to the bladder and causing urinary tract infection.
Craniosacral therapy	Light-touch massage and acupuncture.
Creatine supplement	Dietary supplement of creatine, an amino acid involved in cellular energy production in skeletal muscle.
Dolphin-assisted therapy	Interaction of dolphins and humans that includes sonar echolocation.
Flower-essence therapy	The use of a mixture of flower petals that do not contain biologically active molecules.
Homeopathy	The use of natural substances found in plants, minerals, or animals. Homeopathy is based on the premise that low doses can stimulate the body's defense mechanisms.
Laserpuncture	A therapy that combines elements of acupuncture and laser therapy by using a laser beam of infrared light for acupuncture needles on the patient's torso.
Magnetic therapy	Therapy that involves the use of magnets.
D-Mannose	Simple sugar used as a supplement to prevent urinary tract infection.
Massage	Manipulation of soft tissues to increase circulation and to stimulate relaxation.
Mimosa pudica	A plant native of tropical America.
Omental therapy	Surgical lengthening and placement of the omentum, a vascular, fatty membranous tissue that surrounds the lower abdomen, over the site of injury.
Peripheral nerve rerouting	Surgical rerouting of peripheral nerves from above the site of injury and connecting them to peripheral nerves below the site of injury.
Qigong	Physical and mental training in gentle movements, breathing, and meditative practices.

Shark embryo cell transplantation	Surgical procedure involving decompression surgery, removal of bone fragments, drainage of cysts, and injection of blue shark embryo cells and growth factors, followed by physical therapy.
St. John's wort	Herbal medicine that may treat mild cases of depression.

SOURCES: Johnston, L. 2002. *Alternative & Innovative Therapies for Physical Disability*. [Online]. Available: http://healingtherapies.info/ [accessed August 5, 2004]; Spinal Cord Injury Information Network. 1998. *Alternative Therapies*. [Online]. Available: http://www.spinalcord.uab.edu/show.asp?durki=21745 [accessed November 10, 2004]; Northwest Regional Spinal Cord Injury System. 2002. *Complementary and Alternative Medicine*. [Online]. Available: http://www.depts.washington.edu/rehab/sci/comp_alt_med.html [accessed February 25, 2005].

G

SPINAL CORD INJURY CLINICAL TRIALS PUBLISHED FROM 1998 TO 2003

To identify the spinal cord injury clinical trials that were published from 1998 to 2003, Institute of Medicine staff searched Medline using the relevant medical subject headings as search terms and limiting the searches by publication types relevant to clinical trials. Additional clinical trial terms, namely, "randomized controlled trial," "controlled," "placebo," "double-blind," and "prospective," were also used in the search strategy.

The titles and abstracts were reviewed to determine the clinical conditions and outcomes that were addressed in each article. Table G-1 categorizes the clinical trials by the primary outcome(s) examined and secondarily is organized in chronological order. The majority of clinical trials targeted secondary complications that arise as a result of a spinal cord injury and did not directly test therapies to improve lost function. Articles that addressed multiple conditions (e.g., the effects of bowel and bladder functions on the quality of life) were counted once in each category and are designated with an asterisk.

TABLE G-1 Spinal Cord Injury Clinical Trials, 1998 to 2003

Topic and Author(s)	Study Title	Journal Reference
Acute Care		
Spinal Cord Injury Thromboprophylaxis Investigators (2003)*	Prevention of venous thromboembolism in the acute treatment phase after spinal cord injury: A randomized, multicenter trial comparing low-dose heparin plus intermittent pneumatic compression with enoxaparin.	*Journal of Trauma: Injury Infection & Critical Care* 54(6): 1116-1124
Geisler et al. (2001)	The Sygen multicenter acute spinal cord injury study.	*Spine* 26(24 Suppl): S87-98
Matsumoto et al. (2001)	Early complications of high-dose methylpred-nisolone sodium succinate treatment in the follow-up of acute cervical spinal cord injury.	*Spine* 26(4): 426-430
McIlvoy et al. (2000)	Use of an acute spinal cord injury clinical pathway.	*Critical Care Nursing Clinics of North America* 12(4): 521-530
Pointillart et al. (2000)	Pharmacological therapy of spinal cord injury during the acute phase.	*Spinal Cord* 38(2): 71-76
Prasad et al. (1999)	Characteristics of injuries to the cervical spine and spinal cord in polytrauma patient population: Experience from a regional trauma unit.	*Spinal Cord* 37(8): 560-568
Selden et al. (1999)*	Emergency magnetic resonance imaging of cervical spinal cord injuries: Clinical correlation and prognosis.	*Neurosurgery* 44(4): 785-792
Shepard et al. (1999)*	Magnetic resonance imaging and neurological recovery in acute spinal cord injury: Observations from the National Acute Spinal Cord Injury Study 3.	*Spinal Cord* 37(12): 833-837

Continued

TABLE G-1 Continued

Topic and Author(s)	Study Title	Journal Reference
Bracken et al. (1998)*	Methylprednisolone or tirilazad mesylate administration after acute spinal cord injury: 1-year follow up. Results of the third National Acute Spinal Cord Injury randomized controlled trial.	*Journal of Neurosurgery* 89(5): 699-706
Petitjean et al. (1998)	Medical treatment of spinal cord injury in the acute stage.	*Annales Francaises d Anesthesie et de Reanimation* 17(2): 114-122
Segal et al. (1998)	Methylprednisolone disposition kinetics in patients with acute spinal cord injury.	*Pharmacotherapy* 18(1): 16-22
Xiong et al. (1998)	Manipulation for cervical spinal dislocation under general anesthesia: Serial review for 4 years.	*Spinal Cord* 36(1): 21-24
Alternative Therapy		
Wong et al. (2003)	Clinical trial of acupuncture for patients with spinal cord injuries.	*American Journal of Physical Medicine & Rehabilitation* 82(1): 21-27
Zemper et al. (2003)	Assessment of a holistic wellness program for persons with spinal cord injury.	*American Journal of Physical Medicine & Rehabilitation* 82(12): 957-968
Diego et al. (2002)	Spinal cord patients benefit from massage therapy.	*International Journal of Neuroscience* 112(2): 133-142
Dyson-Hudson et al. (2001)*	Acupuncture and Trager psychophysical integration in the treatment of wheelchair user's shoulder pain in individuals with spinal cord injury.	*Archives of Physical Medicine and Rehabilitation* 82(8): 1038-1046
Honjo et al. (2000)*	Acupuncture on clinical symptoms and urodynamic measurements in spinal-cord-injured patients with detrusor hyperreflexia.	*Urologia Internationalis* 65(4): 190-195

TABLE G-1 Continued

Topic and Author(s)	Study Title	Journal Reference
Cheng et al. (1998)*	A therapeutic trial of acupuncture in neurogenic bladder of spinal cord injured patients: A preliminary report.	*Spinal Cord* 36(7): 476-480
Bladder-Bowel		
Abrams et al. (2003)	Tamsulosin: Efficacy and safety in patients with neurogenic lower urinary tract dysfunction due to suprasacral spinal cord injury.	*Journal of Urology* 170 (4 Pt 1): 1242-1251
Kim et al. (2003)	Intravesical resiniferatoxin for refractory detrusor hyperreflexia: A multicenter, blinded, randomized, placebo-controlled trial.	*Journal of Spinal Cord Medicine* 26(4): 358-363
Laessoe et al. (2003)*	Effects of ejaculation by penile vibratory stimulation on bladder capacity in men with spinal cord lesions.	*Journal of Urology* 169(6): 2216-2219
Lazzeri et al. (2003)	Urodynamic effects of intravesical nociceptin/ orphanin FQ in neurogenic detrusor overactivity: A randomized, placebo-controlled, double-blind study.	*Urology* 61(5): 946-950
O'Leary et al. (2003)	Effect of controlled-release oxybutynin on neurogenic bladder function in spinal cord injury.	*Journal of Spinal Cord Medicine* 26(2): 159-162
Reitz et al. (2003)	Afferent fibers of the pudendal nerve modulate sympathetic neurons controlling the bladder neck.	*Neurourology & Urodynamics* 22(6): 597-601
Schmid et al. (2003)*	Clinical value of combined electrophysiological and urodynamic recordings to assess sexual disorders in spinal cord injured men.	*Neurourology & Urodynamics* 22(4): 314-321

Continued

TABLE G-1 Continued

Topic and Author(s)	Study Title	Journal Reference
Xiao et al. (2003)	An artificial somatic-central nervous system-autonomic reflex pathway for controllable micturition after spinal cord injury: Preliminary results in 15 patients.	*Journal of Urology* 170(4 Pt 1): 1237-1241
Chartier-Kastler et al. (2002)	Intrathecal catheter with subcutaneous port for clonidine test bolus injection. A new route and type of treatment for detrusor hyperreflexia in spinal cord-injured patients.	*European Urology* 37(1): 1 4-17
Cosman et al. (2002)	Topical lidocaine does not limit autonomic dysreflexia during anorectal procedures in spinal cord injury: A prospective, double-blind study.	*International Journal of Colorectal Disease* 17(2): 104-108
Krogh et al. (2002)	Efficacy and tolerability of prucalopride in patients with constipation due to spinal cord injury.	*Scandinavian Journal of Gastroenterology* 37(4): 431-436
Rodic et al. (2002)*	Magnetic stimulation of sacral roots for assessing the efferent neuronal pathways of lower urinary tract.	*Muscle & Nerve* 26(4): 486-491
Sesay et al. (2002)*	Autonomic hyperreflexia induced by sacral root stimulation is detected by spectral analysis of the EEG.	*Canadian Journal of Anaesthesia* 49(9): 936-941
Tsai et al. (2002)	Treatment of detrusor-sphincter dyssynergia by pudendal nerve block in patients with spinal cord injury.	*Archives of Physical Medicine and Rehabilitation* 83(5): 714-717
Creasey et al. (2001)	An implantable neuro-prosthesis for restoring bladder and bowel control to patients with spinal cord injuries: A multicenter trial.	*Archives of Physical Medicine and Rehabilitation* 82(11): 1512-1519

TABLE G-1 Continued

Topic and Author(s)	Study Title	Journal Reference
Giannantoni et al. (2001)	Intermittent catheterization with a prelubricated catheter in spinal cord injured patients: A prospective randomized crossover study.	*Journal of Urology* 166(1): 130-133
Hohenfellner et al. (2001)	Sacral bladder denervation for treatment of detrusor hyperreflexia and autonomic dysreflexia.	*Urology* 58(1): 28-32
Kirkham et al. (2001)	The acute effects of continuous and conditional neuromodulation on the bladder in spinal cord injury.	*Spinal Cord* 39(8): 420-428
Reid et al. (2001)	Cranberry juice consumption may reduce biofilms on uroepithelial cells: Pilot study in spinal cord injured patients.	*Spinal Cord* 39(1): 26-30
Chen et al. (2000)	Current trend and risk factors for kidney stones in persons with spinal cord injury: A longitudinal study.	*Spinal Cord* 38(6): 346-353
Christensen et al. (2000)	Neurogenic colorectal dysfunction—use of new antegrade and retrograde colonic wash-out methods.	*Spinal Cord* 38(4): 255-261
Haferkamp et al. (2000)	Dosage escalation of intravesical oxybutynin in the treatment of neurogenic bladder patients.	*Spinal Cord* 38(4): 250-254
Honjo et al. (2000)*	Acupuncture on clinical symptoms and urodynamic measurements in spinal-cord-injured patients with detrusor hyperreflexia.	*Urologia Internationalis* 65(4): 190-195
Hull et al. (2000)	Urinary tract infection prophylaxis using *Escherichia coli* 83972 in spinal cord injured patients.	*Journal of Urology* 163(3): 872-877

Continued

TABLE G-1 Continued

Topic and Author(s)	Study Title	Journal Reference
Kao et al. (2000)	Using technetium-99M dimercaptosuccinic acid renal cortex scintigraphy to differentiate acute pyelonephritis from other causes of fever in patients with spinal cord injury.	*Urology* 55(5): 658-662
Pannek et al. (2000)	Combined intravesical and oral oxybutynin chloride in adult patients with spinal cord injury.	*Urology* 55(3): 358-362
Reid et al. (2000)	Ofloxacin for the treatment of urinary tract infections and biofilms in spinal cord injury.	*International Journal of Antimicrobial Agents* 13(4): 305-307
Sakakibara et al. (2000)	Pressure-flow study as an evaluating method of neurogenic urethral relaxation failure.	*Journal of the Autonomic Nervous System* 80(1-2): 85-88
Biering-Sorensen et al. (1999)	Urethral epithelial cells on the surface on hydrophilic catheters after intermittent catheterization: Cross-over study with two catheters.	*Spinal Cord* 37(4): 299-300
Chancellor et al. (1999)	Sphincteric stent versus external sphincterotomy in spinal cord injured men: Prospective randomized multicenter trial.	*Journal of Urology* 161(6): 1893-1898
Chancellor et al. (1999)	Long-term follow-up of the North American multicenter UroLume trial for the treatment of external detrusor-sphincter dyssynergia.	*Journal of Urology* 161(5): 1545-1550
Chiou-Tan et al. (1999)	Increased norepinephrine levels during catheterization in patients with spinal cord injury.	*American Journal of Physical Medicine & Rehabilitation* 78(4): 350-353
Juan Garcia et al. (1999)	Intraurethral stent prosthesis in spinal cord injured patients with sphincter dyssynergia.	*Spinal Cord* 37(1): 54-57

TABLE G-1 Continued

Topic and Author(s)	Study Title	Journal Reference
Michielsen et al. (1999)	Management of false passages in patients practicing clean intermittent self catheterization.	*Spinal Cord* 37(3): 201-203
Plancke et al. (1999)	Indiana pouch in female patients with spinal cord injury.	*Spinal Cord* 37(3): 208-210
Stohrer et al. (1999)	Efficacy and safety of propiverine in SCI-patients suffering from detrusor hyperreflexia—a double-blind, placebo-controlled clinical trial.	*Spinal Cord* 37(3): 196-200
Virseda Chamorro et al. (1999)	Evidence-based medicine. Usefulness of isolated cystomanometry for the diagnosis of periurethral detrusor-sphincter dyssynergia in patients with suprasacral lesion.	*Archivos Espanoles de Urologia* 52(10): 1073-1078
Walter et al. (1999)	Bioavailability of trospium chloride after intravesical instillation in patients with neurogenic lower urinary tract dysfunction: A pilot study.	*Neurourology & Urodynamics* 18(5): 447-453
Cheng et al. (1998)*	A therapeutic trial of acupuncture in neurogenic bladder of spinal cord injured patients—A preliminary report.	*Spinal Cord* 36(7): 476-480
Dasgupta et al. (1998)	Treating the human bladder with capsaicin: Is it safe?	*European Urology* 33(1): 28-31
De Looze et al. (1998)	Constipation and other chronic gastrointestinal problems in spinal cord injury patients.	*Spinal Cord* 36(1): 63-66
Denys et al. (1998)	Intrathecal clonidine for refractory detrusor hyperreflexia in spinal cord injured patients: A preliminary report.	*Journal of Urology* 160(6 Pt 1): 2137-2138

Continued

TABLE G-1 Continued

Topic and Author(s)	Study Title	Journal Reference
de Seze et al. (1998)	Capsaicin and neurogenic detrusor hyperreflexia: A double-blind placebo-controlled study in 20 patients with spinal cord lesions.	*Neurourology & Urodynamics* 17(5): 513-523
Everaert et al. (1998)	Diagnosis and localization of a complicated urinary tract infection in neurogenic bladder disease by tubular proteinuria and serum prostate specific antigen.	*Spinal Cord* 36(1): 33-38
Giannantoni et al. (1998)	Clean intermittent catheterization and prevention of renal disease in spinal cord injury patients.	*Spinal Cord* 36(1): 29-32
Hamamci et al. (1998)	A quantitative study of genital skin flora and urinary colonization in spinal cord injured patients.	*Spinal Cord* 36(9): 617-620
Horton et al. (1998)	Does refrigeration of urine alter culture results in hospitalized patients with neurogenic bladders?	*Journal of Spinal Cord Medicine* 21(4): 342-347
Kajio et al. (1998)	Clinical features of transurethral anterior sphincterotomy and urological management of patients with cervical spinal cord injury.	*Nippon Hinyokika Gakkai Zasshi (Japanese Journal of Urology)* 89(11): 885-893
Low et al. (1998)	Use of the Memokath for detrusor-sphincter dyssynergia after spinal cord injury: A cautionary tale.	*Spinal Cord* 36(1): 39-44
Moser et al. (1998)	Antibodies to urinary tract pathogens in patients with spinal cord lesions.	*Spinal Cord* 36(9): 613-616
Previnaire et al. (1998)	Is there a place for pudendal nerve maximal electrical stimulation for the treatment of detrusor hyperreflexia in spinal cord injury patients?	*Spinal Cord* 36(2): 100-103

TABLE G-1 Continued

Topic and Author(s)	Study Title	Journal Reference
Stiens et al. (1998)	Polyethylene glycol versus vegetable oil based bisacodyl suppositories to initiate side-lying bowel care: A clinical trial in persons with spinal cord injury.	*Spinal Cord* 36(11): 777-781
Sutton et al. (1998)	Continent ileocecal augmentation cystoplasty.	*Spinal Cord* 36(4): 246-251
Vaidyananthan et al. (1998)	Effect of intermittent urethral catheterization and oxybutynin bladder instillation on urinary continence status and quality of life in a selected group of spinal cord injury patients with neuropathic bladder dysfunction.	*Spinal Cord* 36(6): 409-414
Bone Density		
Jones et al. (2002)*	Intensive exercise may preserve bone mass of the upper limbs in spinal cord injured males but does not retard demineralisation of the lower body.	*Spinal Cord* 40(5): 230-235
Banovac et al. (2001)	Prevention of heterotopic ossification after spinal cord injury with indomethacin.	*Spinal Cord* 39(7): 370-374
Warden et al. (2001)	Efficacy of low-intensity pulsed ultrasound in the prevention of osteoporosis following spinal cord injury.	*Bone* 29(5): 431-436
de Bruin et al. (2000)	Estimation of geometric properties of cortical bone in spinal cord injury.	*Archives of Physical Medicine and Rehabilitation* 81(2): 150-156
Kiratli et al. (2000)	Bone mineral and geometric changes through the femur with immobilization due to spinal cord injury.	*Journal of Rehabilitation Research & Development* 37(2): 225-233

Continued

TABLE G-1 Continued

Topic and Author(s)	Study Title	Journal Reference
Liu et al. (2000)*	Quantitative computed tomography in the evaluation of spinal osteoporosis following spinal cord injury.	*Osteoporosis International* 11(10): 889-896
Sautter-Bihl et al. (2000)	Radiotherapy as a local treatment option for heterotopic ossifications in patients with spinal cord injury.	*Spinal Cord* 38(1): 33-36
Middleton et al. (1999)*	Postural control during stance in paraplegia: Effects of medially linked versus unlinked knee-ankle-foot orthoses.	*Archives of Physical Medicine and Rehabilitation* 80(12): 1558-1565
Nance et al. (1999)	Intravenous pamidronate attenuates bone density loss after acute spinal cord injury.	*Archives of Physical Medicine and Rehabilitation* 80(3): 243-251
Jaovisidha et al. (1998)	Influence of heterotopic ossification of the hip on bone densitometry: A study in spinal cord injured patients.	*Spinal Cord* 36(9): 647-653
Low et al. (1998)	Bone mineral status after pediatric spinal cord injury.	*Spinal Cord* 36(9): 641-646
Wing et al. (1998)	Risk of avascular necrosis following short term megadose methylpred-nisolone treatment.	*Spinal Cord* 36(9): 633-636
Cardiovascular		
Chiou-Tan et al. (2003)	Comparison of dalteparin and enoxaparin for deep venous thrombosis prophylaxis in patients with spinal cord injury.	*American Journal of Physical Medicine & Rehabilitation* 82(9): 678-685
Ethans et al. (2003)*	The effects of sildenafil on the cardiovascular response in men with spinal cord injury at or above the sixth thoracic level.	*Journal of Spinal Cord Medicine* 26(3): 222-226

TABLE G-1 Continued

Topic and Author(s)	Study Title	Journal Reference
Spinal Cord Injury Thromboprophylaxis Investigators (2003)	Prevention of venous thromboembolism in the rehabilitation phase after spinal cord injury: Prophylaxis with low-dose heparin or enoxaparin.	*Journal of Trauma: Injury Infection & Critical Care* 54(6): 1111-1115
Spinal Cord Injury Thromboprophylaxis Investigators (2003)*	Prevention of venous thromboembolism in the acute treatment phase after spinal cord injury: A randomized, multicenter trial comparing low-dose heparin plus intermittent pneumatic compression with enoxaparin.	*Journal of Trauma: Injury Infection & Critical Care* 54(6): 1116-1124
Wakana et al. (2003)	Effects of 4-aminopyridine on cardiac repolarization, PR interval, and heart rate in patients with spinal cord injury.	*Pharmacotherapy* 23(2): 133-136
Yoo et al. (2003)	Cardiovascular responses to endotracheal intubation in patients with acute and chronic spinal cord injuries.	*Anesthesia & Analgesia* 97(4): 1162-1167
Gates et al. (2002)*	Absence of training-specific cardiac adaptation in paraplegic athletes.	*Medicine & Science in Sports & Exercise* 34(11): 1699-1704
Sesay et al. (2002)*	Autonomic hyperreflexia induced by sacral root stimulation is detected by spectral analysis of the EEG.	*Canadian Journal of Anaesthesia* 49(9):936-941
Cooke et al. (2001)	Cardiovascular effects of vasopressin following V(1) receptor blockade compared to effects of nitroglycerin.	*American Journal of Physiology—Regulatory Integrative & Comparative Physiology* 281(3): R887-893
Gerrits et al. (2001)*	Peripheral vascular changes after electrically stimulated cycle training in people with spinal cord injury.	*Archives of Physical Medicine and Rehabilitation* 82(6): 832-839

Continued

TABLE G-1 Continued

Topic and Author(s)	Study Title	Journal Reference
Houtman et al. (2001)	Changes in cerebral oxygenation and blood flow during LBNP in spinal cord-injured individuals.	*Journal of Applied Physiology* 91(5): 2199-2204
Legramante et al. (2001)*	Positive and negative feedback mechanisms in the neural regulation of cardiovascular function in healthy and spinal cord-injured humans.	*Circulation* 103(9): 1250-1255
Lohmann et al. (2001)	Prevention of thrombo-embolism in spinal fractures with spinal cord injuries. Standard heparin versus low-molecular-weight heparin in acute paraplegia.	*Zentralblatt für Chirurgie* 126(5): 385-390
Tsuji et al. (2001)*	Evaluation of spinal cord blood flow during prostaglandin E1-induced hypotension with power Doppler ultrasonography.	*Spinal Cord* 39(1): 31-36
Averill et al. (2000)*	Blood pressure response to acupuncture in a population at risk for autonomic dysreflexia.	*Archives of Physical Medicine and Rehabilitation* 81(11): 1494-1497
Sipski et al. (2000)*	Sildenafil effects on sexual and cardiovascular responses in women with spinal cord injury.	*Urology* 55(6): 812-815
Yamasaki et al. (2000)	Effect of acute heat exposure on skin blood flow of the paralyzed thigh in persons with spinal cord injury.	*Spinal Cord* 38(4): 224-228
Kjaer et al. (1999)*	Heart rate during exercise with leg vascular occlusion in spinal cord-injured humans.	*Journal of Applied Physiology* 86(3): 806-811
Roussi et al. (1999)	Contribution of D-dimer determination in the exclusion of deep venous thrombosis in spinal cord injury patients.	*Spinal Cord* 37(8): 548-552

TABLE G-1 Continued

Topic and Author(s)	Study Title	Journal Reference
Hopman et al. (1998)*	Blood redistribution and circulatory responses to submaximal arm exercise in persons with spinal cord injury.	*Scandinavian Journal of Rehabilitation Medicine* 30(3): 167-174
Pruitt et al. (1998)*	Health behavior in persons with spinal cord injury: Development and initial validation of an outcome measure.	*Spinal Cord* 36(10): 724-731
Schmid et al. (1998)*	Physical performance and cardiovascular and metabolic adaptation of elite female wheelchair basketball players in wheelchair ergometry and in competition.	*American Journal of Physical Medicine & Rehabilitation* 77(6): 527-533
Cough		
Lin et al. (1999)	Cough threshold in people with spinal cord injuries.	*Physical Therapy* 79(11): 1026-1031
Lin et al. (1998)*	Effects of an abdominal binder and electrical stimulation on cough in patients with spinal cord injury.	*Journal of the Formosan Medical Association* 97(4): 292-295
Lin et al. (1998)*	Functional magnetic stimulation for restoring cough in patients with tetraplegia.	*Archives of Physical Medicine and Rehabilitation* 79(5): 517-522
Exercise and Locomotion		
Eser et al. (2003)*	Influence of different stimulation frequencies on power output and fatigue during FES-cycling in recently injured SCI people.	*IEEE Transactions on Neural Systems & Rehabilitation Engineering* 11(3): 236-240
Gagnon et al. (2003)*	Biomechanical analysis of a posterior transfer maneuver on a level surface in individuals with high and low-level spinal cord injuries.	*Clinical Biomechanics* 18(4): 319-331

Continued

TABLE G-1 Continued

Topic and Author(s)	Study Title	Journal Reference
Goldfarb et al. (2003)*	Preliminary evaluation of a controlled-brake orthosis for FES-aided gait.	*IEEE Transactions on Neural Systems & Rehabilitation Engineering* 11(3): 241-248
Harvey et al. (2003)	Randomised trial of the effects of four weeks of daily stretch on extensibility of hamstring muscles in people with spinal cord injuries.	*Australian Journal of Physiotherapy* 49(3): 176-181
Hicks et al. (2003)*	Long-term exercise training in persons with spinal cord injury: Effects on strength, arm ergometry performance and psychological well-being.	*Spinal Cord* 41(1): 34-43
Schalow et al. (2003)	High-load coordination dynamics in athletes, physiotherapists, gymnasts, musicians and patients with CNS injury.	*Electromyography & Clinical Neurophysiology* 43(6): 353-365
Scivoletto et al. (2003)	A prototype of an adjustable advanced reciprocating gait orthosis (ARGO) for spinal cord injury (SCI).	*Spinal Cord* 41(3): 187-191
Stein et al. (2003)*	A wheelchair modified for leg propulsion using voluntary activity or electrical stimulation.	*Medical Engineering & Physics* 25(1): 11-19
Davoodi et al. (2002)*	Development of an indoor rowing machine with manual FES controller for total body exercise in paraplegia.	*IEEE Transactions on Neural Systems & Rehabilitation Engineering* 10(3): 197-203
Gates et al. (2002)*	Absence of training-specific cardiac adaptation in paraplegic athletes.	*Medicine & Science in Sports & Exercise* 34(11): 1699-1704
Gerasimenko et al. (2002)	Control of locomotor activity in humans and animals in the absence of supraspinal influences.	*Neuroscience & Behavioral Physiology* 32(4): 417-423

TABLE G-1 Continued

Topic and Author(s)	Study Title	Journal Reference
Jones et al. (2002)*	Intensive exercise may preserve bone mass of the upper limbs in spinal cord injured males but does not retard demineralisation of the lower body.	*Spinal Cord* 40(5): 230-235
Kilkens et al. (2002)*	The wheelchair circuit: Reliability of a test to assess mobility in persons with spinal cord injuries.	*Archives of Physical Medicine and Rehabilitation* 83(12): 1783-1788
Knikou et al. (2002)*	Hip angle induced modulation of H reflex amplitude, latency and duration in spinal cord injured humans.	*Clinical Neurophysiology* 113(11): 1698-1708
Mirbagheri et al. (2002)*	The effects of long-term FES-assisted walking on intrinsic and reflex dynamic stiffness in spastic spinal-cord-injured subjects.	*IEEE Transactions on Neural Systems & Rehabilitation Engineering* 10(4): 280-289
Reft et al. (2002)	Trajectories of target reaching arm movements in individuals with spinal cord injury: Effect of external trunk support.	*Spinal Cord* 40(4): 186-191
Cooper et al. (2001)	Evaluation of a pushrim-activated, power-assisted wheelchair.	*Archives of Physical Medicine and Rehabilitation* 82(5): 702-708
Cooper et al. (2001)*	Physiological responses to two wheelchair-racing exercise protocols.	*Neurorehabilitation & Neural Repair* 15(3): 191-195
Field-Fote (2001)*	Combined use of body weight support, functional electric stimulation, and treadmill training to improve walking ability in individuals with chronic incomplete spinal cord injury.	*Archives of Physical Medicine and Rehabilitation* 82(6): 818-824
Gerrits et al. (2001)*	Peripheral vascular changes after electrically stimulated cycle training in people with spinal cord injury.	*Archives of Physical Medicine and Rehabilitation* 82(6): 832-839

TABLE G-1 Continued

Topic and Author(s)	Study Title	Journal Reference
Gharooni et al. (2001)	A new hybrid spring brake orthosis for controlling hip and knee flexion in the swing phase.	*IEEE Transactions on Neural Systems & Rehabilitation Engineering* 9(1): 106-107
Mohr et al. (2001)*	Insulin action and long-term electrically induced training in individuals with spinal cord injuries.	*Medicine & Science in Sports & Exercise* 33(8): 1247-1252
Protas et al. (2001)	Supported treadmill ambulation training after spinal cord injury: A pilot study.	*Archives of Physical Medicine and Rehabilitation* 82(6): 825-831
Rodgers et al. (2001)	Influence of training on biomechanics of wheelchair propulsion.	*Journal of Rehabilitation Research & Development* 38(5): 505-511
Seelen et al. (2001)*	Motor preparation in postural control in seated spinal cord injured people.	*Ergonomics* 44(4): 457-472
Brissot et al. (2000)*	Clinical experience with functional electrical stimulation-assisted gait with Parastep in spinal cord-injured patients.	*Spine* 25(4): 501-508
Ditunno et al. (2000)*	Walking index for spinal cord injury (WISCI): An international multicenter validity and reliability study.	*Spinal Cord* 38(4): 234-243
Gerrits et al. (2000)*	Altered contractile properties of the quadriceps muscle in people with spinal cord injury following functional electrical stimulated cycle training.	*Spinal Cord* 38(4): 214-223
Harvey et al. (2000)	A randomized trial assessing the effects of 4 weeks of daily stretching on ankle mobility in patients with spinal cord injuries.	*Archives of Physical Medicine and Rehabilitation* 81(10): 1340-1347

TABLE G-1 Continued

Topic and Author(s)	Study Title	Journal Reference
Petrofsky et al. (2000)*	The relationship between exercise work intervals and duration of exercise on lower extremity training induced by electrical stimulation in humans with spinal cord injuries.	*European Journal of Applied Physiology* 82(5-6): 504-509
Rodgers et al. (2000)	Influence of trunk flexion on biomechanics of wheelchair propulsion.	*Journal of Rehabilitation Research & Development* 37(3): 283-295
Beekman et al. (1999)	Energy cost of propulsion in standard and ultralight wheelchairs in people with spinal cord injuries.	*Physical Therapy* 79(2): 146-158
Chilibeck et al. (1999)*	Histochemical changes in muscle of individuals with spinal cord injury following functional electrical stimulated exercise training.	*Spinal Cord* 37(4): 264-268
Curtis et al. (1999)*	Effect of a standard exercise protocol on shoulder pain in long-term wheelchair users.	*Spinal Cord* 37(6): 421-429
Houtman et al. (1999)	Effect of a pulsating anti-gravity suit on peak exercise performance in individual with spinal cord injuries.	*European Journal of Applied Physiology & Occupational Physiology* 79(2): 202-204
Kamper et al. (1999)	Preliminary investigation of the lateral postural stability of spinal cord-injured individuals subjected to dynamic perturbations.	*Spinal Cord* 37(1): 40-46
Kjaer et al. (1999)*	Heart rate during exercise with leg vascular occlusion in spinal cord-injured humans.	*Journal of Applied Physiology* 86(3): 806-811
Lajoie et al. (1999)	Attentional requirements of walking in spinal cord injured patients compared to normal subjects.	*Spinal Cord* 37(4): 245-250

Continued

TABLE G-1 Continued

Topic and Author(s)	Study Title	Journal Reference
Middleton et al. (1999)*	Postural control during stance in paraplegia: Effects of medially linked versus unlinked knee-ankle-foot orthoses.	*Archives of Physical Medicine and Rehabilitation* 80(12): 1558-1565
Newsam et al. (1999)	Three-dimensional upper extremity motion during manual wheelchair propulsion in men with different levels of spinal cord injury.	*Gait & Posture* 10(3): 223-232.
Sarver et al. (1999)	A study of shoulder motions as a control source for adolescents with C4 level SCI.	*IEEE Transactions on Rehabilitation Engineering* 7(1): 27-34
Hopman et al. (1998)*	Blood redistribution and circulatory responses to submaximal arm exercise in persons with spinal cord injury.	*Scandinavian Journal of Rehabilitation Medicine* 30(3): 167-174
Klokker et al. (1998)*	The natural killer cell response to exercise in spinal cord injured individuals.	*European Journal of Applied Physiology & Occupational Physiology* 79(1): 106-109
Lamontagne et al. (1998)*	Evaluation of reflex- and nonreflex-induced muscle resistance to stretch in adults with spinal cord injury using hand-held and isokinetic dynamometry.	*Physical Therapy* 78(9): 964-975
Norman et al. (1998)	Effects of drugs on walking after spinal cord injury.	*Spinal Cord* 36(10): 699-715
Schmid et al. (1998)	Catecholamines, heart rate, and oxygen uptake during exercise in persons with spinal cord injury.	*Journal of Applied Physiology* 85(2): 635-641
Schmid et al. (1998)*	Physical performance and cardiovascular and metabolic adaptation of elite female wheelchair basketball players in wheelchair ergometry and in competition.	*American Journal of Physical Medicine & Rehabilitation* 77(6): 527-533

TABLE G-1 Continued

Topic and Author(s)	Study Title	Journal Reference
Segal et al. (1998)	4-Aminopyridine alters gait characteristics and enhances locomotion in spinal cord injured humans.	*Journal of Spinal Cord Medicine* 21(3): 200-204
Silva et al. (1998)*	Effect of aerobic training on ventilatory muscle endurance of spinal cord injured men.	*Spinal Cord* 36(4): 240-245

Functional Electrical Stimulation and Functional Magnetic Stimulation

Capel et al. (2003)	The amelioration of the suffering associated with spinal cord injury with subperception transcranial electrical stimulation.	*Spinal Cord* 41(2): 109-117
Eser et al. (2003)*	Influence of different stimulation frequencies on power output and fatigue during FES-cycling in recently injured SCI people.	*IEEE Transactions on Neural Systems & Rehabilitation Engineering* 11(3): 236-240
Goldfarb et al. (2003)*	Preliminary evaluation of a controlled-brake orthosis for FES-aided gait.	*IEEE Transactions on Neural Systems & Rehabilitation Engineering* 11(3): 241-248
Stein et al. (2003)*	A wheelchair modified for leg propulsion using voluntary activity or electrical stimulation.	*Medical Engineering & Physics* 25(1): 11-19
Birch et al. (2002)	Initial on-line evaluations of the LF-ASD brain-computer interface with able-bodied and spinal-cord subjects using imagined voluntary motor potentials.	*IEEE Transactions on Neural Systems & Rehabilitation Engineering* 10(4): 219-222
Craig et al. (2002)	The effectiveness of a hands-free environmental control system for the profoundly disabled.	*Archives of Physical Medicine and Rehabilitation* 83(10): 1455-1458
Davoodi et al. (2002)*	Development of an indoor rowing machine with manual FES controller for total body exercise in paraplegia.	*IEEE Transactions on Neural Systems & Rehabilitation Engineering* 10(3): 197-203

Continued

TABLE G-1 Continued

Topic and Author(s)	Study Title	Journal Reference
Ioannides et al. (2002)	Brain activation sequences following electrical limb stimulation of normal and paraplegic subjects.	*Neuroimage* 16(1): 115-129
Lin et al. (2002)	Functional magnetic stimulation facilitates gastric emptying.	*Archives of Physical Medicine and Rehabilitation* 83(6): 806-810
Mirbagheri et al. (2002)*	The effects of long-term FES-assisted walking on intrinsic and reflex dynamic stiffness in spastic spinal-cord-injured subjects.	*IEEE Transactions on Neural Systems & Rehabilitation Engineering* 10(4): 280-289
Rodic et al. (2002)*	Magnetic stimulation of sacral roots for assessing the efferent neuronal pathways of lower urinary tract.	*Muscle & Nerve* 26(4): 486-491
Taylor et al. (2002)	The functional impact of the Freehand System on tetraplegic hand function. Clinical results.	*Spinal Cord* 40(11): 560-566
Field-Fote (2001)*	Combined use of body weight support, functional electric stimulation, and treadmill training to improve walking ability in individuals with chronic incomplete spinal cord injury.	*Archives of Physical Medicine and Rehabilitation* 82(6): 818-824
Mela et al. (2001)	Excessive reflexes in spinal cord injury triggered by electrical stimulation.	*Archives of Physiology & Biochemistry* 109(4): 309-315
Misawa et al. (2001)*	The effects of therapeutic electric stimulation on acute muscle atrophy in rats after spinal cord injury.	*Archives of Physical Medicine and Rehabilitation* 82(11): 1596-1603
Mohr et al. (2001)*	Insulin action and long-term electrically induced training in individuals with spinal cord injuries.	*Medicine & Science in Sports & Exercise* 33(8): 1247-1252

TABLE G-1 Continued

Topic and Author(s)	Study Title	Journal Reference
Petrofsky (2001)*	The use of electromyogram biofeedback to reduce Trendelenburg gait.	*European Journal of Applied Physiology* 85(5): 491-495
Brissot et al. (2000)*	Clinical experience with functional electrical stimulation-assisted gait with Parastep in spinal cord-injured patients.	*Spine* 25(4): 501-508
Crameri et al. (2000)	Effects of electrical stimulation leg training during the acute phase of spinal cord injury: A pilot study.	*European Journal of Applied Physiology* 83(4-5): 409-415
Gerrits et al. (2000)*	Altered contractile properties of the quadriceps muscle in people with spinal cord injury following functional electrical stimulated cycle training.	*Spinal Cord* 38(4): 214-223
Petrofsky et al. (2000)*	The relationship between exercise work intervals and duration of exercise on lower extremity training induced by electrical stimulation in humans with spinal cord injuries.	*European Journal of Applied Physiology* 82(5-6): 504-509
Riess et al. (2000)	Adaptive neural network control of cyclic movements using functional neuromuscular stimulation.	*IEEE Transactions on Rehabilitation Engineering* 8(1): 42-52
Sampson et al. (2000)	Functional electrical stimulation effect on orthostatic hypotension after spinal cord injury.	*Archives of Physical Medicine and Rehabilitation* 81(2): 139-143
van Beekvelt et al. (2000)	The effect of electrical stimulation on leg muscle pump activity in spinal cord-injured and able-bodied individuals.	*European Journal of Applied Physiology* 82(5-6): 510-516

Continued

TABLE G-1 Continued

Topic and Author(s)	Study Title	Journal Reference
Borgens et al. (1999)	An imposed oscillating electrical field improves the recovery of function in neurologically complete paraplegic dogs.	*Journal of Neurotrauma* 16(7): 639-657
Chilibeck et al. (1999)*	Histochemical changes in muscle of individuals with spinal cord injury following functional electrical stimulated exercise training.	*Spinal Cord* 37(4): 264-268
Hillegass et al. (1999)*	Surface electrical stimulation of skeletal muscle after spinal cord injury.	*Spinal Cord* 37(4): 251-257
Murphy et al. (1999)	Salbutamol effect in spinal cord injured individuals undergoing functional electrical stimulation training.	*Archives of Physical Medicine and Rehabilitation* 80(10): 1264-1267
Baldi et al. (1998)*	Muscle atrophy is prevented in patients with acute spinal cord injury using functional electrical stimulation.	*Spinal Cord* 36(7): 463-469
Byers et al. (1998)*	An electromechanical testing device for assessment of hand motor function.	*IEEE Transactions on Rehabilitation Engineering* 6(1): 88-94
Lin et al. (1998)*	Functional magnetic stimulation for restoring cough in patients with tetraplegia.	*Archives of Physical Medicine and Rehabilitation* 79(5): 517-522
Lin et al. (1998)*	Effects of an abdominal binder and electrical stimulation on cough in patients with spinal cord injury.	*Journal of the Formosan Medical Association* 97(4): 292-295

Imaging

Epstein et al. (2003)*	Documenting fusion following anterior cervical surgery: A comparison of roentgenogram versus two-dimensional computed tomographic findings.	*Journal of Spinal Disorders & Techniques* 16(3): 243-247

TABLE G-1 Continued

Topic and Author(s)	Study Title	Journal Reference
Tsuji et al. (2001)*	Evaluation of spinal cord blood flow during prostaglandin E1-induced hypotension with power Doppler ultrasonography.	*Spinal Cord* 39(1): 31-36
Liu et al. (2000)*	Quantitative computed tomography in the evaluation of spinal osteoporosis following spinal cord injury.	*Osteoporosis International* 11(10): 889-896
Brugieres et al. (1999)*	Dynamic MRI in the evaluation of syringomyelic cysts.	*Neuro-Chirurgie* 45(Suppl 1): 115-129
Selden et al. (1999)*	Emergency magnetic resonance imaging of cervical spinal cord injuries: Clinical correlation and prognosis.	*Neurosurgery* 44(4): 785-792
Shepard et al. (1999)*	Magnetic resonance imaging and neurological recovery in acute spinal cord injury: Observations from the National Acute Spinal Cord Injury Study 3.	*Spinal Cord* 37(12): 833-837
Splavski et al. (1998)	Computed tomography of the spine as an important diagnostic tool in the management of war missile spinal trauma.	*Archives of Orthopaedic & Trauma Surgery* 117(6-7): 360-363
Immunology		
Edwards et al. (2001)	Modified cotton gauze dressings that selectively absorb neutrophil elastase activity in solution.	*Wound Repair & Regeneration* 9(1): 50-58
Ersoz et al. (1999)	Platelet aggregation in traumatic spinal cord injury.	*Spinal Cord* 37(9): 644-647
Klokker et al. (1998)*	The natural killer cell response to exercise in spinal cord injured individuals.	*European Journal of Applied Physiology & Occupational Physiology* 79(1): 106-109
Waites et al. (1998)	Immunogenicity of pneumococcal vaccine in persons with spinal cord injury.	*Archives of Physical Medicine and Rehabilitation* 79(12): 1504-1509

Continued

TABLE G-1 Continued

Topic and Author(s)	Study Title	Journal Reference
Mental Health, Behavior, and Patient Well-Being		
Hicks et al. (2003)*	Long-term exercise training in persons with spinal cord injury: Effects on strength, arm ergometry performance and psychological well-being.	*Spinal Cord* 41(1): 34-43
Kennedy et al. (2003)	Coping effectiveness training reduces depression and anxiety following traumatic spinal cord injuries.	*British Journal of Clinical Psychology* 42(Pt 1): 41-52
Alexander et al. (2002)	Mothers with spinal cord injuries: Impact on marital, family, and children's adjustment.	*Archives of Physical Medicine and Rehabilitation* 83(1): 24-30
Phillips et al. (2001)	Telehealth: Reaching out to newly injured spinal cord patients.	*Public Health Reports* 116(Suppl 1): 94-102
Unalan et al. (2001)	Quality of life of primary caregivers of spinal cord injury survivors living in the community: Controlled study with short form-36 questionnaire.	*Spinal Cord* 39(6): 318-322
Hultling et al. (2000)*	Quality of life in patients with spinal cord injury receiving Viagra (sildenafil citrate) for the treatment of erectile dysfunction.	*Spinal Cord* 38(6): 363-370
Kreuter et al. (1998)	Partner relationships, functioning, mood and global quality of life in persons with spinal cord injury and traumatic brain injury.	*Spinal Cord* 36(4): 252-261
Potter et al. (1998)*	Randomized double-blind crossover trial of Fampridine-SR (sustained release 4-aminopyridine) in patients with incomplete spinal cord injury.	*Journal of Neurotrauma* 15(10): 837-849

TABLE G-1 Continued

Topic and Author(s)	Study Title	Journal Reference
Radnitz et al. (1998)	A comparison of post-traumatic stress disorder in veterans with and without spinal cord injury.	*Journal of Abnormal Psychology* 107(4): 676-680
Muscle and Spasticity		
Gagnon et al. (2003)*	Biomechanical analysis of a posterior transfer maneuver on a level surface in individuals with high and low-level spinal cord injuries.	*Clinical Biomechanics* 18(4): 319-331
Gregory et al. (2003)	Effects of testosterone replacement therapy on skeletal muscle after spinal cord injury.	*Spinal Cord* 41(1): 23-28
Grijalva et al. (2003)	Efficacy and safety of 4-aminopyridine in patients with long-term spinal cord injury: A randomized, double-blind, placebo-controlled trial.	*Pharmacotherapy* 23(7): 823-834
Hayes et al. (2003)	Pharmacokinetics of an immediate-release oral formulation of Fampridine (4-aminopyridine) in normal subjects and patients with spinal cord injury.	*Journal of Clinical Pharmacology* 43(4): 379-385
Hicks et al. (2003)*	Long-term exercise training in persons with spinal cord injury: effects on strength, arm ergometry performance and psychological well-being.	*Spinal Cord* 41(1): 34-43
Faghri et al. (2002)	Electrically induced and voluntary activation of physiologic muscle pump: A comparison between spinal cord-injured and able-bodied individuals.	*Clinical Rehabilitation* 16(8): 878-885
Godfrey et al. (2002)*	Differential fatigue of paralyzed thenar muscles by stimuli of different intensities.	*Muscle & Nerve* 26(1): 122-131

Continued

TABLE G-1 Continued

Topic and Author(s)	Study Title	Journal Reference
Hidler et al. (2002)	Frequency response characteristics of ankle plantar flexors in humans following spinal cord injury: Relation to degree of spasticity.	*Annals of Biomedical Engineering* 30(7): 969-981
Jacobs et al. (2002)	Oral creatine supplementation enhances upper extremity work capacity in persons with cervical-level spinal cord injury.	*Archives of Physical Medicine and Rehabilitation* 83(1): 19-23
Kakebeeke et al. (2002)	The importance of posture on the isokinetic assessment of spasticity.	*Spinal Cord* 40(5): 236-243
Raynor et al. (2002)	Can triggered electromyograph thresholds predict safe thoracic pedicle screw placement?	*Spine* 27(18): 2030-2035
Thomas et al. (2002)	Motor unit activation order during electrically evoked contractions of paralyzed or partially paralyzed muscles.	*Muscle & Nerve* 25(6): 797-804
Burns et al. (2001)	Intrathecal baclofen in tetraplegia of spinal origin: Efficacy for upper extremity hypertonia.	*Spinal Cord* 39(8): 413-419
Misawa et al. (2001)*	The effects of therapeutic electric stimulation on acute muscle atrophy in rats after spinal cord injury.	*Archives of Physical Medicine and Rehabilitation* 82(11): 1596-1603
Petrofsky (2001)*	The use of electromyogram biofeedback to reduce Trendelenburg gait.	*European Journal of Applied Physiology* 85(5): 491-495
Seelen et al. (2001)*	Motor preparation in postural control in seated spinal cord injured people.	*Ergonomics* 44(4): 457-472
van der Bruggen et al. (2001)	Randomized trial of 4-aminopyridine in patients with chronic incomplete spinal cord injury.	*Journal of Neurology* 248(8): 665-671

TABLE G-1 Continued

Topic and Author(s)	Study Title	Journal Reference
Wolfe et al. (2001)	Effects of 4-aminopyridine on motor evoked potentials in patients with spinal cord injury: A double-blinded, placebo-controlled crossover trial.	*Journal of Neurotrauma* 18(8): 757-771
Castro et al. (2000)	Muscle fiber type-specific myofibrillar Ca^{2+} ATPase activity after spinal cord injury.	*Muscle & Nerve* 23(1): 119-121
Donovan et al. (2000)*	Intravenous infusion of 4-AP in chronic spinal cord injured subjects.	*Spinal Cord* 38(1): 7-15
Elokda et al. (2000)	Effect of functional neuromuscular stimulation on postural related orthostatic stress in individuals with acute spinal cord injury.	*Journal of Rehabilitation Research & Development* 37(5): 535-542
Gerrits et al. (2000)*	Altered contractile properties of the quadriceps muscle in people with spinal cord injury following functional electrical stimulated cycle training.	*Spinal Cord* 38(4): 214-223
Halter et al. (2000)	Intrathecal administration of 4-aminopyridine in chronic spinal injured patients.	*Spinal Cord* 38(12): 728-732
Hiersemenzel et al. (2000)*	From spinal shock to spasticity: Neuronal adaptations to a spinal cord injury.	*Neurology* 54(8): 1574-1582
Segal et al. (2000)	Absorption characteristics of sustained-release 4-aminopyridine (Fampridine SR) in patients with chronic spinal cord injury.	*Journal of Clinical Pharmacology* 40(4): 402-409
Sherwood et al. (2000)	Altered motor control and spasticity after spinal cord injury: Subjective and objective assessment.	*Journal of Rehabilitation Research & Development* 37(1): 41-52

Continued

TABLE G-1 Continued

Topic and Author(s)	Study Title	Journal Reference
Akman et al. (1999)	Assessment of spasticity using isokinetic dynamometry in patients with spinal cord injury.	*Spinal Cord* 37(9): 638-643
Castro et al. (1999)	Influence of complete spinal cord injury on skeletal muscle cross-sectional area within the first 6 months of injury.	*European Journal of Applied Physiology & Occupational Physiology* 80(4): 373-378
Castro et al. (1999)	Influence of complete spinal cord injury on skeletal muscle within 6 mo of injury.	*Journal of Applied Physiology* 86(1): 350-358
Chilibeck et al. (1999)*	Histochemical changes in muscle of individuals with spinal cord injury following functional electrical stimulated exercise training.	*Spinal Cord* 37(4): 264-268
Dudley et al. (1999)	A simple means of increasing muscle size after spinal cord injury: A pilot study.	*European Journal of Applied Physiology & Occupational Physiology* 80(4): 394-396
Gaviria et al. (1999)*	Variability of the fatigue response of paralyzed skeletal muscle in relation to the time after spinal cord injury: Mechanical and electrophysiological characteristics.	*European Journal of Applied Physiology & Occupational Physiology* 80(2): 145-153
Hillegass et al. (1999)*	Surface electrical stimulation of skeletal muscle after spinal cord injury.	*Spinal Cord* 37(4): 251-257
Potten et al. (1999)	Postural muscle responses in the spinal cord injured persons during forward reaching.	*Ergonomics* 42(9): 1200-1215
Segal et al. (1999)	Safety and efficacy of 4-aminopyridine in humans with spinal cord injury: A long-term, controlled trial.	*Pharmacotherapy* 19(6): 713-723

TABLE G-1 Continued

Topic and Author(s)	Study Title	Journal Reference
Baldi et al. (1998)*	Muscle atrophy is prevented in patients with acute spinal cord injury using functional electrical stimulation.	*Spinal Cord* 36(7): 463-469
Bracken et al. (1998)*	Methylprednisolone or tirilazad mesylate administration after acute spinal cord injury: 1-year follow up. Results of the third National Acute Spinal Cord Injury randomized controlled trial.	*Journal of Neurosurgery* 89(5): 699-706
Dalyan et al. (1998)	Factors associated with contractures in acute spinal cord injury.	*Spinal Cord* 36(6): 405-408
Geisler (1998)	Clinical trials of pharma-cotherapy for spinal cord injury.	*Annals of the New York Academy of Sciences* 845: 374-381
Konishi et al. (1998)	Electrophysiologic evaluation of denervated muscles in incomplete paraplegia using macro electromyography.	*Archives of Physical Medicine and Rehabilitation* 79(9): 1062-1068
Lamontagne et al. (1998)*	Evaluation of reflex- and nonreflex-induced muscle resistance to stretch in adults with spinal cord injury using hand-held and isokinetic dynamometry.	*Physical Therapy* 78(9): 964-975
Noreau et al. (1998)	Comparison of three methods to assess muscular strength in individuals with spinal cord injury.	*Spinal Cord* 36(10): 716-723
Potter et al. (1998)*	Randomized double-blind crossover trial of Fampridine-SR (sustained release 4-aminopyridine) in patients with incomplete spinal cord injury.	*Journal of Neurotrauma* 15(10): 837-849
Seelen et al. (1998)	Development of new muscle synergies in postural control in spinal cord injured subjects.	*Journal of Electromyography & Kinesiology* 8(1): 23-34

Continued

TABLE G-1 Continued

Topic and Author(s)	Study Title	Journal Reference
Seelen et al. (1998)	Postural motor programming in paraplegic patients during rehabilitation.	*Ergonomics* 41(3): 302-316
Neurological Responses		
Horlocker et al. (2003)	Small risk of serious neurologic complications related to lumbar epidural catheter placement in anesthetized patients.	*Anesthesia & Analgesia* 96(6): 1547-1552
Cariga et al. (2002)	Segmental recording of cortical motor evoked potentials from thoracic paravertebral myotomes in complete spinal cord injury.	*Spine* 27(13): 1438-1443
Knikou et al. (2002)*	Hip angle induced modulation of H reflex amplitude, latency and duration in spinal cord injured humans.	*Clinical Neurophysiology* 113(11): 1698-1708
Collins et al. (2001)	Large involuntary forces consistent with plateau-like behavior of human motoneurons.	*Journal of Neuroscience* 21(11): 4059-4065
Legramante et al. (2001)*	Positive and negative feedback mechanisms in the neural regulation of cardiovascular function in healthy and spinal cord-injured humans.	*Circulation* 103(9): 1250-1255
Hiersemenzel et al. (2000)*	From spinal shock to spasticity: Neuronal adaptations to a spinal cord injury.	*Neurology* 54(8): 1574-1582
Houtman et al. (2000)	Sympathetic nervous system activity and cardiovascular homeostatis during head-up tilt in patients with spinal cord injuries.	*Clinical Autonomic Research* 10(4): 207-212

TABLE G-1 Continued

Topic and Author(s)	Study Title	Journal Reference
Tran et al. (2000)	Increased threshold sural amplitude after upper limb isometric contraction in complete paraplegics.	*American Journal of Physical Medicine & Rehabilitation* 79(6): 542-546
Lacourse et al. (1999)	Cortical potentials during imagined movements in individuals with chronic spinal cord injuries.	*Behavioural Brain Research* 104(1-2): 73-88
Baba et al. (1998)	Cervical myelo-radiculopathy with entrapment neuropathy: A study based on the double-crush concept.	*Spinal Cord* 36(6): 399-404
Levander et al. (1998)	Are there any mild interhemispheric effects after moderately severe closed head injury?	*Brain Injury* 12(2): 165-173
Maurer et al. (1998)	Usefulness and diagnostic value of evoked potentials in patients with neurologic diseases in postoperative intensive care.	*Anasthesiologie, Intensivmedizin, Notfallmedizin, Schmerztherapie* 33(7): 430-440
Vaidyanathan et al. (1998)*	Pathophysiology of autonomic dysreflexia: Long-term treatment with terazosin in adult and paediatric spinal cord injury patients manifesting recurrent dysreflexic episodes.	*Spinal Cord* 36(11): 761-770

Outcome Measures and Health Assessment

Gillette et al. (2002)	Center of pressure measures to assess standing performance.	*Biomedical Sciences Instrumentation* 38: 239-244
Ishida et al. (2002)	Predictors of neurologic recovery in acute central cervical cord injury with only upper extremity impairment.	*Spine* 27(15): 1652-1658
Kilkens et al. (2002)*	The wheelchair circuit: Reliability of a test to assess mobility in persons with spinal cord injuries.	*Archives of Physical Medicine and Rehabilitation* 83(12): 1783-1788

Continued

TABLE G-1 Continued

Topic and Author(s)	Study Title	Journal Reference
Tobimatsu et al. (2001)	The order of re-acquirement of activity of daily living functions in people with spinal cord injury during rehabilitation after initial medical treatment and its affecting factors.	*Tohoku Journal of Experimental Medicine* 194(3): 181-190
Ditunno et al. (2000)*	Walking index for spinal cord injury (WISCI): An international multicenter validity and reliability study.	*Spinal Cord* 38(4): 234-243
Taricco et al. (2000)	Functional status in patients with spinal cord injury: A new standardized measurement scale. Gruppo Interdisciplinare Valutazione Interventi Riabilitativi.	*Archives of Physical Medicine and Rehabilitation* 81(9): 1173-1180
Craig et al. (1999)	Improving the long-term adjustment of spinal cord injured persons.	*Spinal Cord* 37(5): 345-350
Mulcahey et al. (1999)	Evaluation of the lower motor neuron integrity of upper extremity muscles in high level spinal cord injury.	*Spinal Cord* 37(8): 585-591
Vaccaro et al. (1999)	Magnetic resonance evaluation of the inter-vertebral disc, spinal ligaments, and spinal cord before and after closed traction reduction of cervical spine dislocations.	*Spine* 24(12): 1210-1217
Byers et al. (1998)*	An electromechanical testing device for assessment of hand motor function.	*IEEE Transactions on Rehabilitation Engineering* 6(1): 88-94
Cheliout-Heraut et al. (1998)	Evaluation of early motor and sensory evoked potentials in cervical spinal cord injury.	*Neurophysiologie Clinique* 28(1): 39-55
Claxton et al. (1998)*	Predictors of hospital mortality and mechanical ventilation in patients with cervical spinal cord injury.	*Canadian Journal of Anaesthesia* 45(2): 144-149

TABLE G-1 Continued

Topic and Author(s)	Study Title	Journal Reference
Pruitt et al. (1998)*	Health behavior in persons with spinal cord injury: Development and initial validation of an outcome measure.	*Spinal Cord* 36(10): 724-731
Toh et al. (1998)	Functional evaluation using motor scores after cervical spinal cord injuries.	*Spinal Cord* 36(7): 491-496
Pain		
Ahn et al. (2003)	Gabapentin effect on neuropathic pain compared among patients with spinal cord injury and different durations of symptoms.	*Spine* 28(4): 341-346
Finnerup et al. (2003)	Sensory function above lesion level in spinal cord injury patients with and without pain.	*Somatosensory & Motor Research* 20(1): 71-76
Malinovsky et al. (2003)	Sedation caused by clonidine in patients with spinal cord injury.	*British Journal of Anaesthesia* 90(6): 742-745
Cardenas et al. (2002)	Efficacy of amitriptyline for relief of pain in spinal cord injury: Results of a randomized controlled trial.	*Pain* 96(3): 365-373
Finnerup et al. (2002)	Lamotrigine in spinal cord injury pain: A randomized controlled trial.	*Pain* 96(3): 375-383
Kuesgen et al. (2002)	Decreased cutaneous sensory axon-reflex vasodilatation below the lesion in patients with complete spinal cord injury.	*Somatosensory & Motor Research* 19(2): 149-152
Tai et al. (2002)	Gabapentin in the treatment of neuropathic pain after spinal cord injury: A prospective, randomized, double-blind, crossover trial.	*Journal of Spinal Cord Medicine* 25(2): 100-105

Continued

TABLE G-1 Continued

Topic and Author(s)	Study Title	Journal Reference
Turner et al. (2002)	Blinding effectiveness and association of pretreatment expectations with pain improvement in a double-blind randomized controlled trial.	*Pain* 99(1-2): 91-99
Defrin et al. (2001)	Characterization of chronic pain and somatosensory function in spinal cord injury subjects.	*Pain* 89(2-3): 253-263
Dyson-Hudson et al. (2001)*	Acupuncture and Trager psychophysical integration in the treatment of wheelchair user's shoulder pain in individuals with spinal cord injury.	*Archives of Physical Medicine and Rehabilitation* 82(8): 1038-1046
Sindou et al. (2001)*	Microsurgical DREZotomy for pain due to spinal cord and/or cauda equina injuries: Long-term results in a series of 44 patients.	*Pain* 92(1-2): 159-171
Attal et al. (2000)	Intravenous lidocaine in central pain: A double-blind, placebo-controlled, psychophysical study.	*Neurology* 54(3): 564-574
Averill et al. (2000)*	Blood pressure response to acupuncture in a population at risk for autonomic dysreflexia.	*Archives of Physical Medicine and Rehabilitation* 81(11): 1494-1497
Donovan et al. (2000)*	Intravenous infusion of 4-AP in chronic spinal cord injured subjects.	*Spinal Cord* 38(1): 7-15
Siddall et al. (2000)	The efficacy of intrathecal morphine and clonidine in the treatment of pain after spinal cord injury.	*Anesthesia & Analgesia* 91(6): 1493-1498
Curtis et al. (1999)*	Effect of a standard exercise protocol on shoulder pain in long-term wheelchair users.	*Spinal Cord* 37(6): 421-429

TABLE G-1 Continued

Topic and Author(s)	Study Title	Journal Reference
Saddiki-Traki et al. (1999)	Differences between the tactile sensitivity on the anterior torso of normal individuals and those having suffered complete transection of the spinal cord.	*Somatosensory & Motor Research* 16(4): 391-401
Demirel et al. (1998)	Pain following spinal cord injury.	*Spinal Cord* 36(1): 25-28
Vaidyanathan et al. (1998)*	Pathophysiology of autonomic dysreflexia: Long-term treatment with terazosin in adult and paediatric spinal cord injury patients manifesting recurrent dysreflexic episodes.	*Spinal Cord* 36(11): 761-770
Physiological Responses		
Jacobs et al. (2003)	Physiologic responses to electrically assisted and frame-supported standing in persons with paraplegia.	*Journal of Spinal Cord Medicine* 26(4): 384-389
Spungen et al. (2003)	Factors influencing body composition in persons with spinal cord injury: A cross-sectional study.	*Journal of Applied Physiology* 95(6): 2398-2407
Cooper et al. (2001)*	Physiological responses to two wheelchair-racing exercise protocols.	*Neurorehabilitation & Neural Repair* 15(3): 191-195
Apstein et al. (1998)	Serum lipids during the first year following acute spinal cord injury.	*Metabolism: Clinical & Experimental* 47(4): 367-370
Bauman et al. (1998)	The effect of residual neurological deficit on serum lipoproteins in individuals with chronic spinal cord injury.	*Spinal Cord* 36(1): 13-17
Klefbeck et al. (1998)	Obstructive sleep apneas in relation to severity of cervical spinal cord injury.	*Spinal Cord* 36(9): 621-628
Schmid et al. (1998)	Free plasma catecholamines in spinal cord injured persons with different injury levels at rest and during exercise.	*Journal of the Autonomic Nervous System* 68(1-2): 96-100

Continued

TABLE G-1 Continued

Topic and Author(s)	Study Title	Journal Reference
Respiration		
Koga et al. (2001)	Comparison of no airway device, the Guedel-type airway and the cuffed oropharyngeal airway with mask ventilation during manual in-line stabilization.	*Journal of Clinical Anesthesia* 13(1): 6-10
Liaw et al. (2000)	Resistive inspiratory muscle training: Its effectiveness in patients with acute complete cervical cord injury.	*Archives of Physical Medicine and Rehabilitation* 81(6): 752-756
Singas et al. (1999)	Inhibition of airway hyperreactivity by oxybutynin chloride in subjects with cervical spinal cord injury.	*Spinal Cord* 37(4): 279-283
Claxton et al. (1998)*	Predictors of hospital mortality and mechanical ventilation in patients with cervical spinal cord injury.	*Canadian Journal of Anaesthesia* 45(2): 144-149
Estenne et al. (1998)	Effects of abdominal strapping on forced expiration in tetraplegic patients.	*American Journal of Respiratory & Critical Care Medicine* 157(1): 95-98
Fein et al. (1998)	The effects of ipratropium bromide on histamine-induced bronchoconstriction in subjects with cervical spinal cord injury.	*Journal of Asthma* 35(1): 49-55
Silva et al. (1998)*	Effect of aerobic training on ventilatory muscle endurance of spinal cord injured men.	*Spinal Cord* 36(4): 240-245
Tromans et al. (1998)	The use of the BiPAP biphasic positive airway pressure system in acute spinal cord injury.	*Spinal Cord* 36(7): 481-484
Sexual Function		
Dalmose et al. (2003)	Conditional stimulation of the dorsal penile/clitoral nerve may increase cystometric capacity in patients with spinal cord injury.	*Neurourology & Urodynamics* 22(2): 130-137

TABLE G-1 Continued

Topic and Author(s)	Study Title	Journal Reference
Ethans et al. (2003)*	The effects of sildenafil on the cardiovascular response in men with spinal cord injury at or above the sixth thoracic level.	*Journal of Spinal Cord Medicine* 26(3): 222-226
Laessoe et al. (2003)*	Effects of ejaculation by penile vibratory stimulation on bladder capacity in men with spinal cord lesions.	*Journal of Urology* 169(6): 2216-2219
Schmid et al. (2003)*	Clinical value of combined electrophysiological and urodynamic recordings to assess sexual disorders in spinal cord injured men.	*Neurourology & Urodynamics* 22(4): 314-321
Brackett et al. (2002)	Semen retrieval in men with spinal cord injury is improved by interrupting current delivery during electroejaculation.	*Journal of Urology* 167(1): 201-203
Mirbagheri et al. (2002)*	The effects of long-term FES-assisted walking on intrinsic and reflex dynamic stiffness in spastic spinal-cord-injured subjects.	*IEEE Transactions on Neural Systems & Rehabilitation Engineering* 10(4): 280-289
Trabulsi et al. (2002)	Leukocyte subtypes in electroejaculates of spinal cord injured men.	*Archives of Physical Medicine and Rehabilitation* 83(1): 31-34
Lebib Ben Achour et al. (2001)	Intracavernous injections in the treatment of erectile dysfunction in spinal cord injured patients: Experience with 36 patients.	*Annales de Readaptation et de Medecine Physique* 44(1): 35-40
Sanchez et al. (2001)	Efficacy, safety and predictive factors of therapeutic success with sildenafil for erectile dysfunction in patients with different spinal cord injuries.	*Spinal Cord* 39(12): 637-643
Hultling et al. (2000)*	Quality of life in patients with spinal cord injury receiving Viagra (sildenafil citrate) for the treatment of erectile dysfunction.	*Spinal Cord* 38(6): 363-370

Continued

TABLE G-1 Continued

Topic and Author(s)	Study Title	Journal Reference
Mallidis et al. (2000)	Necrospermia and chronic spinal cord injury.	*Fertility & Sterility* 74(2): 221-227
Schmid et al. (2000)	Sildenafil in the treatment of sexual dysfunction in spinal cord-injured male patients.	*European Urology* 38(2): 184-193
Sipski et al. (2000)*	Sildenafil effects on sexual and cardiovascular responses in women with spinal cord injury.	*Urology* 55(6): 812-815
Bodner et al. (1999)	Intraurethral alprostadil for treatment of erectile dysfunction in patients with spinal cord injury.	*Urology* 53(1): 199-202
Giuliano et al. (1999)	Randomized trial of sildenafil for the treatment of erectile dysfunction in spinal cord injury. Sildenafil Study Group.	*Annals of Neurology* 46(1): 15-21
Giuliano et al. (1999)	Sildenafil citrate (Viagra): A novel oral treatment for erectile dysfunction caused by traumatic spinal cord injury.	*International Journal of Clinical Practice Supplement* 102: 24-26
Hultling (1999)	Partners' perceptions of the efficacy of sildenafil citrate (Viagra) in the treatment of erectile dysfunction.	*International Journal of Clinical Practice Supplement* 102: 16-18
Jackson et al. (1999)	A multicenter study of women's self-reported reproductive health after spinal cord injury.	*Archives of Physical Medicine and Rehabilitation* 80(11): 1420-1428
Maytom et al. (1999)	A two-part pilot study of sildenafil (Viagra) in men with erectile dysfunction caused by spinal cord injury.	*Spinal Cord* 37(2): 110-116
Brackett et al. (1998)	An analysis of 653 trials of penile vibratory stimulation in men with spinal cord injury.	*Journal of Urology* 159(6): 1931-1934

TABLE G-1 Continued

Topic and Author(s)	Study Title	Journal Reference
Courtois et al. (1998)	Sympathetic skin responses and psychogenic erections in spinal cord injured men.	*Spinal Cord* 36(2): 125-131
Derry et al. (1998)	Efficacy and safety of oral sildenafil (Viagra) in men with erectile dysfunction caused by spinal cord injury.	*Neurology* 51(6): 1629-1633
Le Chapelain et al. (1998)	Ejaculatory stimulation, quality of semen and reproductive aspects in spinal cord injured men.	*Spinal Cord* 36(2): 132-136
Surgery		
Brodke et al. (2003)	Comparison of anterior and posterior approaches in cervical spinal cord injuries.	*Journal of Spinal Disorders & Techniques* 16(3): 229-235
Epstein et al. (2003)*	Documenting fusion following anterior cervical surgery: A comparison of roentgenogram versus two-dimensional computed tomographic findings.	*Journal of Spinal Disorders & Techniques* 16(3): 243-247
Papadopoulos et al. (2002)	Immediate spinal cord decompression for cervical spinal cord injury: Feasibility and outcome.	*Journal of Trauma: Injury Infection & Critical Care* 52(2): 323-332
Sustic et al. (2002)	Surgical tracheostomy versus percutaneous dilational tracheostomy in patients with anterior cervical spine fixation: Preliminary report.	*Spine* 27(17): 1942-1945
Sindou et al. (2001)*	Microsurgical DREZotomy for pain due to spinal cord and/or cauda equina injuries: Long-term results in a series of 44 patients.	*Pain* 92(1-2): 159-171
Tator et al. (1999)	Current use and timing of spinal surgery for management of acute spinal cord injury in North America: Results of a retrospective multicenter study.	*Journal of Neurosurgery* 91(1 Suppl): 12-18

Continued

TABLE G-1 Continued

Topic and Author(s)	Study Title	Journal Reference
Syringomyelia		
Wirth et al. (2001)	Feasibility and safety of neural tissue transplantation in patients with syringomyelia.	*Journal of Neurotrauma* 18(9): 911-929
Brugieres et al. (1999)*	Dynamic MRI in the evaluation of syringomyelic cysts.	*Neuro-Chirurgie* 45(Suppl 1): 115-129
Hort-Legrand et al. (1999)	Evoked motor and sensory potentials in syringomyelia.	*Neuro-Chirurgie* 45(Suppl 1): 95-104
Perrouin-Verbe et al. (1999)	Post-traumatic syringomyelia.	*Neuro-Chirurgie* 45(Suppl 1): 58-66
Perrouin-Verbe et al. (1998)	Post-traumatic syringomyelia and post-traumatic spinal canal stenosis: A direct relationship: Review of 75 patients with a spinal cord injury.	*Spinal Cord* 36(2): 137-143
Ulcers and Pressure Sores		
Sprigle et al. (2003)	Relationships among cushion type, backrest height, seated posture, and reach of wheelchair users with spinal cord injury.	*Journal of Spinal Cord Medicine* 26(3): 236-243
Han et al. (2002)	The value of Jamshidi core needle bone biopsy in predicting postoperative osteomyelitis in grade IV pressure ulcer patients.	*Plastic & Reconstructive Surgery* 110(1): 118-122
Adegoke et al. (2001)	Acceleration of pressure ulcer healing in spinal cord injured patients using interrupted direct current.	*African Journal of Medicine & Medical Sciences* 30(3): 195-197
Brienza et al. (1999)	A method for custom-contoured cushion design using interface pressure measurements.	*IEEE Transactions on Rehabilitation Engineering* 7(1): 99-108

TABLE G-1 Continued

Topic and Author(s)	Study Title	Journal Reference
Krause (1998)	Skin sores after spinal cord injury: Relationship to life adjustment.	*Spinal Cord* 36(1): 51-56
Ljungberg (1998)	Comparison of dextranomer paste and saline dressings for management of decubital ulcers.	*Clinical Therapeutics* 20(4): 737-743

H

LEGISLATION SPONSORING STATE SPINAL CORD INJURY RESEARCH

Administrative Structure	Source of Program Funding	Budget and Types of Awards
California In 2000, funds were established for spinal cord and nerve regeneration research through collaborative projects carried out at Reeve-Irvine Research Center Core Laboratory, and research projects throughout the University of California system and the state.	Private and public funding	2004-2005: $1.4 million 2003-2004: $1.6 million Individual or collaborative projects
Connecticut In 1999, 6-member board was established to develop funding streams and solicit organizations for potential research funding.	Not yet available	Information not available
Florida A 1989 law created a 16-member Advisory Council and established trust fund whereby 5% of designated revenue is given to the University of Miami for spinal cord injury research.	DUI charges	2003: $1.4 million

Administrative Structure	Source of Program Funding	Budget and Types of Awards
Illinois In 2000, the Department of Public Health distributed funds to research facilities.	Traffic surcharges, donations, gifts	Information not available
Indiana In 1998, 6-member board was established at Purdue University and Indiana University to oversee head and spinal cord injury research centers.	State funds, federal funds, donations	$1 million/year University-based research centers
Kentucky In 1994, a 7-member board was established to support grants, fellowships, and develop a 5-year strategic plan for research at the University of Kentucky and the University of Louisville.	Traffic violation surcharge	2004: $2.9 million Competitive grants; endowed chairs and professorships; postdoctoral and graduate fellowships; lecture series and research symposia
Maryland In 2000, 11-member board was established to solicit, review, and award research funds.	Health insurer taxes	$1 million/year Basic, preclinical, and clinical research, fellowships
Massachusetts In 2004, 3-member board was established to review grant proposals.	Licensing reinstatement fees	Information not available
Missouri In 2001, 8-member board was created under the authority of the University of Missouri to solicit, review, and award research grants.	Traffic surcharges, donations, federal grants	2004-2005: $375,000 Individual research awards
New Jersey In 1999, 11-member board was established to solicit and approve research projects, compile a directory of state-based spinal cord injury research projects, and establish a central registry of individuals with spinal cord injuries.	$1 surcharge on traffic or motor vehicle fines or penalties, donations, gifts	2005: $7 million 2004: $6.5 million Senior and junior faculty grants; one-time grants for startup costs; individual research grants; fellowship grants

Administrative Structure	Source of Program Funding	Budget and Types of Awards
New York In 1998, 13-member board was established to solicit, review, and administer grants.	Traffic surcharges, gifts, donations	Up to $8.5 million/year Three types of research grants: Collaborations to Achieve Research Translation; Innovative, Development, or Exploratory Activities; and Center of Research Excellence grants
Oregon In 1999, 11-member board was created to solicit, review, and fund research initiatives.	Private (gifts, grants) and public sources	2001-2003: $1[a]
South Carolina In 2000, 7-member board was created to recruit researchers to serve as reviewers for applications for research funds; staff and administrative support provided by the Medical University of South Carolina.	$100 surcharges on fines for DUI	FY 2004-2005: $1.4 million Primary research grants for junior faculty, career development awards, faculty recruitment initiative, small pilot grant funds, research dissemination funds
Virginia In 1997, a 7-member board was established to solicit, review, and administer research funds.	Licensing reinstatement fees; donations; grants	2003: $3.2 million[b] Research on the mechanisms and treatment of neurotrauma; community-based rehabilitation services

[a]The legislature passed House Bill HB 5041, which stated that the maximum amount to be provided to the program was $50,000, although the legislature appropriated $1.

[b]Brain and spinal cord injury grants and community rehabilitation service grants awarded in alternate years. There is a 5% cap on administrative costs.

NOTE: The information in this table is limited to state enacted laws (as of October 2004) that establish funds for research on spinal cord injuries. This does not include legislation that allocates monies toward rehabilitation expenses or legislation under consideration. The information was largely derived from Lexis-Nexis searches of legislation, literature reviews, and a review of state websites. Information was verified with state officials, individuals, and award recipients when possible. Abbreviations: DUI = driving under the influence of alcohol; FY = fiscal year.

I

COMMITTEE AND STAFF BIOGRAPHIES

COMMITTEE

Richard T. Johnson, M.D. (*Chair*), is Distinguished Service Professor of Neurology, Microbiology and Neuroscience at Johns Hopkins University School of Medicine and Bloomberg School of Public Health. His clinical and research work is focused on infections and inflammatory and degenerative diseases of the nervous system. He authored the highly cited book *Viral Infections of the Nervous System* and edited a widely used biennial volume *Current Therapy in Neurological Diseases.* Dr. Johnson has published more than 300 articles and chapters. He is currently the editor of *Annals of Neurology.* Dr. Johnson has been active in the National Multiple Sclerosis Society since 1970, serving as the chair of its Research Programs Advisory Committee from 1981 to 1983 and the Medical Advisory Board from 1985 to 1900. Dr. Johnson was awarded the Jean Martin Charcot Award from the International Federation of Multiple Sclerosis Societies in 1985 and was the first recipient, in 1989, of the Association of British Neurologists' Multiple Sclerosis Society Medal. He was elected an Honorary Fellow of the Royal College of Physicians in 2003 and has been an member of the Institute of Medicine (IOM) since 1987. He has chaired several IOM committees, including a committee that studied prion disease (2003) and a committee that reviewed the connection between childhood vaccinations and neurological illness (2001).

Albert J. Aguayo, M.D., is university professor and former director of the Center for Research in Neuroscience at McGill University in Montreal,

Quebec, Canada. Dr. Aguayo was among the first to demonstrate that spinal cord regeneration is possible in the mature, mammalian central nervous system. Most recently, his research has uncovered methods to promote the regeneration of damaged optic nerves. Dr. Aguayo is secretary-general of the International Brain Research Organization and serves on the Consortium Advisory Panel of the Christopher Reeve Paralysis Foundation and several other agencies and foundations. Among other awards, he is a past recipient of one of Canada's most prestigious scientific awards, the Killam Prize, for his "distinguished lifetime achievement and outstanding contribution to the advancement of knowledge in the fields of natural sciences, health sciences, and engineering." He has served as president of the Society for Neuroscience, the Canadian Association of Neuroscience, and the Canadian Neurological Society. He was elected to the Institute of Medicine in 1990 and is an Officer of the Order of Canada.

Jeremiah A. Barondess, M.D., is president of the New York Academy of Medicine (NYAM) and professor emeritus of clinical medicine at Cornell University. Dr. Barondess has written extensively on various topics in internal medicine, clinical ethics, and physician training. At NYAM he oversees programs aimed at exploring the interrelationship among medicine, science, and society; the improvement of the biomedical research enterprise; and a broad agenda of research and interventions on issues in urban health. Dr. Barondess is the founder of the coalition Doctors Against Handgun Injury. He serves as a member of the Board of Trustees of the Johns Hopkins University, the Board of Trustees of the Associates of the Yale Medical Library, and the Johns Hopkins Society of Scholars. Dr. Barondess is a fellow of the American Academy of Arts and Sciences and serves on the Board of Directors of the American Federation for Aging Research. He was elected to the Institute of Medicine (IOM) in 1971. He has chaired three IOM studies: one on musculoskeletal injury in the workplace (2001), another on health care systems and rheumatic disease (1997), and a third on technology assessment in medicine (1983).

Mary Bartlett Bunge, Ph.D., is professor of cell biology and anatomy and neurological surgery and the Christine E. Lynn Distinguished Professor of Neuroscience at the University of Miami Leonard M. Miller School of Medicine and works in the Miami Project to Cure Paralysis. Dr. Bunge was a pioneer in elucidating the structure and function of cells that insulate nerve projections and, more recently, in developing a new spinal cord injury model and novel combination strategies to improve repair of the injured spinal cord. Her laboratory conducts preclinical studies aimed at developing neuroprotective or neuroregenerative therapies for spinal cord injuries. These therapies include the transplantation of genetically modified cells to facilitate regeneration in seriously damaged spinal cords. She has served on National Institutes of Health study sections and the National Advisory Neurological Disorders and Stroke Council. She received the Wakeman Award (1996) for her seminal contributions to the field of spinal cord injury repair, the Christopher Reeve Research Medal for Spinal Cord Repair (2001), and the Javits Neuroscience Investigator Award (1998) and was the first recipient of the Mika Salpeter Women in Neuroscience Lifetime Achievement Award (2000). From 1996 to 1997 she served as interim scientific director of the Miami Project to Cure Paralysis. She is a member of the research consortium of the Christopher Reeve Paralysis Foundation and the Dana Alliance for Brain Initiatives.

Fred H. Gage, Ph.D., is the Vi and John Adler Professor of the Laboratory of Genetics at the Salk Institute in San Diego, California. Dr. Gage's research focuses on the structural plasticity in the adult nervous system. In addition to studying the mechanism and function of adult neurogenesis, his research efforts also focus on genetic engineering and cell transplantation strategies to reverse or restore function lost as a result of neurodegeneration or neurotrauma. In 1998 he led the team that discovered neural stem cells in the human brain. His professional activities have included service on the National Institutes of Health (NIH) Advisory Council on Aging, the NIH Working Group on Guidelines for the Use of Human Embryonic Stem Cells, the Research Consortium of the Christopher Reeve Paralysis Foundation, and the Advisory Board of the American Society of Gene Therapy. Dr. Gage has also served on the editorial boards of more than two dozen scientific journals and as president of the Society for Neuroscience. He has received numerous awards and honors, including the NIH Merit Award, and the Decade of the Brain Medal. He was elected to the Institute of Medicine (IOM) in 2001 and the National Academy of Sciences in 2003 and served on an IOM committee that studied the biological impact of exposure to electromagnetic fields (1996).

Suzanne T. Ildstad, M.D., is director of the Institute for Cellular Therapeutics (ICT), the Jewish Hospital Distinguished Professor of Transplantation, and professor of surgery at the University of Louisville. ICT is a multidisciplinary translational research program designed to develop cellular therapies and rapidly transfer them from the laboratory to the clinic. Dr. Ildstad's research focuses on developing methods to make bone marrow transplantation safe enough for widespread application for the treatment of autoimmune diseases, the induction of tolerance to organ and islet cell transplants, and the treatment of hemoglobinopathies such as sickle cell disease and thalassemia. She is credited with being the first to discover "facilitator cells," which are bone marrow cells that enhance engraftment of bone marrow stem cells while avoiding graft-versus-host reactivity. She also pioneered the use of mixed chimerism to induce tolerance to allografts and xenografts. More recently, Dr. Ildstad's research has focused on stem cell plasticity for the regeneration of damaged organs, including cardiac and retinal tissue. She holds numerous patents related to her research and is the founding scientist of Regenerex, L.L.C., a biotechnology company whose vision is to provide an engineered bone marrow graft to improve the safety of bone marrow transplantation. She was elected to the Institute of Medicine (IOM) in 1997 and has served on IOM committees studying organ transplantation policies (1999), multiple sclerosis research strategies (2001), and the challenges of small clinical trials (2001), a committee that she chaired.

John A. Jane, Sr., M.D., Ph.D., F.R.C.S.(C.), is professor of neurosurgery and chair of the Department of Neurosurgery at the University of Virginia Health Sciences Center. Dr. Jane's clinical and research efforts focus on the surgical treatment of severe spine and head injuries. His clinic treated nearly 400 individuals with spinal cord injuries in the year 2002, and he treated Christopher Reeve in the immediate aftermath of the actor's 1995 horseback riding accident. He is widely known for his seminal research characterizing cranial aneurysms, for his development of modern craniofacial surgical techniques, and as an educator of many of the nation's leading neurosurgeons. Dr. Jane is a recipient of the Grass Foundation Award for his outstanding commitment to neurosurgical research. He has served as director of the American Board of Neurological Surgery and president of the Society of Neurological Surgeons. Since 1992 he has been the editor of the *Journal of Neurosurgery*, and since 1999 he has been the editor of *Journal of Neurosurgery: Spine*.

Lynn T. Landmesser, Ph.D., is the Arline H. and Curtis F. Garvin Professor and Chair of the Department of Neurosciences at Case Western Research University. Dr. Landmesser's research involves characterization of the cellular and molecular mechanisms responsible for the guidance of growing nerve projections, specifically, of spinal motor neurons, and for the formation of functional motor circuits in the developing spinal cord. Her professional activities include service as president of the Society for Developmental Biology, chair of the Neuroscience Section of the American Association for the Advancement of Science, member of the National Advisory Council of the National Institute of Neurological Disorders and Stroke, and a fellow of the American Academy of Arts and Sciences. Dr. Landmesser was elected to the National Academy of Sciences (NAS) in 2001. She is a member of the NAS committee responsible for evaluating national workforce needs in the biomedical and behavioral sciences.

Linda B. Miller, OTR, M.S., is president of the Volunteer Trustees Foundation in Washington, D.C., a consortium of not-for-profit health facility governing boards. Ms. Miller has extensive experience with advocacy and funding mechanisms and the processes of health care institutions and foundations across the nation. She has taught orthotics and prosthetics and for 5 years served as an occupational therapist at the Rusk Institute of Rehabilitation Medicine in New York, specializing in spinal cord injury and early biomechanical attempts at function restoration. Ms. Miller served as a member of the National Institutes of Health Consensus Panel on Liver Transplantation, she has advocated and written extensively on issues of not-for-profit health care, and her writings have been published in both the medical and the popular press. Ms. Miller was elected to the Institute of Medicine in 1997.

P. Hunter Peckham, Ph.D., is a professor of biomedical engineering at Case Western Reserve University and is the director of the Functional Electrical Stimulation Center, a consortium of the Cleveland Veterans Association Medical Center, Metro Health Center, and Case Western Reserve University. Dr. Peckham's research focuses on the use of electrical currents and neural implants to stimulate nerve and muscular function in individuals with central nervous system paralysis. His work has earned him numerous awards, including special recognition from the Food and Drug Administration for his role in the multicenter clinical development of a hand-grasp prosthesis for patients with spinal cord dysfunction. In 2001, he received the Paul B. Magnuson Award, "in recognition of outstanding rehabilitation research dedicated to seeking new knowledge to benefit the nation's veterans." Dr. Peckham holds multiple patents related to his work. In 1996-1997 he chaired the National Institutes of Health National Advisory Board to the National Center for Medical Rehabilitation Research. Dr. Peckham was elected to the National Academy of Engineering in 2002.

Robert T. Schimke, M.D., is emeritus professor of biological sciences and emeritus research professor of the American Cancer Society at Stanford University in Palo Alto. In 1995 he had a bicycling accident that damaged his spinal cord at level C5-C6, rendering him paralyzed from the waist down and with limited upper-extremity function. He is well known for his work in gene amplification and DNA replication and repair. He is credited with opening the field of protein degradation. Dr. Schimke received the W. C. Rose Award in Biochemistry in 1983 and the Sloan Prize from the General Motors Cancer Research Foundation. He was elected to the National Academy of Sciences in 1976 and to the Institute of Medicine in 1983.

Christopher B. Shields, M.D., F.R.C.S.(C.), is a professor and department chair at the Norton Hospital and the clinical director of the Kentucky Spinal Cord Injury Research Center, Department of Neurological Surgery, University of Louisville School of Medicine. Dr. Shields has extensive experience treating and advocating for individuals with spinal cord injuries. He was instrumental in the development of legislation in the state of Kentucky to provide increased support for spinal cord injury research. His work involves numerous animal and clinical studies aimed at treating spinal cord injuries using such techniques as intraoperative imaging, stem cell grafts, and hypothermia. Dr. Shields is a past president of the Congress of Neurological Surgeons, and he has served on numerous scientific editorial boards and as the chair of the Cerebrovascular Section of the American Association of Neurological Surgeons.

Stephen G. Waxman, M.D., Ph.D., is a professor and chair of the Department of Neurology and director of the Center for Neuroscience and Regeneration Research, a collaboration of the Paralyzed Veterans of America and the United Spinal Association with Yale University. He is a professor of neurobiology and pharmacology and neurologist-in-chief at Yale University. His laboratory focuses on the molecular processes that underlie functional recovery in spinal cord injuries and multiple sclerosis. He has served on numerous scientific advisory committees, including advisory boards of the U.S. Department of Veterans Affairs, the Spinal Cord Research Foundation, the Board of Scientific Counselors of the National Institute of Neurological Disorders and Stroke, and Acorda Therapeutics, Inc., a biotechnology firm that develops drugs to treat spinal cord injuries and several other neurological disorders. He has received the Wartenberg Award, the highest honor awarded by the American Academy of Neurology (AAN), and the Dystel Prize for MS research, awarded by the AAN and the National Multiple Sclerosis Society. He has edited and written several books on basic and clinical neuroscience, including *Spinal Cord Compression*; *Diseases of the Spine and Spinal Cord*; and *The Axon: Structure, Function, and Pathophysiology*. He is also the editor of *The Neuroscientist* and serves on the editorial boards of more than a dozen scientific journals. Dr. Waxman was elected to the Institute of Medicine (IOM) in 1996 and served on an IOM committee that reviewed the state of research in multiple sclerosis (2001).

BOARD LIAISON

Sid Gilman, M.D., F.R.C.P., is the William J. Herdman Professor and chair of the Department of Neurology at the University of Michigan Medical School. He has held the position of professor and chair of the Department of Neurology since 1977. His research work is in vestibular and cerebellar physiology and in the pathophysiological processes underlying neurodegenerative disorders, notably, cerebellar ataxias, Parkinson's disease, parkinsonian syndromes, and Alzheimer's disease. From 1988 to 2000 he served as director of the state of Michigan's program in the dementias, currently designated the Michigan Dementia Program. In 1991 he became director of the Michigan Alzheimer's Disease Research Center. He has received numerous honors and awards. In 1997 he became the William J. Herdman Professor of Neurology and remained chair of the Department of Neurology. In 1997 he was designated an honorary member of the American Neurological Association, and in 2000 he was elected a fellow of the American Association for the Advancement of Science. He was named the Henry Russel Lecturer at the University of Michigan for 2001, the highest honor that the university bestows upon a senior faculty member. In 2001 he was elected a fellow of the Royal College of Physicians, and in the same year, he was elected a fellow of the American Academy of Arts and Sciences. He is a member of the Institute of Medicine of the National Academy of Sciences and a past president of the American Neurological Association. Before going to the University of Michigan, Dr. Gilman held faculty and hospital appointments at Harvard Medical School and Columbia Presbyterian Medical Center. He is editor-in-chief of the *Contemporary Neurology Series* and *MedLink Neurology* and a member of the editorial boards of seven other neurological journals. He became editor-in-chief of the journal *Experimental Neurology* in January 2003. Dr. Gilman has published about 400 scientific papers, book chapters, and abstracts, including seven books that he coauthored or edited. He earned an undergraduate degree in 1954 and an M.D. degree in 1957, both from the University of California, Los Angeles.

STAFF

Andrew Pope, Ph.D., is director of the Board on Health Sciences Policy and the Board on Neuroscience and Behavioral Health at the Institute of Medicine. With a Ph.D. in physiology and biochemistry, his primary interests focus on environmental and occupational influences on human health. Dr. Pope's previous research activities focused on the neuroendocrine and reproductive effects of various environmental substances in food-producing animals. During his tenure at the National Academies and since 1989 at the Institute of Medicine, Dr. Pope has directed numerous studies; topics include injury control, disability prevention, biological markers, neurotoxicology, indoor allergens, and the enhancement of environmental and occupational health content in medical and nursing school curricula. Most recently, Dr. Pope directed studies on National Institutes of Health priority-setting processes, organ procurement and transplantation policy, and the role of science and technology in countering terrorism.

Catharyn T. Liverman, M.L.S., is a senior program officer at the Institute of Medicine (IOM). In her 12 years at IOM, she has worked on studies addressing a range of topics, primarily focused on public health and science policy. Most recently she was the study director for the IOM committee that produced the report *Preventing Childhood Obesity: Health in the Balance.* Other recent studies include *Testosterone and Aging: Clinical Research Directions, Gulf War and Health,* and *Reducing the Burden of Injury.* Her background is in medical library science, with previous positions at the National Agricultural Library and the Naval War College Library. She received a B.A. from Wake Forest University and an M.L.S. from the University of Maryland.

Janet Joy, Ph.D., served as a senior program officer at the Institute of Medicine (IOM) from 1994 through August 2004. She has directed a number of IOM studies, including *Multiple Sclerosis: Current Status and Strategies for the Future* (2001), *Stem Cells and the Promise of Regenerative Medicine* (2002), and, most recently, *Integration and Innovation: A Framework for Progress in Early Detection and Diagnosis of Breast Cancer* (2004). Dr. Joy received a Ph.D. in neuroscience from the University of Toronto in 1983, after which she did postdoctoral work at the University of Texas and Northwestern University and then spent 5 years at the National Institute of Mental Health as a senior staff fellow. She is coauthor with Alison Mack of the book *Marijuana as Medicine?: The Science Beyond the Controversy.*

Michael Abrams, M.P.H., served as a program officer with the Board on Neuroscience and Behavioral Health of the Institute of Medicine (IOM). He directed the IOM study that resulted in the report *Incorporating Research into Psychiatry Residency Training.* Mr. Abrams earned a master's in public health degree from Johns Hopkins University (2000), in which he focused his studies on childhood mental health disorders. From 1997 to 2001 he served as a junior faculty member in the Department of Psychiatry and Behavioral Sciences at the Johns Hopkins University School of Medicine. From 1994 to 2001 he was involved in and managed structural and functional neuroimaging experiments aimed at the elucidation of neuropathologies that underlie various genetic disorders affecting learning and language in children. From 1990 to 1994 he worked as a research assistant on a behavioral genetics investigation that focused on fragile X and Turner syndromes. He has written 25 peer-reviewed publications.

Bruce M. Altevogt, Ph.D., is a program officer at the Institute of Medicine. In 2004 he received his doctorate from Harvard University's Program in Neuroscience. Since joining the Board on Neuroscience and Behavioral Health, he has worked on the spinal cord injury study and is currently directing the IOM study *Sleep Disorders: Research, Education, Training, and Practice.* While at Harvard, Dr. Altevogt studied how glial cells in the central and peripheral nervous systems form a network of cells through intracellular communication, and the role this network plays in maintaining myelin. In addition to Dr. Altevogt's work at Harvard, he also has performed research at the National Institutes of Health and the University of Virginia. He received a B.A. from the University of Virginia, where he majored in biology and minored in South Asian studies.

Kathleen M. Patchan is a research associate at the Institute of Medicine (IOM). In addition to her work on the spinal cord injury study, she has worked on a study on health literacy and assisted with staffing IOM's Sarnat Award. She recently worked on the IOM study that resulted in the report *Incorporating Research into Psychiatry Residency Training.* Previously, at the Congressional Research Service and the Center on Budget and Policy Priorities, she conducted research and wrote reports on Medicaid, the State Children's Health Insurance Program (SCHIP), and state-funded immigrant health care. She has also worked at the Institute for Health Policy Solutions, where she developed reports on SCHIP and employer-sponsored health insurance. Ms. Patchan graduated from the University of Maryland at College Park with a B.S. in cell and molecular biology and a B.A. in history.

Lora K. Taylor is a senior project assistant for the Board on Neuroscience and Behavioral Health at the Institute of Medicine. She has 11 years of experience working at the National Academies and before joining the Institute of Medicine served as the administrative associate for the Report Review Committee and the Division on Life Sciences' Ocean Studies Board. Ms. Taylor has a B.A. from Georgetown University with a double major in psychology and fine arts.

Index